ESSENTIALS OF
Perioperative Nursing

Terri Goodman, PhD, RN, CNOR
Terri Goodman & Associates
Dallas, Texas

Cynthia Spry, MA, MS, RN, CNOR, CSIT
Independent Clinical Consultant
New York, New York

JONES & BARTLETT
L E A R N I N G

World Headquarters
Jones & Bartlett Learning
5 Wall Street
Burlington, MA 01803
978-443-5000
info@jblearning.com
www.jblearning.com

Jones & Bartlett Learning books and products are available through most bookstores and online booksellers. To contact Jones & Bartlett Learning directly, call 800-832-0034, fax 978-443-8000, or visit our website, www.jblearning.com.

Substantial discounts on bulk quantities of Jones & Bartlett Learning publications are available to corporations, professional associations, and other qualified organizations. For details and specific discount information, contact the special sales department at Jones & Bartlett Learning via the above contact information or send an email to specialsales@jblearning.com.

15799-4

Production Credits
VP, Executive Publisher: David D. Cella
Executive Editor: Amanda Martin
Acquisitions Editor: Teresa Reilly
Editorial Assistant: Danielle Bessette
Vendor Manager: Nora Menzi
Marketing Communications Manager: Katie Hennessy
VP, Manufacturing and Inventory Control: Therese Connell
Composition: S4Carlisle Publishing Services
Cover Design: Michael O'Donnell
Rights & Media Specialist: Wes DeShano
Media Development Editor: Troy Liston
Cover Image: © cluckva/Shutterstock
Printing and Binding: Edwards Brothers Malloy
Cover Printing: Edwards Brothers Malloy

Library of Congress Cataloging-in-Publication Data
Names: Goodman, Terri, author. | Spry, Cynthia, author.
Title: Essentials of perioperative nursing / Terri Goodman, Cynthia Spry.
Description: Sixth edition. | Burlington, MA : Jones & Bartlett Learning, [2017] | Includes
    bibliographical references and index.
Identifiers: LCCN 2016001282 | ISBN 9781284079821
Subjects: | MESH: Perioperative Nursing | Programmed Instruction
Classification: LCC RD32.3 | NLM WY 18.2 | DDC 617.9/17—dc23 LC record available at http://lccn.loc.gov/2016001282

6048

Printed in the United States of America
20 19 18 17 16   10 9 8 7 6 5 4 3 2 1

Contents

CHAPTER 4   Aseptic Practices: Preparing the Sterile Field and the Patient for Surgery   93

CHAPTER 5   Positioning the Patient for Surgery   141

CHAPTER 9   Wound Management: Wound Closure   241

CHAPTER 10   Anesthesia and Medication Safety   265

CHAPTER 11   Environment of Care and Life Safety   315

Introduction

Essentials of Perioperative Nursing provides the knowledge and skills required to navigate safely and effectively in an aseptic environment. It is a valuable text for a basic nursing curriculum as well as for personnel working in a perioperative setting. Competencies required to prevent infections apply to treating patients throughout the healthcare system. Creating and maintaining a sterile field requires the same knowledge, skills, and commitment to patient safety, whether that sterile field is created in the operating room for a surgical procedure, in interventional radiology, or for the insertion of a central line, a dressing change, or the insertion of a urinary catheter.

With the increase in the number and complexity of surgical procedures being undertaken in both inpatient and outpatient settings, managers and educators must orient a growing number of nurses to the perioperative arena quickly and efficiently. *Essentials of Perioperative Nursing* can be used by nurses independently or as an adjunct to a formal orientation process. The text can also be instrumental in preparing in-service programs for the entire perioperative nursing staff, for reference and review, and for preparing for the CNOR certification exam.

Essentials of Perioperative Nursing is an introductory text designed to teach and reinforce essential knowledge and skills necessary to navigate a sterile environment and to deliver entry-level patient care. The text does not address surgical specialties or specific procedures. It does, however, prepare the new perioperative nurse to pursue competence in the wide variety of surgical specialties—a process that may take several years of exposure and hands-on experience.

Each chapter contains objectives, a lesson plan, study questions, a post-test, and a competency checklist that will help the perioperative educator or the individual nurse organize, assess, and reinforce learning.

Objectives

Following mastery of the content, the learner will be able to do the following:

- Describe essential elements of perioperative practice

- Discuss application of the Perioperative Nursing Data Set (PNDS)
- List nursing diagnoses commonly applicable to surgical patients
- Identify desired patient outcomes relative to surgical intervention
- Discuss the responsibility of the perioperative nurse in achieving desired patient outcomes
- Demonstrate understanding of basic principles and concepts of perioperative nursing by responding correctly to the section questions and post-test questions in each chapter
- Identify the behavioral skills necessary to demonstrate competency in essential perioperative practice

Assumptions about the Learner

The learner is assumed to have the following characteristics:

- Is a registered nurse
- May have no perioperative experience or may have varied clinical experience
- Is self-motivated
- Does not yet function at the expert level
- Views knowledge of perioperative nursing practice as desirable and useful
- Demonstrates competency in nursing practice

The first edition of *Essentials of Perioperative Nursing* was published in 1987, followed by revisions in 1997, 2005, 2009, and 2013. Although the basic principles have not changed markedly since the last edition, practice changes have occurred as the body of knowledge related to desired patient outcomes grows. Evidence-based practice continues to be a key phrase in the current literature, meaning that practice decisions should be supported by research or empirical evidence demonstrating that the practice contributes to desired patient outcomes. This *Sixth Edition* has been revised to reflect the most current research findings, literature reviews, and the most recent Association of periOperative Registered Nursing (AORN) perioperative guidelines. In addition, the section questions and post-test questions throughout the book are new.

I am honored that the original author of *Essentials of Perioperative Nursing*, Cynthia Spry, MSN, MA, RN, CNOR, chose me to provide new editions of the text. For nearly thirty years, this text has been used by countless appreciative readers. It has been a valuable teaching tool, a source of reference and review, and an excellent resource for preparing for the certification exam. I hope that we will continue to hear "I use your book all the time."

Every surgical patient deserves the caring and competent services of a registered nurse, whether the procedure is performed in an acute care or an ambulatory setting, an interventional site, or as a sterile procedure done at the bedside. I hope that *Essentials of Perioperative Nursing* will continue to be a premier text for perioperative nurses and for all nurses who will deliver aseptic care to patients regardless of the setting.

Terri Goodman

Acknowledgments

Cynthia Spry, MA, MS, RN, CNOR, CSIT
Independent Clinical Consultant
New York, New York

Steven Dean, DNP, CRNA
Certified Registered Nurse Anesthetist
McKinney, Texas

Jennifer Bertault, BSN, RN, CASC, CNOR, CRCST
Manager, Sterile Processing and Surgical Support
Medical City/Medical City Children's Hospital
Dallas, Texas

Introduction to Perioperative Nursing

LEARNER OBJECTIVES

1. Define the three phases of the surgical experience.
2. Describe the scope of perioperative nursing practice.
3. Discuss application of the *Perioperative Nursing Data Set* (PNDS).
4. Discuss the outcomes a patient can be expected to achieve following a surgical intervention.
5. Describe the role of each of the members of the surgical team.

Phases of the Surgical Experience

1. The perioperative period begins when the patient is informed of the need for surgery, includes the surgical procedure and recovery, continues with discharge, and ends when the patient achieves his or her optimal level of postsurgical function.

2. Perioperative nurses provide care for surgical patients during the three distinct phases of the surgical experience: (1) preoperative, (2) intraoperative, and (3) postoperative. The word "perioperative" is used to encompass all three phases. In larger facilities, it is common for perioperative nurses to care for the patient during only one phase; in smaller facilities and in ambulatory settings the same nurse may provide patient care during all three phases.

Preoperative

3. The preoperative phase begins when the patient, or someone acting on the patient's behalf, is informed of the need for surgery and makes the decision to have the procedure. This phase includes preparation for surgery before and after admission to the surgical facility and ends when the patient is transferred to the operating room bed.

4. During the preoperative phase, the patient is prepared physically and psychologically for surgery. The length of the preoperative period varies. For the patient whose surgery is elective, the period may be lengthy. For the patient whose surgery is urgent, the period is brief, and the patient may have no awareness of this phase.

5. The results of diagnostic studies initiated during the preoperative period should be available to the nurse who does the immediate preoperative assessment. Nurses use information obtained from the chart review, preoperative assessment, and interview to prepare a plan of care for the patient.

6. Nursing activities in the preoperative phase are directed toward patient support, teaching, and preparation for the procedure.

Intraoperative

7. The intraoperative phase begins when the patient is transferred to the operating room bed and ends with transfer to the postanesthesia care unit (PACU) or other area where immediate postsurgical recovery care is given.

8. During the intraoperative period, the patient is monitored, anesthetized, prepped, draped, and the procedure is performed.

9. Nursing activities in the intraoperative period focus on patient safety, emotional support, facilitation of the procedure, prevention of infection, and the patient's satisfactory physiologic response to anesthesia and the surgical intervention.

Postoperative

10. The postoperative phase begins with the patient's transfer to the recovery unit and ends with return to an optimal level of functioning. The postoperative period may be brief or extensive and most commonly includes a period of time following discharge from the surgical facility.

11. The perioperative nurse must provide complete and concise information when transferring the patient to the postop caregiver.
    - Most surgical patients go from surgery into the PACU. Any information that can assist the postop caregiver in customizing interventions to meet the patient's specific needs should be included in the handoff report.
    - Critically ill patients may be transferred immediately to the intensive care unit (ICU) following surgery. In this case, the perioperative nurse may not provide care beyond the intraoperative phase. The circulating nurse must advise the ICU as soon as possible of the plan to transfer the patient immediately following the procedure and make the necessary arrangements (e.g., ICU bed, appropriate transport personnel, portable oxygen and monitoring equipment) for a safe and efficient patient transfer.
    - Depending upon the complexity of the surgery, ambulatory surgery patients may be nearly ready for discharge when admitted to the PACU.

12. In an effort to better utilize nursing resources and increase efficiency, particularly in smaller hospitals and in ambulatory surgery, many perioperative nurses assume responsibility for providing care in both the operating room and in the PACU. Care at home, if required, is provided by family or other primary caregivers.

13. Nursing activities in the immediate postoperative phase center on support of the patient's physiologic systems. In the later stages of recovery, much of the focus is on reinforcing the essential information that the patient and other caregivers require in preparation for discharge.

Nursing Process Throughout the Perioperative Period

14. With advances in technology, surgical techniques, and anesthesia care, the percentage of surgical procedures done on a same-day basis increases each year. In 2013, more than 65% of all surgeries performed in hospitals were done as outpatient procedures (American Hospital Association, 2015).

15. Perioperative nursing was formerly referred to as "operating room nursing," a term that historically referred to patient care provided

in the intraoperative period and administered within the operating room itself. However, as the responsibilities of the operating room nurse expanded to include care in the preoperative and postoperative periods, the term "perioperative" was recognized as more appropriate. In 1999, the organization that represents perioperative nurses, once known as the Association of Operating Room Nurses (AORN), changed its name to the Association of periOperative Registered Nurses (AORN). Today, the terms "perioperative" and "perioperative nursing" are accepted and utilized in nursing and medical literature.

16. The perioperative nurse provides for the surgical patient throughout the continuum of care. The AORN Perioperative Patient-Focused Model identifies four specific domains—patient safety, physiologic response, behavioral responses, and the health system—that are the focus of concern for the perioperative nurse.

17. The domains of safety, physiologic response, and behavioral responses of patients reflect the nature of the surgical experience for the patient and serve as a guide for providing care.

18. The fourth domain represents other members of the healthcare team and the healthcare system. Perioperative nurses work collaboratively with other healthcare team members to formulate nursing diagnoses, identify desired outcomes, and provide care within the context of the healthcare system to achieve desirable patient outcomes (AORN, 2011, pp. 3–4).

19. Perioperative nurses provide patient care within the framework of the nursing process. They use the tools of patient assessment, care planning, intervention, and evaluation of patient outcomes to meet the needs of patients who are undergoing operative or other invasive procedures. Every patient is unique, and the plan of care is tailored to meet the patient's specific needs. The plan addresses physiologic, psychological, sociocultural, and spiritual aspects of care.

20. Much of perioperative nursing involves familiarity with technology and technical expertise, including responsibility for equipment, instrumentation, and surgical techniques. Much of the nurse's time during the intraoperative phase is spent managing technology and documenting patient care; however, the patient must remain the focus of the perioperative nurse's attention.

21. The goal of perioperative nursing is to provide care to patients and support to their families, using the nursing process to assist patients and their families in making decisions and to meet and support the needs of patients undergoing surgical or other invasive procedures. The overall desired outcome is that the patient will achieve a level of wellness equal to or greater than the level prior to surgery.

22. Perioperative nursing care is provided in a variety of settings, including acute care facilities, ambulatory settings, and physician-based office settings. Perioperative nurses provide care to patients, their families, and others who support the patient. The perioperative nurse focuses on three major activities: providing direct care, coordinating comprehensive care, and educating patients and their families.

Assessment

23. Nursing assessment of the patient may take place in a number of settings and timeframes. Assessment may be performed a week or more before surgery or just prior to the procedure. It may occur in the patient's inpatient hospital unit, the surgeon's office, the preadmission testing unit of the surgical facility, or the same-day/ambulatory surgery unit.

24. In some instances, the assessment process is initiated in a telephone conversation with the patient prior to surgery and completed on the day of surgery at the surgical facility. Often, the initial nursing assessment is performed by a nurse who is not a perioperative nurse.

25. It is more likely that the perioperative nurse's assessment of the patient will take place just prior to bringing the patient into the operating room. This assessment will include a brief interview, a quick physical inspection of the patient, and a review of the patient's record, including the results of diagnostic testing and assessment data obtained previously by other caregivers.

Nursing Diagnoses

26. Assessment data provide information that the perioperative nurse uses to formulate nursing diagnoses and identify desired outcomes. Several nursing diagnoses, such as knowledge deficit and high risk for infection, are typical for the surgical patient. Assessment data form the foundation for patient-specific nursing diagnoses and planning individualized care tailored to meet each patient's individual and unique needs (AORN, 2011).

Planning

27. The perioperative nurse uses knowledge of the patient, the proposed procedure, identified patient needs, related nursing diagnoses, and desired outcomes to plan care for each patient.

28. The perioperative nurse begins care planning before seeing the patient. Initial planning is based on knowledge of the planned procedure, the resources required, and the common nursing diagnoses related to surgical intervention.

29. Knowledge of the individual patient obtained during the assessment process is combined with this previous planning to prepare for meeting the unique needs of the patient and providing care that is individually tailored to each patient.

Intervention

30. In the intervention stage of the nursing process, the perioperative nurse provides, coordinates, supervises, and documents care within the framework of accepted standards of nursing care, as identified by the AORN (2015) guidelines for perioperative practice.

Evaluation

31. In the final evaluation stage of the nursing process, the perioperative nurse evaluates the results of nursing care in relation to the extent that expected patient outcomes have been met.

Section Questions

1. Define the perioperative experience. [Ref 1]

2. Identify the primary nursing focus and desired outcomes in the preoperative phase of the perioperative experience. [Refs 3–6]

3. Identify the primary nursing focus and desired outcomes in the intraoperative phase of the perioperative experience. [Refs 7–9]

4. Identify the primary nursing focus and desired outcomes in the postoperative phase of the perioperative experience. [Refs 10–13]

5. Discuss the significance of the term "perioperative." [Ref 15]

6. Identify the four domains of the AORN Perioperative Patient-Focused Model. [Ref 16]

7. Identify the four aspects of patient care addressed in the plan for each patient. [Ref 19]

8. In which settings is perioperative nursing provided? [Ref 22]

9. Where and when does the assessment of the surgical patient take place? [Refs 23–25]

10. When does planning for the surgical patient begin? [Ref 28]

Perioperative Nursing Data Set

32. In 2000, AORN published the first *Perioperative Nursing Data Set* (PNDS). The PNDS is a controlled, structured nursing vocabulary that can be used to describe perioperative nursing practice. Following revisions, the PNDS, 3rd Edition, now includes 40 nurse-sensitive patient outcomes, 44 nursing diagnoses, and 53 interventions (AORN, 2011).

33. The PNDS may be used for the following purposes:
    - Provide a framework to standardize documentation.
    - Provide a universal language for perioperative nursing practice and education.
    - Assist in the measurement and evaluation of patient care outcomes.
    - Provide a foundation for perioperative nursing research and evaluation of patient outcomes.

34. A primary benefit in day-to-day practice is the use of a universal language for nursing diagnoses, interventions, and expected outcomes.

35. In some facilities, the PNDS has been incorporated into the electronic health record, allowing nurses to manage data using a common language. Even when the documentation is not computerized, the perioperative nurse should refer to the PNDS when planning patient care.

36. Examples of nursing diagnoses using the PNDS include the following:
    - Risk of infection
    - Impaired transfer ability
    - Imbalanced nutrition: more than body requirement

37. Examples of desired patient outcomes include the following:
    - The patient is free of signs and symptoms of infection.
    - The patient is free of signs and symptoms of injury related to transfer/transport.
    - The patient demonstrates knowledge of nutritional requirements related to operative or other invasive procedures.

38. Examples of implementation include the following:
    - Implements aseptic technique, protects from cross-contamination
    - Evaluates for signs and symptoms of skin and tissue injury as a result of transfer or transport
    - Provides instruction regarding dietary needs
    - (AORN, 2015, pp. 693–710)

39. Perioperative nursing is patient centric, not task oriented. Perioperative nurses focus on preventive practice rather than on the identification of problems. They must use knowledge, judgment, and skill based on the principles of biological, physiologic, behavioral, social, and nursing sciences to plan and implement care to achieve desired patient outcomes.

40. AORN (2015) has identified patient outcomes that describe the results a patient can expect to achieve during surgical interventions. These guidelines reflect the responsibilities of the perioperative nurse and may serve as a framework with which to evaluate patient response to perioperative nursing interventions.

41. The PNDS describes 39 outcome relationships (AORN, 2011, pp. 139–391):
    - The patient's procedure is performed on the correct site, side, and level.
    - The patient's current status is communicated throughout the continuum of care.
    - The patient is free from signs and symptoms of electrical injury.
    - The patient is free from signs and symptoms of injury related to thermal sources.
    - The patient is free from signs or symptoms of unintended retained foreign objects.
    - The patient is free from signs and symptoms of injury related to positioning.
    - The patient is free from signs and symptoms of laser injury.
    - The patient is free from signs and symptoms of chemical injury.
    - The patient is free from signs and symptoms of radiation injury.
    - The patient is free from signs and symptoms of injury caused by extraneous objects.
    - The patient is free from signs and symptoms of injury related to transfer/transport.
    - The patient receives appropriately administered medication(s).
    - The patient's specimen(s) is managed in the appropriate manner.
    - The patient has wound perfusion consistent with or improved from baseline levels.
    - The patient has tissue perfusion consistent with or improved from baseline levels.
    - The patient's gastrointestinal status is maintained at or improved from baseline levels.
    - The patient's genitourinary status is maintained at or improved from baseline levels.
    - The patient's musculoskeletal status is maintained at or improved from baseline levels.
    - The patient's endocrine status is maintained at or improved from baseline levels.
    - The patient is free from signs and symptoms of infection.
    - The patient is at or returning to normothermia at the conclusion of the immediate postoperative period.
    - The patient's fluid, electrolyte, and acid–base balances are maintained at or improved from baseline levels.
    - The patient's respiratory status is maintained at or improved from baseline levels.
    - The patient's cardiovascular status is maintained at or improved from baseline levels.
    - The patient demonstrates and/or reports adequate pain control.

- The patient's neurological status is maintained at or improved from baseline levels.
- The patient or designated support person demonstrates knowledge of expected psychosocial responses to the procedure.
- The patient or designated support person demonstrates knowledge of nutritional management related to the operative or other invasive procedure.
- The patient or designated support person demonstrates knowledge of medication management.
- The patient or designated support person demonstrates knowledge of pain management.
- The patient or designated support person demonstrates knowledge of wound management.
- The patient or designated support person demonstrates knowledge of expected responses to the operative or invasive procedure.
- The patient or designated support person participates in decisions affecting his or her perioperative plan of care.
- The patient or designated support person participates in the rehabilitation process.
- The patient's value system, lifestyle, ethnicity, and culture are considered, respected, and incorporated in the perioperative plan of care.
- The patient's care is consistent with the individualized perioperative plan of care.
- The patient's right to privacy is maintained.
- The patient is the recipient of competent and ethical care within legal standards of practice.
- The patient is the recipient of consistent and comparable care regardless of the setting.

42. Other desired patient outcomes not specifically listed in the AORN outcome standards may be identified by the perioperative nurse and included in the plan of care. New knowledge regarding patient responses to surgery and the effects of nursing interventions may lead to the identification of new desired patient outcomes that have implications for perioperative nursing practice. The perioperative nurse who plans patient care should be guided by, but not limited by, established patient outcome standards.

Roles of the Perioperative Nurse

43. Perioperative nurses function in various roles, including those of manager/director, clinical practitioner (e.g., scrub nurse, circulating nurse, clinical nurse specialist, registered nurse first assistant [RNFA]), educator, and researcher. In these roles, the perioperative nurse's responsibilities include, but are not limited to, the following:

- Patient assessment before, during, and after surgery
- Patient and family teaching
- Patient and family support and reassurance
- Patient advocacy
- Performing as scrub or circulating nurse during surgery
- Control of the environment
- Efficient provision of resources
- Coordination of activities related to patient care
- Communication, collaboration, and consultation with other healthcare team members
- Maintenance of asepsis
- Ongoing monitoring of the patient's physiologic and psychological status
- Supervision of ancillary personnel

44. Additional responsibilities that promote personal and professional growth and contribute to the profession of perioperative nursing include, but are not limited to, the following:

- Participation in professional organization activities
- Participation in research activities that support the profession of perioperative nursing
- Exploration and validation of current and future practice; pursuing evidence to support practice
- Participation in continuing education programs to enhance personal knowledge and to promote the profession of perioperative nursing
- Certification to validate excellence in nursing practice
- Functioning as a role model for nursing students and perioperative nursing colleagues
- Mentoring, precepting, and instructing other perioperative nurses

Expanded and Advanced Practice Roles

45. The RNFA is an expanded role of perioperative nursing. The RNFA practices under the direction of the surgeon and assists the surgeon during the intraoperative phase of the surgical experience. A more complete definition of the RNFA and the qualifications for this role are outlined in the revised "AORN Position Statement on RN First Assistants" (AORN, 2013).

46. The perioperative nurse may pursue an advanced practice nursing (APRN) graduate degree. The four categories of advanced practice nursing include clinical nurse specialist (CNS), certified nurse practitioner (CNP), certified registered nurse anesthetist (CRNA), or certified nurse midwife (CNM). Responsibilities and job descriptions vary with employment settings and individual state legislation (AORN, 2014).

Section Questions

1. Explain the purpose of the PNDS. [Ref 33]

2. Describe one primary benefit of the PNDS. [Ref 34]

3. Give examples of nursing diagnoses using the PNDS. [Ref 36]

4. Describe some of the desired patient outcomes defined in the PNDS. [Ref 37]

5. How does the perioperative nurse achieve patient outcomes? [Ref 38]

6. Explain the concept of patient-centric perioperative nursing care. [Ref 39]

7. Give examples of patient outcomes described in the PNDS. [Ref 41]

8. How are additional desired patient outcomes identified? [Ref 42]

9. Identify activities that promote personal and professional growth and development as a nurse. [Ref 44]

10. What distinguishes an expanded role in nursing from an advanced practice role? [Refs 45–46]

Practice Settings

47. Technological advances in anesthesia and operative techniques have dramatically increased the number of procedures that can be performed on an outpatient basis. Many procedures that once required a hospital-based operating room, that necessitated a large incision, and that involved a hospital stay and an extended recovery can now be performed in same-day, outpatient, or ambulatory settings.

48. Minimally invasive surgery (MIS) refers to surgery performed through small puncture holes with specialized instruments and equipment. Compared to open procedures, this surgical approach minimizes tissue damage and facilitates rapid recovery and same-day discharge.

49. Innovations in technology and surgical technique are making MIS applicable to increasingly more complex procedures. Reimbursement guidelines also encourage same-day surgery and early discharge. As a result, many surgical procedures have moved into settings outside the acute care, hospital-based operating room.

50. Many complex procedures (e.g., anterior cruciate ligament repair, single-level lumbar laminectomy) are performed in freestanding surgical centers, satellite surgery facilities, mobile surgical units, surgeons' office-based operating rooms, and clinics.

51. Some procedures such as the placement of stents, once performed exclusively in the operating room are now performed in the radiology unit using interventional techniques rather than open surgery.

52. As long as reimbursement favors outpatient surgery and technological advances in instrumentation and procedures continue to emerge, the number and type of surgeries performed in physicians' offices will also continue to increase.

53. The needs of the patient undergoing surgery transcend the setting in which the surgery takes place. In every setting, the perioperative nurse brings specialized skills, technical competence, knowledge, and caring that are essential to a successful surgical experience.

Members and Responsibilities of the Surgical Team

54. Safe and effective care of the surgical patient requires a team effort. Desired patient outcomes depend on the effective coordination of the unique skills of each member of the surgical team.

55. Team members are categorized based on their responsibilities during the procedure. Sterile team members are those who scrub their hands and arms, don sterile attire, contact sterile instruments and supplies, and work within the sterile field (i.e., the area immediately surrounding the surgical site). They are referred to as the "scrubbed" members of the team.

56. Members of the sterile surgical team include the primary surgeon, assistants to the surgeon (i.e., other surgeons, residents, physician assistants, and RNFAs), and the scrub person who may be a registered nurse, a licensed practical nurse, or a surgical technologist. Often, more than one scrub person is required in order to hold the camera for laparoscopic surgical procedures, or to hold retractors.

57. Members of the nonsterile surgical team carry out their responsibilities outside the sterile field and do not wear sterile attire. Members of the nonsterile surgical team include the anesthesiologist, the nurse anesthetist, the anesthesia assistant, the circulating nurse, and others such as the perfusionist and the radiology technician.

58. The primary surgeon is responsible for the preoperative diagnosis, selection of the procedure to be performed, and the actual performance of surgery.

59. Surgical assistants work under the direction of the primary surgeon and are responsible for providing assistance during surgery, such as exposing the site, suctioning, handling tissue, and suturing. The nature of the surgery, the state in which the surgery is performed, the medical board and the board of nursing, the surgeon's preference, and hospital policies are factors that determine who may function as an assistant.

60. The scrub person works primarily with instruments and equipment. The scrub person has the following responsibilities:
    - Selecting instruments, equipment, and other supplies appropriate for the surgery
    - Preparing the sterile field and setting up the sterile table(s) with instruments and other sterile supplies needed for the procedure
    - Scrubbing, and then donning a gown and gloves
    - Maintaining the integrity and sterility of the sterile field throughout the procedure
    - Having knowledge of the procedure and anticipating the surgeon's needs throughout the procedure
    - Providing instruments, sutures, and supplies to the surgeon in an appropriate and timely manner
    - Preparing sterile dressings
    - Implementing procedures that contribute to patient safety (e.g., surgical counts for instruments, sponges, and sharps)
    - Cleaning and preparing instruments for terminal sterilization

61. Factors that determine the most appropriate scrub person include the nature of the surgery, the skills required for the procedure, the staffing skill mix, and hospital policy.

62. The anesthesia provider is responsible for assessing the patient prior to surgery and for administering anesthetic agents to facilitate surgery and provide pain relief. Anesthesia providers include anesthesiologists, certified registered nurse anesthetists (CRNAs), and anesthesia assistants (American Association of Nurse Anesthetists, 2015). Each state determines which anesthesia providers will be licensed, who can practice independently, and who administers anesthesia under the direct supervision of the anesthesiologist or surgeon. The role of the perioperative registered nurse in monitoring the patient under conscious sedation is discussed in another chapter.

63. The perioperative nurse in the circulating role coordinates the care of the patient,

serves as the patient's advocate throughout the intraoperative experience, and has responsibility for managing and implementing activities outside the sterile field. Activities are directed toward psychological support of the awake patient, assuring patient safety, and achieving desired patient outcomes. The nursing process is used as a framework for these activities.

64. Examples of activities performed by the perioperative nurse in the circulating role include the following:

    • Providing emotional support to the patient prior to the induction of anesthesia

    • Performing ongoing patient assessment

    • Formulating a nursing diagnosis

    • Developing and implementing a plan of care

    • Documenting patient care

    • Evaluating patient outcomes

    • Teaching patient and family

    • Obtaining appropriate surgical supplies and equipment

    • Creating and maintaining a safe environment

    • Administering medications

    • Implementing and enforcing policies and procedures that contribute to patient safety, such as surgical checklists, "time-out" protocols, surgical counts for instruments, sponges, and sharps, as well as performing equipment checks

    • Preparing and disposing of specimens

    • Communicating relevant information to other team members and to the patient's family

65. All members of the surgical team present at the beginning of the procedure participate in the surgical time-out protocol.

66. Perioperative nurse managers assume a variety of roles. In a very small facility, the perioperative nurse may serve as manager and also scrub or circulate on cases as needed. In very large facilities, it is common to have several clinical and administrative managers. Budgets for surgical care in excess of $20 million are not uncommon and are often administered by a dedicated business financial manager. Surgery is often the largest revenue-producing department in a healthcare facility.

67. In addition to administrative department managers, other leadership/management positions include team leaders and managers or coordinators who assume responsibility for a particular surgical specialty. Such responsibilities may include:

    • Assigning staff

    • Managing and ensuring adequate inventory of specialty supplies

    • Ensuring availability of supplies and equipment needed for scheduled surgeries

    • Maintaining and updating preference cards that identify specific supplies and instruments needed by each surgeon for each procedure

    • Creating preference cards for surgeons new to the service

    • Periodically reviewing the contents of instrument trays for appropriateness

    • Standardizing supplies and trays whenever possible

    • Promoting or providing education

68. The operating room manager, team leader, or charge nurse "runs the desk" or "runs the board," which typically involves assigning surgeries to rooms, assigning staff to procedures, and making adjustments to keep the schedule moving throughout the day. An unanticipated emergency often requires quickly altering the daily schedule.

69. The scheduling coordinator, the person who places a procedure on the operating room schedule, must have knowledge of patient acuity and the resources required for the procedure. When a procedure requires staffing with a specific set of skills and/or unique equipment, it is essential to choose a time and place to ensure their availability.

70. Perfusionists; radiology and laboratory technicians; perioperative educators; pathologists; nurses' aides; clerks; and personnel from materials management, environmental services, and central service are among the personnel necessary to ensure safe patient care and achieve desired patient outcomes. It is the perioperative nurse who coordinates the contributions of each of these team members.

Section Questions

1. What factors have spurred the transition from inpatient surgery to same-day, outpatient, and ambulatory surgery? [Ref 47]

2. Describe the term "minimally invasive surgical techniques." [Ref 48]

3. Where, besides operating rooms, are invasive procedures performed? [Ref 52]

4. Identify members of the sterile and nonsterile components of the surgical team. [Refs 56–57]

5. What determines who may function as an assistant to the surgeon? [Ref 59]

6. Describe the responsibilities of the scrub person. [Ref 60]

7. Discuss the role of the circulating nurse. [Ref 63]

8. Describe the responsibilities of the circulating nurse. [Ref 64]

9. Who participates in the surgical time-out protocol? [Ref 65]

10. Which other activities can be performed by registered nurses in the perioperative setting? [Refs 67–69]

References

American Association of Nurse Anesthetists (AANA). (2015). *Federal supervision rule/opt out information.* Retrieved from http://www.aana.com/advocacy/stategovernmentaffairs/Pages/Federal-Supervision-Rule-Opt-Out-Information.aspx

American Hospital Association. (2015). Utilization and volume. In: *Trends Affecting Hospitals and Health Systems.* Retrieved from http://www.aha.org/research/reports/tw/chartbook/2014/chapter3.pdf

Association of periOperative Registered Nurses (AORN). (2011). *Perioperative nursing data set (PNDS)* (3rd ed.). Denver, CO: AORN.

Association of periOperative Registered Nurses (AORN). (2013). *AORN position statement on RN first assistants.* Retrieved from http://www.aorn.org/WorkArea/DownloadAsset.aspx?id=25934

Association of periOperative Registered Nurses (AORN). (2014). *Position statement on advanced practice registered nurses in the perioperative environment.* Retrieved from http://www.aorn.org/WorkArea/DownloadAsset.aspx?id=26698

Association of periOperative Registered Nurses (AORN). (2015). *Guidelines for perioperative practice.* Denver, CO: AORN.

Post-Test

Read each question carefully. Each question may have more than one correct answer.

1. The perioperative period begins when the patient
   a. arrives in the holding area and ends in PACU.
   b. arrives in the hospital and ends with discharge.
   c. is informed of the need for surgery and ends with discharge from the hospital.
   d. is informed of the need for surgery and ends when the patient achieves an optimal level of postsurgical function.

2. Which of the following is *not* a nursing focus during the preoperative period?
   a. Patient teaching
   b. Patient and family support
   c. Getting informed consent from the patient
   d. Preparation for the procedure

3. Intraoperative phase begins when
   a. the patient arrives at the hospital for surgery.
   b. the patient is transferred to the operating room bed.
   c. the anesthesia provider induces the patient.
   d. the surgeon makes the initial incision.

4. *Initial* nursing focus in the postoperative period focuses on
   a. controlling postoperative pain.
   b. supporting the patient's physiologic systems.
   c. preparing the patient for discharge.
   d. making arrangements for the patient to return to normal activity.

5. Why was the term "operating room nurse" changed to "perioperative nurse"?
   a. AORN decided it sounded more contemporary.
   b. To eliminate the "OR mystique" and encourage more nurses to join the specialty.
   c. The responsibilities of nurses in this specialty have expanded to support and care for the surgical patient through the continuum of care.
   d. Because PACU nurses wanted to be included.

6. AORN's Patient-Focused Model includes which of the following domains?
   a. Patient safety, physiologic response, behavioral responses, the health system
   b. Patient teaching, patient safety, behavioral responses, discharge planning
   c. Patient safety, patient assessment, discharge planning, the health system
   d. Patient assessment, plan of care, discharge planning, the health system

7. Perioperative nurses provide patient care
   a. to assist the surgeon and the anesthesia provider.
   b. that focuses primarily on patient and family education and support.
   c. within the framework of the nursing process: assessment, planning, intervention, and evaluation of patient outcomes.
   d. that is focused primarily on the patient's surgical diagnosis.

8. Nursing assessment of the surgical patient
   a. may take place in a number of settings and timeframes.
   b. may include a telephone call to the patient prior to surgery for teaching, support, and data gathering.
   c. is usually initiated by someone other than the perioperative nurse.
   d. takes place just prior to surgery and includes an interview, chart review, and a quick physical inspection of the patient.

9. Typical nursing diagnoses for the surgical patient include
   a. knowledge deficit and high risk for infection.
   b. prevention of adverse outcomes and patient teaching.
   c. high risk for infection and support of patient and family.
   d. maintenance of normothermia and anatomical body alignment.

10. The perioperative nurse begins the patient's care plan
    a. prior to the procedure, based on information about the patient from the surgeon and other healthcare providers.
    b. in the holding area based on interview and assessment data.
    c. prior to the procedure based on knowledge of the planned procedure, typical related nursing diagnoses, and resources required.
    d. when the patient enters the operating room and all attention is focused on supporting the patient.

11. The framework for the intervention stage of perioperative patient care is based on
    a. the surgeon's preferences related to the surgical procedure.
    b. the patient's medical diagnosis and comorbidities.
    c. the needs of the healthcare team participating in the surgical procedure.
    d. accepted standards of clinical practice and professional performance.

12. The criteria upon which the final evaluation is made is the extent to which
    a. the goals of the surgical procedure were met and the patient was transferred to the appropriate recovery area.
    b. the desired patient outcomes have been achieved.
    c. hospital policy and professional standards were upheld.
    d. the patient and family express satisfaction with the entire surgical experience.

13. The *Perioperative Nursing Data Set* (PNDS) is
    a. standardized nursing vocabulary used to describe perioperative nursing practice.
    b. a collection of recommended practices to guide patient care.
    c. used by all electronic health record systems to standardize patient records.
    d. a set of evaluation tools to determine the extent to which patient care has been successful.

14. Perioperative nursing is
    a. task oriented and designed to care effectively for surgical patients.
    b. nursing science related to surgical patients.
    c. patient oriented and focused on prevention, and uses knowledge, judgment, and skill.
    d. a framework to evaluate patients' responses to surgical and other invasive procedures.

15. Which of the following is not a standard of perioperative care?
    a. The patient is free from signs and symptoms of electrical injury.
    b. The patient receives appropriately administered medications.
    c. The patient's wound perfusion is consistent with or improved from baseline levels.
    d. The patient's comorbidities are managed effectively during the operative or other invasive procedure.

16. Which of the following facilitate(s) personal and professional growth?
    a. Participating in research activities
    b. Participating in professional organization activities
    c. Mentoring and precepting other perioperative nurses
    d. Pursuing certification

17. Which of the following is a true statement about the registered nurse first assistant (RNFA)?
    a. An RNFA is an advanced practice perioperative nurse, regardless of his or her academic level of preparation.
    b. The RNFA position is an expanded role in perioperative nursing.
    c. The RNFA practices under the license of the physician.
    d. The RNFA must have an advanced degree in nursing.

18. The transitioning of complex procedures from the traditional operating room to alternative settings is primarily the result of
    a. reimbursement guidelines.
    b. technological advances in anesthesia and surgical technique.
    c. patient preference.
    d. the nursing shortage.

19. Who may function in the scrub role?
    a. Perioperative registered nurse
    b. Licensed vocational or licensed practice nurse
    c. Surgical technologist
    d. CRNA

20. Who or what determines who may function as an assistant to the surgeon during the procedure?
    a. Surgeon
    b. Facility policy
    c. State board of medicine
    d. State board of nursing

21. What is the *primary* focus of the perioperative nurse?
    a. Managing the operating room environment
    b. Patient safety and achieving the desired patient outcomes
    c. Supervising the scrub person
    d. Documenting intraoperative patient care

22. Which of the following roles is *not* part of the sterile surgical team?
    a. Perfusionist
    b. RNFA
    c. First assistant
    d. Surgical technologist

2

Preparing the Patient for Surgery

LEARNER OBJECTIVES

1. Recognize common nursing diagnoses related to the preoperative phase.
2. Identify desired patient outcomes related to the preoperative phase.
3. Describe the critical factors included in a preoperative patient assessment.
4. Describe interventions to achieve desired preoperative patient outcomes.
5. Identify at least eight factors that may contribute to wrong-site surgery.
6. Describe the three components of The Joint Commission protocol to prevent wrong-site surgery.
7. Discuss the content of preoperative patient teaching.

LESSON OUTLINE

Communication of Relevant Patient Data

1. Continuity of care and planning for appropriate therapeutic interventions depend upon clear, concise, and complete information. Written documentation and verbal communication of patient data and patient responses to interventions are essential components of safe and effective patient care (Wheeler, 2014).

2. The perioperative nurse most often encounters the patient for the first time immediately prior to surgery in the preop holding area. Because there is rarely enough time to carry out a comprehensive history and assessment, the perioperative nurse must rely on information gathered by others.

3. Transfer of care is an essential component of patient safety. The nurse caring for the patient in the preoperative period must provide appropriate hand-off information to the nurse caring for the patient during the intraoperative period.

4. A defined process of communicating among healthcare providers is critical to insuring that assessment information with relevance to the intraoperative and postoperative care reaches the appropriate members of the healthcare team. Standardization in the hand-off process

provides a framework for comprehensive and concise communication. A written tool used consistently is an effective approach to promoting patient safety (Association of peri-Operative Registered Nurses [AORN], 2015, p. 583). See **Exhibits 2-1** and **2-2**.

5. Because a significant number of patient injuries is caused by poor communication or the absence of communication among caregivers, The Joint Commission (TJC) mandated a standardized approach to hand-off communications, including the opportunity to ask and respond to questions, into its National Patient Safety Goals in 2010.

6. Patient assessment and care in the preoperative period may be documented on stand-alone forms or may be part of an integrated form that includes assessment and patient care throughout the preoperative, intraoperative, and postoperative periods.

7. Several hand-off protocols have been used successfully to communicate comprehensive and concise patient-focused information:

    • The SBAR (Situation, Background, Assessment, and Recommendation) technique is an example of a process that can be used for prompt and appropriate communication throughout the perioperative period, including during preoperative assessment, intraoperatively among caregivers, and during hand-off to the postanesthesia care unit (PACU). SBAR is modeled on naval military protocol and was adapted for use in health care by Kaiser Permanente (**Figure 2-1**).

    • I PASS the BATON (Introduction, Patient, Assessment, Situation, Safety concerns, Background, Actions, Timing, Ownership, Next) is a technique used in the U.S. Department of Defense's Patient Safety Program to provide a structure that improves communication during transitions in care. It should include opportunities to confirm receipt, ask questions, clarify information, and verify that the information is understood (**Figure 2-2**).

    • PACE for healthcare (Patient/Problem, Assessment/Actions, Continuing interventions/Changes, Evaluation) is another acronym identifying essential elements in patient care.

    • FIVE Ps (Patient, Plan, Purpose, Problem, Precautions, coordinating Physician). Alliteration often assists us in remembering steps in a process.

    • SHARQ (Situation, History, Assessment, Recommendations/Results, Questions)

    All of the communication tools represent unique acronyms and mnemonics designed to remind us of the essential components of communication about patients.

Nursing Diagnoses

8. The perioperative nurse combines unique knowledge of the surgical procedure with patient assessment data to formulate nursing diagnoses that serve as the basis for the patient's plan of care.

9. The *Perioperative Nursing Data Set* (PNDS) developed by AORN (2011) identifies 93 nursing diagnoses, 151 interventions, and 40 nurse-sensitive patient outcomes specifically related to the patient undergoing a surgical or invasive procedure.

10. NANDA International (2014) has defined 235 evidence-based diagnoses relevant to a broader patient population.

11. The plan of care evolves as the perioperative nurse identifies nursing diagnoses and interventions specific to the patient. Some nursing diagnoses apply to a single phase of the perioperative experience; others might apply to all three phases.

Desired Patient Outcomes

12. While each plan of care must be customized to address the patient's specific diagnoses, several nursing diagnoses, desired outcomes, and associated interventions are common to all surgical patients.

13. For example, the desired outcome, "The patient or designated support person demonstrates knowledge of the expected responses to the operative or invasive procedure" (AORN, 2011, p. 114), applies to all surgical patients.

14. To achieve the desired outcome, the nurse will validate that the patient and support person understand the procedure to be performed and the risks described in the consent form.

Preoperative Assessment and Interventions

15. Nursing interventions during the preoperative period are directed toward preparing the patient psychologically and physiologically for surgery.

Exhibit 2-1 Preoperative Visit Assessment

OR #: _____				**PRE-OP VISIT**		

PERSONAL PHYSICIAN	SURGEON	ANESTHESIOLOGIST	SEX □ M □ F	AGE

DATE	TIME	PROCEDURE		NICKNAME

ALLERGIES	ISOLATION PRECAUTIONS □ TB □ Other

MEDICAL & SURGICAL HISTORY:
_____
_____
_____
_____
_____
_____
_____

	SKIN ASSESSMENT	**MENTAL/ EMOTIONAL**	**VISION**	**PRE-OP TUBES**	**LABORATORY INFORMATION**	**PRE-OP:**
HT:	COLOR:	□ Oriented	□ Adequate	□ Foley		
	□ Pale	□ Disoriented To:	□ Decreased	□ NG		**TIME:**
WT:	□ Flushed	□ Time	□ Blind	□ Other:		
T:	□ Dusky	□ Place	□ Rt □ Lt			
P:	□ Cyanotic	□ Person	□ Glasses	**CHART REQUIREMENTS**		**ROUTINE MEDS:**
	□ Jaundice	□ Lethargic	□ Contacts			
R:	□ Normal	□ Comatose	**HEARING**	□ Permit		
BP RANGE:	□ Other:	□ Dementia/ Alzheimers	□ Adequate	□ H & P		
PERIPHERAL PERFUSION:	CONDITION:	□ Protective Devices	□ Decreased	**DENTURES**	□ BLOOD GLUCOSE MONITORING	
	□ No Problem		□ Deaf	□ Upper	SHA / OR / PACU INSTRUCTIONS:	
PULSES:	□ Rash	□ Calm	□ Rt □ Lt	□ Lower		
RR:	□ Boney Area	□ Apprehensive	□ Hearing Aid	□ Partial	X-RAYS:	
LR:	□ Redness	□ Emotional Disorders	COMMUNICATION BARRIERS:			
RP:	□ Decubiti	UNITS OF BLOOD:			SCANS:	
LP:	□ Contusions/ Abrasions	□ T & C	CONSULTING PHYSICIANS/ SPECIALTY:			
SMOKES:	□ Edema	Number of Units on Hand:			EKG:	
□ Yes	□ Other:					
□ No						
□ PPD ____					FAMILY	
□ Quit ____					□ FWA □ ICU FWA □ HOME □ OTHER:	

COMMENTS:
_____
_____
_____
_____

IVs: □ Central □ Peripheral DATE OF INSERTION: _____	Fluids: _____ Support Meds: Type _____ Rate _____ TPN & Rate: _____	□ OR RN □ PACU RN Signature:

Pilot Draft form courtesy of St. Luke's Medical Center, Milwaukee, Wisconsin.

Exhibit 2-2 Preoperative Flowsheet

Operative Permit Complete ☐ Yes ☐ No	ID Bracelet ☐ Yes ☐ No	Glasses/Contact Lenses ☐ Yes ☐ No	Dentures ☐ Yes ☐ No	Hearing Aid ☐ Yes ☐ No
Chest X-ray on Chart ☐ Yes ☐ No	Allergy Bracelet ☐ Yes ☐ No	Blood Bracelet ☐ Yes ☐ No No. of Units	Preop Bath/Shower ☐ Yes ☐ No	
ECG on Chart ☐ Yes ☐ No	History and Physical ☐ Yes ☐ No	List any abnormalities, blindness, deafness, prosthesis, amputation, paralysis, etc. _____		
Ordered Lab Work on Chart ☐ Yes ☐ No Abnormal Called to:		Isolation Required: ☐ Yes ☐ No Reason:		
General Appearance: Flushed ☐ Yes ☐ No Diaphoretic ☐ Yes ☐ No Pale ☐ Yes ☐ No Skin Intact ☐ Yes ☐ No Cyanotic ☐ Yes ☐ No Other _____ Jaundice ☐ Yes ☐ No		Jewelry Removed ☐ N/A ☐ Yes ☐ No ☐ Rings Tape ☐ Given to Family, Who?_____ Hospital Gown ☐ Yes ☐ No Voided/Foley ☐ Yes ☐ No Time	Level of Consciousness: ☐ Alert ☐ Oriented x3 ☐ Drowsy ☐ Other _____ Patient's Emotional Status ☐ Accepting ☐ Apprehensive	

NURSING INTERVENTION

For SAU Nurse Only		Patient Sent on O₂ Patient ECG Monitored ☐ Yes ☐ No	
☐ Blood Pressure Cuff On	Antibiotic Hanging ☐ Yes ☐ No ☐ N/A	☐ Yes L/m _____ ☐ Nasal Cannula ☐ Mask ☐ Ambu Bag	

Preop Medication/Dosage	Time	Int.		Time	Int.	Transporter's Initial:
1.			4.			
2.			5.			
3.			6.			

Beta Blocker Given: ☐ Yes ☐ No ☐ N/A   Reason held _____

Sending RN	Initial	Receiving RN verifies above information	Initial

MARKING OF OPERATIVE SITE

OR SAU		
☐ ☐	Patient identified using 2 indicators—Name, DOB	
☐ ☐	Correct site verified w/OR schedule, H&P, patient & physician order	

OR SAU		
☐ ☐	Operative site marked "Yes"—Laterality identified ☐ N/A	
☐ ☐	Site marked by ☐ Patient ☐ Nurse ☐ Physician	
☐	Diagnostics available in OR suite for site verification	

PATIENT ASSESSMENT BY OPERATING NURSE		Antibiotic Administration	Time	Int.
		☐ Ancef 1 gm IVPB		
		☐ Zinacef 1.5 gms		
☐ Lab Values Reviewes ☐ Chart Reviewed		☐ Vancomyacin 1 gm IVPB		
Allergies:		☐ Cefotan 2 gms IVPB		
Condition of skin:		☐ Ciproflaxin 400 mg IVPB		
Motor/Sensory impairment		☐ Claforan 2 gms IVPB		
Abnormalities		☐ Clindamyacin 600 mg IVPB		
Operative/Procedure confirmed ☐ Yes ☐ No		☐ Flagyl 500 mg IVPB		
Cardiovascular		☐ Unasyn 3 gms IVPB		
Respiratory		☐ Mefoxin 2 gms IVPB		
Additional Findings		☐ Other		

PATIENT/FAMILY EDUCATION

Relevant information on surgical procedure given to patient. ☐ Yes ☐ No   Family Present ☐ Yes ☐ No
If no, why? _____

NURSING COMMENTS _____

_____ RN
Operating Room Nurse Signature   Date   Time

INTEGRIS BAPTIST MEDICAL CENTER
PREOPERATIVE FLOWSHEET

16. Preoperative preparations focus on a variety of nursing activities, including patient assessment and data collection, patient and family teaching, providing emotional support, planning care for the intraoperative and postoperative periods, and communicating patient information to healthcare team members.

17. Assessment data come from a combination of chart review, patient/family questionnaire and interview, observation, and communication with other healthcare providers. A preoperative assessment/checklist completed prior to transport to the holding area may provide valuable information (**Exhibits 2-1** and **2-2**).

18. Interventions related to providing support during the preoperative period apply to all surgical patients. Encouraging patients to express their feelings about the surgical experience addresses the desired outcome that the patient's level of anxiety or fear will be reduced to a minimum.

19. Nurses want all surgical patients to be able to demonstrate knowledge of the anticipated responses related to the operative or invasive procedure. Assessing the patient's unique learning needs enables the nurse to provide relevant information in a manner appropriate for the patient.

20. Commonly targeted patient outcomes include freedom from infection, freedom from injury, skin integrity, electrolyte balance, and patient participation in the rehabilitation process.

21. The preoperative assessment provides information necessary to address these outcomes effectively. For example, assessment data that reveal limited range of motion in a shoulder would be valuable when planning for patient transfer and patient positioning to ensure that there would be no further injury to the shoulder. Identifying an existing infection might necessitate postponing the surgical procedure.

22. Administration of antibiotics prior to making the incision in certain types of surgery has been shown to significantly reduce the rate of surgical infection and has been incorporated into the Surgical Care Improvement Project (SCIP) sponsored by the Centers for Medicare & Medicaid Services (CMS) in collaboration with a number of other national partners, including the American Hospital Association (AHA), Centers for Disease Control and Prevention (CDC), Institute for Healthcare Improvement (IHI), and TJC.

23. The goal of prophylaxis with antibiotics is to establish bactericidal tissue and serum levels at the time of skin incision. The SCIP performance measure is that antibiotics will be administered within 1 hour prior to the skin incision (TJC, 2015b) (THR, 2015).

24. Vancomycin and fluoroquinolones require a longer infusion time, so it is acceptable to start these antibiotics within 2 hours prior to incision time (TJC, 2015b) (THR, 2015).

25. The perioperative nurse may share the responsibility for ensuring that preoperative antibiotics are administered in a timely fashion prior to surgery.

26. Body mass index (BMI), or percentage of body fat, has emerged as a major risk factor for postoperative surgical site infections (SSIs) for virtually all surgical services. Obese patients (BMI > 30 kg/m²; CDC, 2015) require a larger loading dose of antibiotics to provide consistent tissue concentrations over the duration of the surgical procedure. Currently, studies are underway to determine the most effective weight-based dose for obese patients undergoing surgical procedures (University of Cincinnati, 2011; University of Colorado, Denver, 2014).

27. Obese patients have decreased tissue perfusion and lower levels of tissue oxygen, increasing their risk for SSIs (Pierpont et al., 2014). In addition, obese patients have an increased frequency of comorbid conditions, such as diabetes mellitus, that may increase their risk for SSIs.

28. Knowledge gained through patient assessment contributes to the nurse's ability to advocate for the patient.

29. During surgery, when normal protective reflexes are compromised, patients must rely on members of the healthcare team to advocate for their safety.

30. The protocol for prevention of wrong-site surgery begins preoperatively with identifying the patient; validating the intended procedure with the patient, the informed consent, and the results of diagnostic testing; and marking the operative site.

Section Questions

1. What is the purpose of a defined process of communicating patient information among healthcare professionals? [Refs 1–5]

2. Using either the SBAR or the I PASS the Baton hand-off tool, identify the essential information required when transferring patient care from one caregiver to another. [Ref 7, Figures 2-1 and 2-2]

3. What sources does the perioperative nurse use to formulate nursing diagnoses for the patient? [Refs 8, 17]

4. What is the purpose of AORN's *Perioperative Nursing Data Set* (PNDS)? [Ref 9]

5. How does the plan of care for each surgical patient develop? [Ref 11]

6. Describe four desired outcomes that apply to all surgical patients. [Ref 20]

7. What is the rationale for the specific time of administration of preoperative antibiotic prophylaxis? [Ref 23]

8. What is the ideal timeframe in which to provide most prophylactic antibiotics to ensure that the tissue and serum levels of the antibiotic are sufficient? [Ref 23]

9. Which preoperative antibiotics require a longer infusion period? [Ref 24]

10. How does obesity affect the risk of adverse outcomes of surgery? [Ref 27]

Assessment Parameters

Physiologic

31. Critical physiologic assessment data include:
    - Medical diagnosis, chronic diseases, and treatment
    - Medications, especially antibiotics; herbal medications; anticoagulants, including aspirin; diuretics that deplete potassium; over-the-counter medications; history of chemotherapy
    - Surgery to be performed and verification of the surgical site
    - Previous surgeries and any complications, including anesthesia complications
    - Vital signs, diagnostic data, and laboratory data as ordered—abnormalities
      - Hemoglobin and hematocrit
      - White blood cell count
      - Platelet count
      - Serum electrolytes
      - Urinalysis
      - Chest X-ray
      - Diagnostic X-rays pertinent to the surgical procedure
      - Electrocardiogram
      - Blood type and cross-match information and availability of replacement blood
      - Results of specific tests or studies specific to the planned procedure
    - Age—very young or very old
    - Substance abuse—smoking, alcohol, drugs
    - Skin condition—color, rashes, lesions
    - Allergies—medication and latex allergies are critical (**Exhibit 2-3**)
    - Potential for malignant hyperthermia—personal history; family history
    - Nutrition and nothing-by-mouth (NPO) status
    - Sensory impairments—presence of lenses, hearing aids, dentures
    - Mobility impairments
    - Presence of prosthetic devices—orthopedic implants, pacemaker, vascular prosthesis
    - Weight/height/BMI—extreme underweight and overweight; height greater than length of the operating room table; implications for medication dosage
    - Preoperative medication as ordered has been given; timing of prophylactic antibiotics

Exhibit 2-3 Parma Community General Hospital Latex Allergy Patient Questionnaire

NOTE: These questions are not intended to be all-inclusive. Individuals who are potentially latex allergic should seek additional testing through their primary care physician. This questionnaire is merely a collection of relevant data to be passed onto your physician for further evaluation/testing for confirmation of allergy.

1. Have you ever been told that you have a latex allergy?   **Yes**   **No**
   If so, do you have documented laboratory tests to confirm this?   **Yes**   **No**

2. What specifically are you allergic to that contains latex?
   _____

3. Have you ever had any reaction to any of the following sources of latex?

Balloons	☐	Rubber gloves	☐	Rubber balls	☐	Rubber bands	☐
Adhesive tape	☐	Ace bandages	☐	Dental bite blocks	☐	Belts	☐
Brassieres	☐	Carpet backing	☐	Clothing with elastic	☐	Rubber cement	☐
Suspenders	☐	Teething rings	☐	Condoms	☐	Corsets	☐
Erasers	☐	Face masks	☐	Foam pillows	☐	Garden hoses	☐
Latex cuffs	☐	Ostomy bags	☐	Milking machines	☐	Tennis grips	☐
Dental masks	☐	Pacifiers	☐	Weather stripping	☐	IV tubing	☐
Golf grips	☐	Poinsettias	☐	Elastic bandages	☐	Other	☐

4. Do you have a history of any symptoms as stated below, following the use of latex products as stated above?

"Contact dermatitis" (redness, itching, cracked skin)	**Yes**	**No**
Rhinitis/allergic rhinitis (nasal congestion, sneezing, runny nose)	**Yes**	**No**
Conjunctivitis (red swollen itchy/sore eyes)	**Yes**	**No**
Hay fever (sneezing)	**Yes**	**No**
Eczema (flaky, itchy, red skin)	**Yes**	**No**
Auto-immune disease	**Yes**	**No**
Asthma (wheezing-type breathing, difficulty with breathing)	**Yes**	**No**
Fatigue/drowsiness	**Yes**	**No**
Facial swelling/redness	**Yes**	**No**
Reactions to bandages/tape	**Yes**	**No**
Hives/unexplained rash	**Yes**	**No**
Sudden onset of bronchitis/sinusitis following contact with above products	**Yes**	**No**

Please describe

_____

_____

5. Do you have any food allergies?   **Yes**   **No**

   List: _____

   Are you allergic to any of the following?

   Banana   Avocado   Potato   Milk   Kiwi   Chestnuts   Peaches
   Tomato   Papaya   Passion fruit   Other tropical fruit

   Describe your allergic reaction: _____

continues

Exhibit 2-3 Parma Community General Hospital Latex Allergy Patient Questionnaire (continued)

6. After handling any latex products have you experienced any of the following:

Chapping/cracking of skin on hands	**Yes No**		Redness	**Yes**	**No**
Swelling	**Yes No**		Hives	**Yes**	**No**
Runny nose or nasal congestion	**Yes No**		Itching	**Yes**	**No**

7. Have you ever had previous surgery?   **Yes   No**
If so how many surgical procedures: _____

Types: _____

_____

8. Do you suffer from any congenital abnormalities (e.g., spina bifida)?   **Yes   No**

Name: _____

9. Does your occupation require you to have frequent contact with latex products?   **Yes   No**

List: _____

10. Have you ever had an anaphylactic reaction to latex or latex-containing products? **Yes   No**
Explain/describe the circumstances:

_____

Questionnaire developed and provided by Ruth Bakst, RN, CNOR, RNFA, Perioperative and Emergency Room Clinical Instructor, Parma Community General Hospital, Parma, Ohio.

Psychosocial

32. Critical psychosocial assessment data include the following:

- Understanding and perception of the procedure to be performed
- Coping ability/support system
- Ability to comprehend
- Readiness to learn
- Anxiety related to the surgical intervention or surgical outcome
- Knowledge of perioperative routines
- Cultural or spiritual beliefs relevant to the surgical intervention

Nursing Diagnoses and Interventions

Preoperative Period

33. The most common nursing diagnoses in the preoperative period are knowledge deficit and anxiety.

34. Knowledge deficit may be related to perioperative routines, surgical interventions, or outcome expectations.

35. Knowledge deficit may be the result of a lack of information regarding the surgical procedure, poor understanding of information shared prior to admission, impaired communication ability, a language barrier, or diminished mental capacity. Nursing interventions for patient teaching must take into account the reason for the patient's knowledge deficit and the patient's learning needs.

36. Anxiety is a general uneasiness, ranging from mild to severe, that may have a variety of etiologies. Patients who are anxious, uneasy, or nervous cannot always identify the exact cause of their anxiety.

37. For some patients, anxiety is most acute at the time the decision to have surgery is made. Others experience the greatest anxiety just prior to surgery.

38. Anxiety differs from fear, which is defined as dread of something specific; the fearful patient can identify the focus of his or her fear.

39. Fear may be related to the surgical intervention, surgical outcome, anesthesia, impact of surgery on lifestyle, loss of control, pain, or death. It is more common for patients to be anxious than fearful.

40. Anticipatory grieving is another related preoperative nursing diagnosis; it is related to possible changes in body image.

41. Increased heart and respiratory rates and an elevated blood pressure can be signs of anxiety or fear.

42. A patient who is nervous or tense may not be able to concentrate or retain information.

43. The desired outcome related to anxiety is that anxiety and fear will be lessened through increased knowledge and the ability to express feelings about the surgical intervention. It is important to assess readiness to learn, because providing more information than the patient desires or can handle can exacerbate anxiety.

44. The following nursing interventions are ways to address anxiety and fear:
    - Listen attentively.
    - Provide information as needed and desired. (Providing information that the patient does not wish to know can increase the patient's anxiety.)
    - Solicit the patient's description of anxiety or fear.
    - Provide emotional support and reassurance.

45. The desired outcome related to a knowledge deficit is that the patient will demonstrate knowledge of the physiologic and psychological responses to surgery.

46. The following nursing interventions are essential to promote patient safety, assess knowledge, and address any knowledge deficits:
    - Confirm the patient's identity.
    - Verify the surgical site and procedure.
    - Verify the patient's consent for surgery.
    - Solicit the patient's perception of the planned procedure.
    - Solicit the patient's questions about the surgery.
    - Identify the patient's learning needs as well as readiness and ability to learn.

- Describe what the patient will experience.
- Explain the procedures that must be followed postoperatively upon discharge (especially critical for patients who will be discharged on the day of their surgery, which limits the time available for teaching).
- Provide information with consideration for the patient's level of understanding, ability to comprehend, desire for information, culture, and religious beliefs. Refer the patient's medical concerns to the surgeon.
- Solicit feedback regarding perioperative procedures.

47. Evaluate achievement of desired outcomes based on the patient's ability to:
    - Confirm the consent.
    - Describe the expected sequence of events.
    - Express feelings about the surgical experience.
    - Demonstrate awareness of the expected surgical outcomes.
    - Confirm procedures to be followed upon discharge.

48. Each patient is unique; many nursing diagnoses will apply to some patients but not to others. Individual patient assessment will determine which nursing diagnoses are applicable, and interventions must be individualized for each patient.

Intraoperative Period

49. The intraoperative period begins when the patient enters the actual operating room and is transferred to the operating room bed. At that point, the room is considered "contaminated to the patient." Should the procedure be canceled, the setup cannot be used for another case.

50. During the intraoperative period, the patient is at high risk for injury related to:
    - Transport and transfer
    - Positioning
    - Equipment such as a pneumatic tourniquet
    - Chemical agents such as skin-prep solutions
    - Use of X-ray, electrosurgery, or laser
    - Fluid deficit
    - Impaired gas exchange related to general anesthesia

• Retained surgical items (e.g., sponge, instrument, or miscellaneous item inadvertently left in the body)

Nursing interventions to prevent these injuries are presented elsewhere.

51. The patient is also at risk for infection related to surgical intervention. Interventions to reduce endogenous flora and prevent exposure to exogenous flora are discussed elsewhere.

Section Questions

1. Give examples of physiologic patient assessment data collected by the perioperative nurse. [Ref 31]

2. Other than medication allergies, what type of allergy might have significance for the intraoperative phase of surgery? [Ref 31]

3. Describe psychosocial assessment data. [Ref 32]

4. What are the two most common nursing diagnoses in the preoperative period? [Ref 33]

5. Differentiate *anxiety* from *fear*. [Refs 36–39]

6. What is the most common focus of *anticipatory grieving*? [Ref 40]

7. What implications do anxiety and fear have for the preparation of the patient for surgery? [Refs 41–42]

8. What interventions help the perioperative nurse to assess and validate the patient's knowledge related to the surgical experience? [Refs 44, 46–47]

9. When does the intraoperative period begin? [Ref 49]

10. What factors in the intraoperative period place the patient at risk for injury? [Refs 50–51]

Prevention of Wrong-Site Surgery

52. In 1999, the Institute of Medicine (IOM, 2000), in *To Err Is Human: Building a Safer Health System*, reported that as many as 98,000 patients die in hospitals each year as a result of preventable medical errors (p. 1). This publication focused the attention of healthcare facilities, professional organizations, the CMS, the CDC, and TJC on initiatives to improve patient safety.

53. TJC (2014a) defines *sentinel events* or *never events* as preventable situations, not primarily related to the natural course of the patient's illness or underlying condition, that result in death, permanent harm, or severe temporary harm, and require intervention to sustain life. They are described as *sentinel* because they signal the need for immediate investigation and response and *never* because they can and should be prevented.

54. One never event is wrong-site surgery, which includes surgery on the wrong patient, wrong body part, wrong side, wrong level, or wrong site; or, it may be the wrong surgical procedure altogether (TJC, 2014a).

55. TJC (2014b) reviewed 8,275 sentinel events between 2004 and June 2014, of which 1,072 were cases of wrong-site surgery. Reporting is voluntary, so actual numbers are likely to be much higher.

56. The following factors, among others, have been identified as contributors to wrong-site surgery (Center for Transforming Healthcare [CTH], 2013, p. 7):

• Unapproved abbreviations, cross-outs, and illegible handwriting

• Missing consent, history, and physical examination, or surgeon's operative orders

• Inconsistent use of site-marking protocol

• Inconsistent or absent time-out process

• Rushing during patient verification

• Change of patient position

• Inadequate patient verification by surgical team

• Lack of intraoperative site verification when multiple procedures are performed by the same surgeon

• Ineffective hand-off communication or briefing process

- Site markings removed during prep or draping
- Distractions and rushing during the time-out process
- Time-out occurs before all staff are ready or before prep and drape
- Time-out performed without full participation
- Time-outs do not occur when there are multiple procedures performed by multiple surgeons in a single operative case
- Inconsistent organizational focus on patient safety; senior leadership not actively engaged
- Staff members are passive or not empowered to speak up
- Marketplace competition and pressure to increase surgical volume leading to shortcuts and variation in practice

57. Since 2004, though individual institutional policies and procedures may vary, all healthcare organizations must comply with The Joint Commission's (2015c) universal protocol for preventing wrong-site surgery. This protocol includes the following three steps which are included in the TJC's National Patient Safety Goals (TJC, 2015a):

    - *Conduct a pre-procedure verification process.* All documents and studies available prior to the procedure should be reviewed and should be consistent with each other, with the patient's expectations, and with the team's understanding of the intended patient, procedure, site, and, as applicable, any implants. Missing information or discrepancies must be addressed before starting the procedure.

    - *Mark the procedure site.* Unambiguously identify the intended site of incision or insertion (for all procedures involving right/left distinction or multiple structures such as fingers and multiple levels such as the spine).

    - *Perform a time-out.* The procedure is not started until all questions or concerns are resolved.

58. In the preoperative period, the nurse performing the patient assessment should verify the patient's identity and the procedure. This should be done verbally with the patient and by checking the patient's name band.

59. Chart review should begin by ascertaining that the patient, the chart, and the name band refer to the same person. If the patient is unable to communicate, verification should be made with the family or an authorized representative and through chart review.

60. Verification of the patient's identity and surgical procedure must be a priority for the perioperative nurse. A patient should never be transferred into the operating room suite without an identification band that has been verified for accuracy.

61. While the surgeon is responsible for determining the patient's need for surgery, identifying the procedure, and delineating the surgical site, verifying the patient's identity and verifying the correct surgical site are the responsibilities of all team members.

62. Most healthcare facilities have policies that identify how verification should occur, who is responsible for verification, and what documentation must be completed. Typically, the surgeon, the anesthesiologist, and the circulating nurse must all participate in verification.

63. For many years, TJC, AORN, and the American College of Surgeons (ACS) have had published guidelines regarding marking the surgical site. These guidelines specify what is marked, how it is marked, and by whom. They also provide guidelines for verifying the surgical site (ACS, 2002; AORN, 2011; CTH, 2013).

64. TJC identifies the following characteristics of the time-out process:

    - It is standardized, as defined by the hospital.
    - It is initiated by a designated member of the team (determined by facility policy).
    - It involves the immediate members of the procedure team, including the individual performing the procedure, the anesthesia providers, the circulating nurse, the scrub person, and other active participants who will be participating in the procedure from the beginning.
    - When two or more procedures are being performed on the same patient, and the person performing the procedure changes, perform a time-out before each procedure is initiated.
    - During the time-out, the team members agree, at a minimum, on the following:
      - Correct patient identity
      - The correct site—site marking is validated
      - The procedure to be done

– Completion of the time-out is documented; the amount and type of documentation are determined by facility policy.

65. Many facilities have developed forms like the *Comprehensive Surgical Checklist* to ensure that all steps are followed and to streamline documentation requirements (**Exhibit 2-4**).

Section Questions

1. What impact did the IOM publication *To Err Is Human* have on the healthcare arena? [Ref 52]
2. What is The Joint Commission's definition of *never events* or *sentinel events*? [Ref 53]
3. What is the definition of *wrong-site surgery*? [Ref 54]
4. What factors have been identified as contributors to wrong-site surgery? [Ref 56]
5. What are the three components for TJC's protocol for preventing wrong-site surgery? [Ref 57]
6. Discuss ways in which the patient's identity is continuously verified during the perioperative process. [Refs 58–62]
7. What should be the first step in reviewing the chart? [Ref 59]
8. What are the characteristics of the time-out process? [Ref 64]
9. Describe the essential elements of the time out. [Ref 64]
10. What is the purpose of the surgical safety checklist? [Ref 65]

Documentation

66. Clear, concise, complete, and accurate documentation is a core responsibility of the perioperative nurse. The patient's record is the only document with complete details of the care received. If information is omitted, it is unavailable to anyone reviewing the record, including caregivers who base decisions about the patient's care on the information available.

67. During a surgical procedure, information must be documented in the patient's record at a time when the circulating nurse is busy delivering direct patient care. That information must be captured so that it can be documented accurately at a later time. Many facilities have developed forms to capture this information. The form is a worksheet that does not become part of the patient's chart (**Exhibit 2-5**).

68. It is essential that the time at which events occurred (e.g., patient in room, anesthesia start time, incision time) that are documented in various places (e.g., electronic health record, anesthesia notes, surgeon's op notes) be consistent. As you record different times on your worksheet, verify with the anesthesia provider that you are both using the same time.

69. The patient's record is a legal document and may be used at some future date to provide information for further care of the patient, or to explore, analyze, or validate the care the patient received during his or her admission. You remain accountable for the information you document.

70. If you did not participate in an activity, document the personnel who did. For instance, if someone else counted with the scrub person, be sure that individual is reflected in the record. If someone else inserted the Foley catheter, provide that information for the record. If the record is used in the future to reconstruct events related to the patient's hospital stay, it is imperative that your documentation leave no room for misinterpretation.

71. Some facilities do a formal post-procedure wrap-up (**Exhibit 2-6**) to assess practices and identify opportunities for improvement in delivering safe and effective patient care (Sadler, 2014).

Exhibit 2-4 Comprehensive Surgical Checklist

PREPROCEDURE: In Holding Area	SIGN-IN: Before Induction of Anesthesia	TIME-OUT: Before Skin Incision	SIGN-OUT: Before the patient leaves the O.R.
Patient Actively Confirms with Registered Nurse (RN):	**RN and Anesthesia Care Provider Confirm:**	**Initiated by designated team member** All other activities to be suspended (unless a life-threatening emergency)	**RN Confirms** **Name of Operative Procedure**
☐ Patient Identity (Name)	☐ Procedure	Introduction of team members ☐ Yes	☐
☐ Birth Date	☐ Procedure site and consents	**All:**	Completion of sponge, sharp, and instrument counts
☐ Check Arm Band (Chart, Sticker)	Site Marked ☐ Yes ☐ NA by person performing the procedure	Confirmation of the following:	☐ Yes ☐ N/A
☐ Allergies	Patient Allergies ☐ Yes ☐ NKA	Identity, procedure, incision site, consent(s) ☐ Yes ☐ No	Specimens identified, numbered, and labeled ☐ Yes ☐ N/A
☐ NPO Status	Difficult Airway or Aspiration Risk	Site marked and visible ☐ Yes ☐ N/A	**All Team Members:** Key concerns for recovery and management of the patient
☐ Teeth, Loose, Dentures, Caps	☐ No	Any equipment concerns:	
☐ Verified with patient: Clothes, Jewelry/Body piercings, Metal inside (pacemaker, AICD, implants)	☐ Yes (preparation confirmed) _____	_____	_____
	SCD Hose or Sequentials Applied	**Anesthesia Provider:** Antibiotic prophylaxis within 1 hour before incision	_____
Procedure: ☐ Correct Site ☐ Site Marked	☐ DVT Protocol	☐ Yes ☐ N/A	_____
☐ History and Physical ☐ Preanesthesia Assessment ☐ Pre-Moderate Sedation Assessment	☐ N/A ☐ Warm Blankets Applied	**Scrub and circulating nurse:** ☐ Sterilization indicators have been confirmed	_____
Consents: ☐ Surgical ☐ Anesthesia	**Briefing:** All members of the team have discussed care plan and addressed concerns ☐ Yes	Additional concerns: _____ _____	
Pregnancy Test ☐ N/A ☐ Diagnostic Tests ☐ X-rays ☐ Blood Products Yes ☐ N/A ☐			

Adapted from Spivey Station Surgery Center, Jonesboro, GA (with permission).

Exhibit 2-4 Comprehensive Surgical Checklist (continued)

Definitions	Fire Risk 0-1	Fire Risk - 2
Oxygen delivery	**Standard Guidelines:**	**Head, Neck, and Chest Guidelines**
Open = Patient receiving oxygen via nasal cannula, face mask, or uncuffed endotracheal tube	☐ Sterile water or saline on field	☐ N/A
	☐ Alcohol base prep dried (at least 3 minutes)	☐ Verbal communication among team about fire risk in time-out
Closed = Patient is intubated	☐ No pooling of prep solution	☐ Use closed oxygen circuit when possible
	☐ ESU holstered when not in use	☐ Verbal communication of oxygen percentage
	☐ Laser safety precautions	☐ Oxygen concentration lowered to 30%
	☐ Fiberoptic light cable safety	☐ Barrier placed between ignition source and oxygen
	☐ NS used when using burrs and/or saw blade	☐ Water soluble eye lubricant
		☐ Use FDA laser safe ET Tube for airway surgery
		☐ Water or N/S on anesthesia machine
		☐ Suction to anesthesia to dissipate gasses
		☐ Coat facial hair with water soluble jelly.
		☐ Keep ESU settings as low as possible
		☐ Use wet sponges when in contact with ignition source (Airway fire)

Include in Preprocedure check-in as per institutional custom:
Beta blocker medication given (SCIP) ☐ Yes ☐ N/A
Venous thromboembolism prophylaxis ordered (SCIP) ☐Yes ☐ N/A
Normothermia measures (SCIP) ☐ Yes ☐N/A

Exhibit 2-5 Nursing Documentation Worksheet

CURRENT PATIENT DATA	TIMES	ANESTHESIA
☐ H&P ☐ Consent	Anesthesia start:	General ☐ Regional ☐ Local ☐
Height: Weight:	Patient in Room	Type of Block
Preop Diagnosis:	Induction	
	Surgeon in Room	
Postop Diagnosis:	Prep	**INTRAOPERATIVE INTERVENTIONS**
	Drape	Actual Procedure
Previous Surgery:	Incision	
	Wound Closed	Positioning
Current Medications	Dressings	
	Out of Room	Repositioning approved by anesthesia/surgeon
Allergies	Time in PACU	☐ Yes ☐ No
	Hand-off to	TIME OUT ☐ Yes ☐ No
Implants	ICU	Preop ABX
BMI	Report called	
Pregnancy Test ☐ N/A	Transfer	Implants–place implant stickers on back (or document implant information there)
MRSA Screen		
		Specimens
PERSONNEL	**EQUIPMENT**	
Anesthesia	☐ SCD #	Drain
Scrub	☐ Knee high ☐ Thigh high ☐ Foot pump	EBL (ml):
Scrub Relief	Activation time:	Foley ☐ N/A ☐ in place ☐ Inserted:
Circulator	☐ Forced Air #:	by
Circ Relief		Urine Output (cc):
Assistant	ESU # ESU Pad #	Counts Correct ☐ Yes ☐ No
	Harmonic #	Dressings
Other (Rep; student, radiology, perfusionist...)	Tourniquet #	Immobilizer ABD Binder C-Collar
	Setting	
	Up Down	
	Up Down	**INTRAOPERATIVE MEDICATIONS**
	Insufflator #	Local: Amt:

Modified from Medical Center of Arlington, Arlington, TX.

Exhibit 2-6 Post-procedure Wrap-up

Topic	Issue		Resolution	Initials
All equipment required for procedure present in the room	☐ Yes ☐ No			
Unneeded equipment removed from room	☐ Yes ☐ No			
Room stock of items sufficient	☐ Yes ☐ No			
Case Cart for procedure complete (according to preference card)	☐ Yes ☐ No			
Changes to preference card required	☐ Yes ☐ No			
Instruments sets complete	☐ Yes ☐ No			
Instruments in good working order	☐ Yes ☐ No			
Equipment functioned as required	☐ Yes ☐ No			
Assistance required for any reason was available in a timely manner	☐ Yes ☐ No			
Breaks for scrub & circulator were provided in a timely fashion	☐ Yes ☐ No			
Assistance with room turnover was available in a timely fashion	☐ Yes ☐ No			
Counts were performed without interruption	☐ Yes ☐ No			
Time out was performed correctly with all required personnel participating	☐ Yes ☐ No			

Initials   Name of individual taking responsibility   Initials   Name of individual taking responsibility   Initials   Name of individual taking responsibility

Modified from Medical Center of Arlington, Arlington, TX.

Patient/Family Teaching

72. Patient/family teaching is especially critical in today's healthcare environment, where patients are often discharged shortly after surgery. Optimal surgical outcomes often depend on how completely the patient understands and complies with instructions for care in the postoperative period.

73. Educating the patient should begin when the prospect of surgery is first discussed—in the physician's office or clinic.

74. Patient teaching during a preadmission workup should be directed toward preparation for surgery and effective participation in the postoperative rehabilitation process. For example, teaching might include instruction on bowel cleansing in preparation for bowel surgery and teaching crutch-walking for the patient whose surgical outcome will be influenced by participation in postoperative rehabilitation.

75. Preoperative teaching content should include the following issues:

    – The procedure, anticipated duration, and expected outcome

    – Specific instructions such as whether to bathe or shower, whether to hold or take medications, and whether to maintain NPO status from a designated time onward

    – An explanation of preoperative events such as diagnostic tests, skin preparation, intravenous (IV) line insertion, sedation, and transfer to holding area

    – An explanation of intraoperative events such as function of the circulating nurse or case manager, application of monitoring equipment, administration of anesthesia, maintenance of privacy and dignity, staff communication with family members during the procedure, and transport to the PACU

‒ An explanation of postoperative events such as expected length of stay; coughing and deep-breathing expectations; turning; presence of lines, drains, and indwelling catheters; pain control; and discharge to a step-down or other unit or to home

76. Patient teaching should continue throughout the preoperative phase. Important information may need to be repeated.

77. Information related to discharge and recovery should be reinforced both in the immediate preop period and following the procedure, before the patient is discharged from the facility.

78. Readiness to learn can be diminished in times of stress. Whenever possible, the patient's family or support persons should be included in the teaching process.

79. Attentive listening, reassurance, and information delivered calmly and candidly can alleviate anxiety and fear. A caring attitude, accompanied by appropriate, reassuring touch, can comfort the patient. Reducing anxiety and fear is a first step in preparing the patient for teaching.

80. Patient teaching must be tailored to the patient's age, learning level, culture, and readiness to learn. Instructional materials and voice level should take possible sight and hearing deficits into consideration.

81. Written instructions, pamphlets, and videos related to preparation for surgery and rehabilitation can be good teaching tools. Teaching materials, however, need to meet the needs of the learner.

82. Printed instructional materials should take into account the patient's level of literacy as well as the patient's level of health literacy. Health literacy is defined as "the degree to which individuals have the capacity to obtain, process, and understand basic health information and services needed to make appropriate health decisions" (National Network of Libraries of Medicine, 2015; U.S. Department of Health and Human Services, 2015).

83. It is critical for the nurse to review printed material with the patient, to solicit feedback to determine whether the patient understands the material, and to provide further instructions as appropriate.

84. Elderly patients' short-term memory may be diminished, so additional time and reinforcement may be necessary for them to comprehend and retain information. Additional time should be planned for instruction when necessary.

85. Other patients who might require additional resources for learning include patients who have minimal education, low socioeconomic status, cultural barriers to health care, or limited proficiency in English.

86. Pediatric patients have special needs.
    • Toddlers are just beginning to gain autonomy, are active, and have short attention spans.
    • Preschoolers are inquisitive and have active imaginations. They may feel that surgery is punishment for bad behavior.
    • School-age children are capable of logic and reasoning and can benefit from learning the steps involved in the surgical process.

87. Patient teaching for pediatric patients may include an opportunity for them to handle simple items that they will encounter during surgery. The ability to touch and manipulate an anesthesia mask, for example, can provide the child with a feeling of control.

88. Sometimes putting an anesthesia mask and dressings on a doll or stuffed animal "patient" can help to distract and calm a child.

89. Teaching in the preoperative holding area will be abbreviated and will reinforce previous teaching.

90. Teaching directed toward discharge will be reinforced in the postoperative period prior to discharge.

Section Questions

1. Explain why documentation in the patient record is so important. [Refs 66, 69]

2. Why is using a paper form to capture information about the procedure so helpful? [Ref 67]

3. Explain the need to check patient in-room time, anesthesia time, and incision time with the anesthesia provider. [Ref 68]

(continues)

Section Questions (continued)

4. How long are you accountable for the information you document in the patient record? [Ref 69]

5. Explain the importance of clear and accurate information in the patient's medical record? [Ref 70]

6. Why is patient and family teaching especially critical in today's healthcare environment? [Ref 72]

7. When should patient teaching begin? [Ref 73]

8. What should early patient teaching address? [Refs 74–75]

9. Explain how teaching needs to be modified when readiness to learn is diminished by stress. [Ref 78]

10. What techniques can be used to alleviate anxiety and fear? [Ref 79]

11. What patient characteristics will impact the nurse's approach to teaching? [Ref 80]

12. What are some important characteristics of printed material? [Ref 82]

13. Define *health literacy*. [Ref 82]

14. What patient populations might require additional time and resources for learning? [Refs 84–86]

15. Describe some special needs related to the pediatric patient population. [Ref 87]

References

American College of Surgeons. (2002). *Statement on ensuring correct patient, correct site, and correct procedure surgery*. Bulletin of the American College of Surgeons, Vol 87 No 12. http://www.facs.org/fellows_info/statements/st-41.html

Association of periOperative Registered Nurses (AORN). (2010). *Preventing wrong-patient, wrong-site, wrong-procedure events*. Denver, CO: AORN. Available at: www.aorn.org/Clinical_Practice/Position_Statements/Position_Statements.aspx Accessed September 2012.

Association of periOperative Registered Nurses (AORN). (2011). *Perioperative nursing data set* (3rd ed.). Denver, CO: AORN.

Association of periOperative Registered Nurses (AORN). (2015). *Guidelines for perioperative practice*. Denver, CO: AORN.

Association of periOperative Registered Nurses (AORNc). (2011). *Preventing wrong-patient, wrong-site, wrong-procedure events*. Denver, CO. http://www.aorn.org/Clinical_Practice/Position_Statements/Position_Statements.aspx

Center for Transforming Healthcare (CTH). (2013). *Reducing the risk of wrong site surgery*. Retrieved from http://www.centerfortransforminghealthcare.org/assets/4/6/CTH_WSS_Storyboard_final_2011.pdf

Centers for Disease Control and Prevention (CDC). (2015). *Defining adult overweight and obesity*. Retrieved from http://www.cdc.gov/obesity/adult/defining.html

The Joint Commission Center for Transforming Healthcare (CTH). (2013). *Reducing the risk of wrong site surgery*. Retrieved from http://www.centerfortransforminghealthcare.org/assets/4/6/CTH_WSS_Storyboard_final_2011.pdf

Edmiston, C. E., Spencer, M., Lewis, B. D., Brown, K. R., Rossi, P. J., Henen, C. R., . . . Seabrook, G. R. (2011). Reducing the risk of surgical site infections: Did we really think SCIP was going to lead us to the promised land? *Surgical Infections,2*(8), 69–77.

Institute of Medicine (IOM). (2000). *To err is human: Building a safer health system*. Washington, DC: National Academy Press.

NANDA International. (2014). *Nursing diagnoses: Definitions and classification, 2015–2017*. Hoboken, NJ: Wiley-Blackwell.

National Network of Libraries of Medicine. (2015). *Health literacy*. Retrieved from http://nnlm.gov/outreach/consumer/hlthlit.html

Pierpont, Y. N., Dinh, T. P., Salas, R. E., Johnson, E. L., Wright, T. G., Robson, M. C., & Payne, W. G. (2014). Obesity and surgical wound healing: A current review. *ISRN Obesity, 2014*(638936). Retrieved from http://www.ncbi.nlm.nih.gov/pmc/articles/PMC3950544/

Sadler, D. (2014). Patient safety and the surgery checklist. *OR Today*. Retrieved from http://ortoday.com/patient-safety-and-the-surgery-checklist/

Texas Health Resources Harris Methodist Hospital Southlake (THR). (2015) *CMS inpatient core measures. surgical care improvement project (SCIP): Tips for physicians*. Retrieved from https://www.texashealthsouthlake.com/files/medicalstaffresources/PhysicianSCIPEducation.pdf

The Joint Commission (TJC). (2014a). *Sentinel event policy and procedures.* Retrieved from http://www .jointcommission.org/Sentinel_Event_Policy_and_Procedures/

The Joint Commission (TJC). (2014b). *Summary data of sentinel events reviewed by The Joint Commission.* Retrieved from http://www.jointcommission.org/ assets/1/18/2004_to_2014_2Q_SE_Stats_-_Summary.pdf

The Joint Commission (TJC). (2015a). 2015 *national patient safety goals.* Retrieved from http://www.joint commission.org/assets/1/6/2015_NPSG_HAP.pdf

The Joint Commission (TJC). (2015b). *Specifications manual for national hospital inpatient quality measures.* Retrieved from http://www.jointcommission.org/ specifications_manual_for_national_hospital_inpatient_ quality_measures.aspx

The Joint Commission (TJC). (2015c). *The universal protocol for preventing wrong site, wrong procedure, and wrong person surgery: Guidance for healthcare professionals (poster).* Retrieved from http://www.joint commission.org/assets/1/18/UP_Poster.pdf

University of Cincinnati. (2011). *Use of 48 hour course of antibiotics to prevent surgical site infection in obese patients undergoing cesarean delivery (SSI).* Retrieved from https://clinicaltrials.gov/ct2/show/NCT01194115? term=antibiotic+dosage+for+obese+surgical+patients& rank=3

University of Colorado, Denver. (2014). *Adequacy of perioperative cefazolin for surgery antibiotic prophylaxis in obese patients.* Retrieved from https://clinicaltrials .gov/ct2/show/record/NCT01886742

U.S. Department of Health and Human Services. (2015). *Quick guide to health literacy.* Retrieved from http:// www.health.gov/communication/literacy/quickguide/ Quickguide.pdf

Wheeler, K. (2014). Effective handoff communication. *OR Nurse, 8*(1)22–26. Retrieved from http://journals .lww.com/ornursejournal/Fulltext/2014/01000/Effective _handoff_communication.5.aspx

Post-Test

Read each question carefully. Each question may have more than one correct answer.

1. Which of the following statements are true about standard hand-off protocols? They
   a. determine which information must be communicated.
   b. provide a framework for comprehensive and concise communication.
   c. are mandated by TJC's National Patient Safety Goals.
   d. become part of the patient's record.

2. What resources does the perioperative nurse use to formulate nursing diagnoses?
   a. AORN's *Perioperative Nursing Data Set* (PNDS)
   b. The nurse's unique knowledge of the surgical procedure
   c. The Joint Commission's list of patient diagnoses for surgery
   d. Patient assessment data

3. Assessment data come from which of the following sources?
   a. Chart review
   b. Observation
   c. Communication with other healthcare providers
   d. The patient and family

4. Commonly targeted patient outcomes include:
   a. The patient will be free of injury.
   b. The patient's skin integrity will be maintained.
   c. The patient will be extubated before transfer to PACU.
   d. The patient will be discharged from PACU within 4 hours.

5. The dose and timing of prophylactic antibiotic administration are determined by
   a. protocol that specifies the drug be given 1 hour before surgery.
   b. the attending surgeon.
   c. the anesthesia provider.
   d. bactericidal tissue and serum level at the time of surgery.

6. What is the exception to administering antibiotics 1 hour prior to the skin incision?
   a. Amoxicillin
   b. Keflex
   c. Vancomycin
   d. Fluoroquinolone

7. Which of the following is true? Obese surgical patients
   a. have an increased frequency of comorbidities.
   b. are at higher risk for surgical-site infection.
   c. do not respond well to antibiotics.
   d. are more fearful of surgery than nonobese patients.

8. Which of the following are considered critical physiologic assessment data?
   a. Previous surgery with complications
   b. Laboratory data
   c. Allergies
   d. Readiness to learn

9. Critical psychosocial assessment data include
    a. knowledge of perioperative routines.
    b. cultural beliefs.
    c. spiritual beliefs.
    d. understanding of the surgical procedure.

10. The most common diagnoses in the preoperative period are
    a. fear and anxiety.
    b. knowledge deficit and hypothermia.
    c. anxiety and knowledge deficit.
    d. fear and sensory impairment.

11. Which of the following best describes anxiety?
    a. General discomfort related to alteration in body image
    b. Uneasiness related to anesthesia and loss of control
    c. Dread of something specific
    d. General uneasiness with no specific etiology

12. Which of the following are considered interventions to address anxiety and fear?
    a. Attentive listening and reassurance
    b. Giving information to the family instead of the patient
    c. Soliciting the patient's description of anxiety or fear
    d. Telling the patient everything he or she needs to know

13. A sentinel event or never event is
    a. a preventable situation that results in death, permanent harm, or severe temporary harm.
    b. an event that should never happen.
    c. an event that requires intervention to sustain life.
    d. an event that isn't reported.

14. Wrong-site surgery as defined by TJC includes
    a. surgery on the wrong side.
    b. surgery on the wrong patient.
    c. the wrong surgical procedure.
    d. surgery at the wrong level.

15. Factors that have been identified as contributors to wrong-site surgery include:
    a. use of unapproved abbreviations.
    b. illegible handwriting.
    c. inconsistent time-out process.
    d. site markings removed during surgical prep.

16. Three protocols that TJC implements in an effort to prevent wrong-site surgery are
    a. site marking, time-out, and better documentation.
    b. time-out, better documentation, and consent form.
    c. pre-procedure verification, site marking, and time-out.
    d. site marking, consent form, and time-out.

17. A priority for the perioperative nurse before bringing the patient into the operating room is
    a. verification of the patient's identity and surgical procedure.
    b. ensuring that the surgeon is in the room.

   c. ensuring the scrub person has completed setting up the sterile field.

   d. ensuring that family members are present in the waiting area.

18. During the time-out, the team agrees on which of the following?

   a. Procedure to be done

   b. Correct site—site marking is validated

   c. Patient identification

   d. Initial counts have been completed

19. For what reason do some facilities use a paper form to capture intraoperative information that will be documented in the patient's record?

   a. The information should be reviewed by another nurse before being officially entered into the record.

   b. The nurse rarely gets to document the information in the record at the time that it occurs.

   c. There should be a backup copy of all information that goes into the patient record.

   d. Notes taken in real time help the nurse enter data accurately into the patient record.

20. Which of the following statements about intervention times is true?

   a. Most facilities have systems that automatically capture the times of important surgical events.

   b. The time of an event that is documented in multiple places in the patient's record must be consistent.

   c. The surgeon is responsible for determining the event time that will be documented in the patient's chart.

   d. When an event time is documented in multiple places in the patient's chart, the nursing documentation takes precedence if the times are not consistent.

21. The focus of patient teaching prior to the day of surgery should focus on

   a. the procedure, length of the procedure, and expected outcome of the procedure.

   b. preoperative events including diagnostic testing and NPO requirement.

   c. postoperative responsibilities related to rehabilitation.

   d. preview of intraoperative events such as monitoring and anesthesia.

22. Patient teaching must be tailored to the patient's

   a. age.

   b. learning level.

   c. culture.

   d. readiness/willingness to learn.

23. Health literacy is the patient's

   a. level of health and wellbeing.

   b. highest level of education.

   c. ability to assimilate information from printed literature.

   d. capacity to obtain, process, and understand health information.

24. Which factor(s) interfere(s) with learning in the elderly?

   a. Elderly patients are more often frightened than anxious.

   b. They have difficulty with written materials.

   c. They do not need as much instruction because others will be caring for them.

   d. Their short-term memory may be impaired.

25. Which of the following statements is *true*?

   a. Toddlers may feel that surgery is punishment for bad behavior.

   b. School-age children have a short attention span.

   c. Becoming familiar with items they will encounter in surgery gives pediatric patients a sense of control.

   d. Preschoolers will benefit from discussing the steps involved in the procedure.

Competency Checklist:
Preparing the Patient for Surgery

Under "Observer's Initials," enter initials upon successful achievement of competency. Enter N/A if competency is not appropriate for institution.

Name _____

	Observer's Initials	Date
1. Patient is identified.	_____	_____
2. Surgical procedure and operative site are verified with the patient.	_____	_____
3. Operative consent is verified with the patient.	_____	_____
4. Patient is assessed (or chart reviewed) for:		
a. Medical diagnosis	_____	_____
b. Medications (prescription, over-the-counter, herbal, prophylactic antibiotic)	_____	_____
c. Lab data (tests ordered, lab results, blood type and cross-match)	_____	_____
d. Previous surgeries	_____	_____
e. Anesthesia complications	_____	_____
f. Substance abuse	_____	_____
g. Skin condition	_____	_____
h. Allergies	_____	_____
i. Nutritional and NPO status		
j. Sensory impairments	_____	_____
k. Dentures	_____	_____
l. Mobility impairments	_____	
m. Presence of prosthesis	_____	_____
n. Weight and height	_____	_____
o. Vital signs	_____	_____
p. Age	_____	_____
5. Patient is assessed for:	_____	_____
a. Level of understanding	_____	_____
b. Ability to comprehend	_____	_____
c. Information desired	_____	_____
d. Cultural and religious beliefs	_____	_____
6. Patient is asked to verbalize understanding of the surgical experience.	_____	_____
7. Patient is encouraged to ask questions regarding the surgical procedure.	_____	_____
8. Patient is encouraged to verbalize concerns about the surgical experience.	_____	_____
9. Intraoperative routines that the patient should expect are explained.	_____	_____
10. Patient teaching takes patient's age and level of understanding into consideration.	_____	_____
11. The Joint Commission universal protocol to prevent wrong-site surgery is implemented.	_____	_____
12. Chart is reviewed for preoperative antibiotic order and action taken as necessary.	_____	_____
13. Postoperative routines are explained to the patient.	_____	_____
14. The above information is communicated to the surgical team.	_____	_____
15. Documentation in the medical record is complete, concise, and clear.	_____	_____

Observer's Signature   Initials   Date

_____

Orientee's Signature

_____

Instrument Processing

LEARNER OBJECTIVES

1. Discuss the responsibilities of the perioperative nurse in processing instruments to prevent patient injury and surgical site infection.
2. Explain the partnership between perioperative personnel and the sterile processing department in instrument processing.
3. Describe responsibilities for cleaning surgical instruments at the point of use and transport to the sterile processing department.
4. Explain the relationship among cleaning, sterilization, and disinfection.
5. Identify the steps associated with inspecting, assembling, and packaging items for sterilization or disinfection.
6. Describe high- and low-temperature sterilization technologies.
7. Discuss responsibilities associated with sterilization monitoring.
8. Explain requirements for storage of sterile items.

LESSON OUTLINE

I. Introduction
II. Managing Instruments at the Point of Use
   A. Instruments Exposed to Prions
   B. Transporting Items from Point of Use to Sterile Processing Department
III. Decontamination: Sterile Processing Department
   A. Manual Cleaning
   B. Mechanical Cleaning
   C. Special Needs Instruments
     i. Eye Instruments
     ii. Flexible Endoscopes
     iii. Robotic Instruments
   D. Ultrasonic Cleaning
   E. Lubrication
IV. Preparation and Packaging
   A. Inspection
   B. Assembly and Packaging
     i. Selection Criteria for Barrier Protection
       1. Woven Fabric
       2. Nonwoven Materials
       3. Pouches: Plastic/Paper, Plastic/Tyvek
       4. Rigid Container Systems
     ii. Packaging Items for Steam Sterilization
     iii. Packaging Items for Low-Temperature Sterilization
   C. Monitoring: Chemical Indicators and Integrators
   D. Labeling

Introduction

1. Postoperative wound infection/surgical site infection (SSI) is a complication of surgery with potentially dire consequences for the patient, including delayed recovery, increased length of stay, increased cost of care, increased pain and suffering, and even death.

2. According to the Centers for Disease Control and Prevention (CDC, 2015c), SSIs are a leading cause of hospital-associated infections (HAIs), accounting for 31% of all HAIs in hospitalized patients in a recent study. SSIs are associated with a 3% mortality rate and 75% of SSI-associated deaths are directly attributable to the SSI.

3. SSI reduction has been identified as a Phase One priority in the U.S. Department of Health and Human Services (HHS, 2013) Action Plan to Prevent Health Care-Associated Infections.

4. Intact skin is the body's first line of defense against infection. Pathogenic microorganisms are capable of causing disease when they invade human tissue.

5. Surgical incisions interrupt skin integrity, providing a portal of entry for pathogenic microorganisms, which increases a patient's risk of getting an infection by giving microorganisms a route into normally sterile areas of the body. Invasive drains, catheters, and monitors also alter skin integrity and contribute to the risk for infection.

6. Contaminated instruments are a known source of infection (Dancer, Stewart, Coulombe, Gregori, & Verdi, 2012; Saito et al., 2014). Every effort must be made to remove microorganisms from any items that contact human tissue during surgical interventions.

7. The nursing diagnoses of "increased risk for infection" and the outcome statement "free from injury" are pertinent when caring for patients undergoing invasive procedures.

8. Most instrument processing is performed in a separate sterile processing department (SPD). The perioperative nurse, however, is a partner in the process of preparing instruments and assumes varying levels of responsibility for cleaning, inspection, packaging, sterilization, and storage of sterile supplies.

9. As the patient's advocate, the perioperative nurse strives to ensure that all instruments delivered to the sterile field have been appropriately prepared and processed and are in good working order. Instruments or supplies improperly prepared or processed can harbor microorganisms that can result in infection. Items that fail to function as intended can cause patient injury.

10. When disinfection and sterilization are accomplished within the operating room department, it is often the perioperative nurse who is responsible for the process.

11. No single method of instrument processing is appropriate for all instruments. Composition and configuration of an instrument determine its compatibility with the sterilization and disinfection processes available within the healthcare facility. Device and equipment manufacturers' instructions for use (IFU) must be considered when purchasing and processing decisions are made.

Definitions

Antiseptics: Chemicals used to destroy microorganisms on body surfaces. The number and type of organisms killed are determined by the composition and concentration of the antiseptic and the amount of time the agent remains active.

Autoclave: A steam sterilizer.

Bioburden: A population of viable microorganisms on an item.

Biofilm: A collection of microscopic organisms that exist in a polysaccharide matrix that adheres to a surface and prevents antimicrobial agents such as sterilants, disinfectants, and antibiotics from reaching the cells.

Biological indicator: A sterilization monitor consisting of a known population of resistant spores that is used to test a sterilizer's ability to kill microorganisms.

Bowie-Dick test: An air-removal test designed to assure that the autoclave can remove air and noncondensable gases from the chamber of a dynamic air-removal autoclave and that steam can penetrate a specified pack.

Cavitation: In an ultrasonic washer, the process by which high-intensity sound waves generate tiny bubbles that expand until they collapse or implode, causing a negative pressure on the surfaces of the instruments that dislodges soil.

Chemical indicator: A device used to monitor one or more process parameters in the sterilization cycle. The device responds with a visible chemical or physical change (usually a color change) to conditions within the sterilizer chamber. Chemical indicators are usually supplied as a paper strip, tape, or label that changes color when the parameter or parameters have been met. Chemical indicators go on the outside and inside of each package to be sterilized.

Contaminated: (1) In the operating room environment, a term referring to items that are not sterile. Items soiled or potentially soiled with microorganisms are considered to be contaminated. Items that were opened for surgery, whether or not they were actually used during surgery and whether or not they are known to contain microorganisms, are also considered to be contaminated. (2) In the regulatory arena, a term referring to an item that has been in contact with an infectious agent.

Decontamination: The process that renders a previously contaminated item safe for handling. Decontamination may be accomplished manually or with an automated system. Decontamination is usually accomplished by cleaning followed with a thermal or chemical disinfection process.

Disinfectant: An antimicrobial agent used to destroy microorganisms on inanimate surfaces. The composition and concentration of the disinfectant and the amount of time an item is exposed to it determine the number and types of organisms that will be killed.

Disinfection: A process that kills all living microorganisms, with the exception of high numbers of spores.
- Low-level disinfection kills vegetative forms of bacteria, lipid viruses, and some fungi.
- Intermediate-level disinfection kills vegetative bacteria, mycobacteria, viruses, and fungi, but not spores.
- High-level disinfection kills vegetative bacteria, mycobacteria, viruses, fungi, and some spores.

Event-related sterility: A sterile item remains sterile until an event happens to render it unsterile.

IFU: Manufacturer's instructions for use; the U.S. Food and Drug Administration (FDA) requires that the manufacturer of every item validated for use in the operating room or sterile processing department must supply written instructions on how to use the item properly.

Immediate-use steam sterilization (IUSS): A steam sterilization process for sterilizing heat- and moisture-stable items that are needed immediately; previously known as "flash sterilization."

Manufacturer's IFU: Written instructions provided by the manufacturer of every validated medical device that details appropriate use and processing of the device.

Prion: An infectious protein particle responsible for rare and fatal diseases of the nervous system.

Spaulding's Classification: A system of categorization that determines the level of processing of an item based on its intended use.

Spore: An inactive or dormant, but viable, state of a microorganism, which is notably resistant to heat, drying, and chemicals and is difficult to kill. Sterilization methods are monitored by assessing their ability to kill a known population of highly resistant spores.

Sterile: Free of all viable microorganisms, including spores.

Sterility assurance level (SAL): The probability of a viable microorganism being present on an item after sterilization.

Sterilization: A process that kills all living microorganisms, including spores. Fiberoptic and robotic instruments costing many thousands of dollars are standard components of many procedures.

Strike-through: Passage of a liquid through a barrier product.

Treated water: Water from which additives such as chlorine, dissolved salts, naturally occurring minerals, organic contaminants, bacteria, and endotoxins have been removed.

Washer-disinfector, washer-decontaminator: Automated processing units used to decontaminate instruments. Cycles within these machines vary but always include washing and rinsing.

12. Selecting the appropriate method of processing instruments requires an understanding of the scientific principles involved in cleaning, inspection, packaging, sterilization, and storage of sterile instruments and supplies.

13. When immediate-use steam sterilization (IUSS) or high-level disinfection is required, the perioperative nurse may assume total responsibility for cleaning, inspection, and packaging, as well as for the sterilization or disinfection process. For instance, the perioperative nurse must understand why no instruments—not even a single instrument intended for IUSS—should ever be cleaned in a scrub sink.

Managing Instruments at the Point of Use

14. All instruments opened for a surgical procedure in the operating room or in an invasive procedure room are considered contaminated whether or not they are used.

15. During a surgical procedure, instruments should be kept as clean as possible; they should be wiped clean with a laparotomy sponge moistened with sterile water or immersed in sterile water to prevent debris from drying in serrations and crevices.

16. Instrument lumens should be flushed free of debris using a syringe filled with sterile water. Irrigation should take place below the surface of the water to prevent aerosolization of particles.

17. Sterile water, not saline, should be used for cleaning items during surgery. Blood and body fluids as well as saline are highly corrosive and can cause rusting and pitting (AORN, 2015, p. 615).

18. Instruments should be cleaned as soon as possible after use to prevent blood and other debris from drying in crevices or the surfaces of an instrument.

19. Bioburden that has been allowed to dry on instruments is difficult to remove and can interfere with the sterilization or disinfection processes by preventing the sterilizing or disinfecting agent from contacting every surface of the item.

20. Once an instrument is opened, it is considered contaminated whether or not it is actually used.

21. Instruments should be returned to their original containers so that sets are complete when they arrive in the SPD for processing.

22. Before instruments leave the operating room:
    - Remove blades and other sharps and discard them in a sharps container.
    - Remove drill bits and saw blades; if disposable, discard in a sharps container; if reusable, wipe clean and segregate them to prevent injury to SPD personnel.
    - Segregate sharp instruments, such as scissors and osteotomes, from other instruments.
    - Open instruments with box locks and joints.
    - Unless contraindicated by the manufacturer's IFU, disassemble devices with multiple components; keep the parts together.
    - Place heavy instruments in the bottom of the tray with lighter ones on top.

23. Preventing bioburden from drying on instruments facilitates effective cleaning in the SPD and helps to prevent corrosion, rusting, and pitting.

24. Instruments should be returned to the SPD as soon after surgery as possible.

25. To prevent the formation of biofilms, particularly within lumens, instruments should not remain in water for lengthy periods of time. Once formed, biofilm cannot be rinsed away and must be removed by mechanical means. If not completely removed, biofilm will prevent the sterilant from contacting all surfaces of the instrument (**Figure 3-1**).

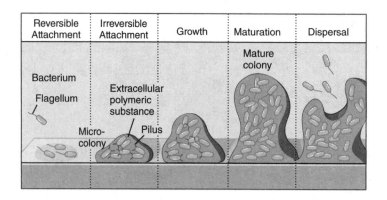

Figure 3-1 Biofilm.

26. Biofilms can pose a serious threat to health. In addition to compromising the disinfection and sterilization processes, biofilm can break free from the surface of a device inside the patient's body, resulting in a massive infusion of bacteria that can cause an infection that is difficult to treat. Because the biofilm lives within a self-made protective glycocalyx, it may be 500 times (or more) resistant to antibiotics (Center for Biofilm Engineering, 2011). Sterilant will not be able to reach the microorganisms protected within the glycocalyx.

27. To prevent the formation of biofilms and to prevent debris from drying on instruments, contaminated instruments should be kept moist until they are cleaned. Coat instruments with an enzymatic spray or gel intended for pretreatment. In some facilities, instruments may be covered with a moist towel or placed inside a package designed to maintain humid conditions.

Instruments Exposed to Prions (American National Standards Institute & AAMI, 2001, Annex C; AORN, 2015, pp. 635–340; Rutala & Weber, 2010)

28. A prion is an infectious protein particle responsible for transmissible spongiform encephalopathies such as Creutzfeldt-Jakob disease (CJD), a rare and always fatal disease of the central nervous system.

29. The brain, spinal cord, dura mater, and eye are considered high-risk tissue for transmission of prion disease.

30. The perioperative nurse should follow institutional policies and procedures, and conduct a patient assessment to identify those patients who are at high risk for prion disease and to identify those procedures with the potential to expose instruments to tissue contaminated with prions.

31. Information and protocols regarding prions are evolving. In addition to the Society for Hospital Epidemiology of America (SHEA) "Guideline for Disinfection and Sterilization of Prion-Contaminated Medical Devices" (Rutala & Weber, 2010), the CDC and the AORN should be consulted when developing protocols for instruments exposed to prions.

32. Unlike bacteria, viruses, and fungi, prions are resistant to routine sterilization and disinfection procedures. Ideally, instruments used on tissue known or suspected to be contaminated with prions should be discarded. When it is not known whether the patient on whom the instruments were used has a prion disease, the instruments should be quarantined until the diagnosis is determined, and, if positive for prion disease, discarded.

33. When a patient has or is suspected of having a prion disease, instruments that are not discarded should be cleaned and sterilized according to special protocols:

    - At the point of use, avoid mixing instruments exposed to high-risk tissue with instruments used on other tissue.

    - Keep instruments moist until cleaned or decontaminated.

    - Clean the instruments as soon as possible to minimize drying of tissue, blood, and body fluids on the instruments.

34. Use the following protocols for decontaminating the instruments:

    - For instruments that are easily cleaned, steam autoclave them after thorough cleaning at 272°F (134°C) for 18 minutes in a prevacuum sterilizer or at 270°F (132°C) for 60 minutes in a gravity-displacement autoclave/cycle.

    - For instruments that are difficult to clean or have small lumens:

        – Discard the instruments

        or

        – Immerse the instruments in 1NaOH for 60 minutes, then remove, rinse with water, and sterilize using one of the cycles already described

    - Once the instruments have been processed, proceed with conventional cleaning, packaging, and sterilizing.

Section Questions

1. What are some of the adverse implications of surgical site infections? [Refs 1–2]

2. How does a surgical procedure place a patient at risk for infection? [Refs 4–6]

(continues)

Section Questions (continued)

3. Describe the perioperative nurse's role in instrument processing. [Refs 8–13]

4. What instrument features influence compatibility with processing technologies? [Ref 11]

5. How does the scrub person reduce bioburden on instruments during a procedure? [Refs 15–16]

6. What is the rationale for choosing sterile water rather than saline to clean instruments on the sterile field? [Ref 17]

7. What is the rationale for keeping instruments clean during a procedure? [Refs 18–19]

8. How should instruments be managed following the procedure in preparation for their return to the sterile processing department? [Refs 21–22, 27]

9. What is a biofilm? [Ref *Definitions*]

10. When should instruments be returned to the sterile processing department? [Ref 24]

11. Why do biofilms present a greater challenge to cleaning than other bioburden? [Refs 25–26]

12. What implication do biofilms have for patient care? [Ref 26]

13. What is a prion? [Ref *Definitions*, 28]

14. What are the high-risk tissues for transmission of prion disease? [Ref 29]

15. What options are available for decontaminating hard-to-clean instruments that have been exposed to prions? [Refs 31–34]

Transporting Items from Point of Use to the Sterile Processing Department

35. Transport items from the point of use to the SPD as soon as possible.

36. Remove all trash and linen from sets. Any items returned to SPD that cannot be processed will be discarded when they arrive in the decontamination area.

37. Contain all instruments in a durable, leak-proof, labeled, or color-coded container that is closed before being removed from the work area to prevent personnel from contacting contaminated items during transfer (AAMI, 2013; Occupational Safety and Health Administration [OSHA], 2012a, 29CFR 1910.1030 (e) (2) (ii) (B)).

38. A biohazard label should be affixed to the cart before it is removed from the work area (OSHA, 2012a, 29CFR 1910.1030(g)(1)(i)(H)).

Decontamination: Sterile Processing Department

Manual Cleaning

39. Instruments are received in the sterile processing department in an area specially designed to contain contamination, often shortened to "decontam" for "decontamination."

40. The "decontam" area is a negative air pressure environment. Negative pressure prevents microorganisms in the air from escaping into surrounding areas. AAMI recommends a minimum of 10 air exchanges per hour (AAMI, 2013, §3.3.6.4); the Facility Guidelines Institute (FGI, 2014) recommends a minimum of 6 air exchanges per hour.

41. In addition, personnel working in the decontamination area should wear the following personal protective equipment (PPE) for protection from exposure to contamination (AAMI, 2013, §4.5.1–4.5.2):

    - A liquid-resistant gown or apron with sleeves
    - Long-cuffed utility gloves
    - A mask
    - Eye protection (goggles or full-face shield)

42. All instruments returned to the SPD are cleaned whether they were used or not. Cleaning is the first and most important step in preparing items for sterilization. If an item is not thoroughly clean, it cannot be sterilized. Any debris remaining on an instrument will prevent sterilant from contacting the surface.

Remember, an item can be clean but not sterile; but no item can be sterile if it is not clean.

43. For instruments and devices that are not sensitive to heat or moisture, mechanical cleaning in an automated system is preferable because the process is consistent. Manual cleaning can be equally effective if performed correctly.

44. Some powered surgical instruments and heat-sensitive, delicate, or specialty items cannot tolerate mechanical washing. These items should be cleaned separately according to the device manufacturer's IFU.

45. When instruments are manually cleaned, regardless of whether they are cleaned in the decontamination section of the SPD or in a decontamination area within the operating room, it is important for the process to be standardized. The following supplies and equipment should be readily available wherever items are processed:

    - Enzymatic detergent
    - Soft-bristle brushes of various sizes
    - Syringes for irrigation of lumens
    - Adaptors and accessories for specific devices as required by the manufacturer's IFU
    - Eyewash station
    - Medical grade compressed air
    - PPE

46. Before washing with a detergent, instruments should be rinsed in cold water to remove gross debris. Hot water coagulates protein and makes the cleaning process more difficult.

47. The detergent, usually containing one or more enzymes, should be specific for instrument cleaning. Detergent should be used strictly according to the manufacturer's IFU. For example, mixing detergents to a higher concentration because of heavy debris is not appropriate and may, in fact, impede rinsing that will subsequently interfere with sterilization or disinfection.

48. Immersible items should be cleaned below the surface of the water to prevent aerosolization of debris. Lumens and cannulas should be flushed while submerged.

49. Items that cannot be immersed should be cleaned in a manner that prevents aerosolization of debris. Soft-bristle brushes or pipe cleaners can remove soil from hard-to-reach places such as hinges and serrations.

50. Abrasive cleaners, scouring pads, metal brushes, or steel wool should not be used on surgical instruments unless indicated in the device's IFU.

Mechanical Cleaning

51. For mechanical cleaning in a washer-disinfector/decontaminator, instruments are arranged in trays with an open-mesh bottom and placed on shelves in the machine.

52. Washer-disinfector/decontaminators usually offer a variety of cycle options. Phases in the cycle may include cool-water rinse, enzymatic soak or rinse, detergent wash, ultrasonic cleaning, hot-water rinse (180–195°F/70–76°C), thermal or chemical disinfection, treated water rinse, and drying.

53. The washer-disinfector/decontaminator is built into the wall between the decontamination area and the clean areas where instruments are assembled and packaged. Instruments are placed into the machine in the decontamination area and are removed from the opposite end in the clean area.

54. Instruments that have been processed in a washer-disinfector/decontaminator or are manually washed and disinfected according to the IFU are considered clean and safe to handle, and are ready to be inspected, assembled, packaged, and prepared for patient use.

Special Needs Instruments
Eye Instruments

55. Although the principles for cleaning are similar for all instruments, eye instruments require special attention. They are delicate and cannot usually be cleaned in automated systems, so special care must be taken to ensure adequate cleaning.

56. It is essential to clean eye instruments in accordance with the manufacturer's IFU. Eye instruments are delicate and have extremely small lumens. Thorough cleaning of lumens immediately following use is essential to ensure the removal of debris that may be responsible for toxic anterior segment syndrome (TASS).

57. Improper processing of eye instruments has been associated with TASS, a noninfectious inflammation of the anterior segment of the eye that can lead to permanent vision impairment (Al-Ghoul et al., 2014).

58. Most cases of TASS occur when foreign material that was not removed during cleaning and sterilization is introduced into the anterior chamber of the eye. Endotoxins from Gram-negative bacteria in ultrasonic cleaners, viscoelastic solution used during eye surgery, and detergent and disinfectant residue have all been associated with TASS (AAMI, 2013, p. 229).

59. Several organizations have established guidelines that should be referenced for detailed instructions on processing ophthalmic instruments:
    - AORN (2015, p. 630)
    - American Society of Cataract and Refractive Surgery (ASCRS) and American Society of Ophthalmic Registered Nurses (ASORN; Henning, 2011)

Flexible Endoscopes

60. Flexible endoscopes are complex instruments; cleaning them is a multistep process. The manufacturers' IFU provide the specific information required to process each device.

61. Personnel responsible for cleaning and disinfecting these devices should refer to the following:
    - American Society for Gastrointestinal Endoscopy (ASGE) and SHEA (Petersen et al., 2011)
    - AORN (2015, p. 589)
    - Society of Gastroenterology Nurses and Associates (SGNA, 2013)
    - CDC (2015b)
    - The endoscope manufacturer's IFU for cleaning and disinfection or sterilization

62. Personnel responsible for endoscope reprocessing should have demonstrated competence for this complex task.

Robotic Instruments

63. Robotic instruments are complex and have lumens and difficult-to-clean components. It is essential to follow the device manufacturer's IFU for cleaning, inspection, and processing.

64. Pay special attention to cleaning the ports and articulating areas on robotic instruments. Flush ports while rotating the articulating component of the device through its full range of motion. Flush until the water runs clear.

Failure to flush effectively may result in incomplete removal of debris that can dry and harden, making cleaning more difficult and impeding effective sterilization.

Ultrasonic Cleaning

65. The purpose of ultrasonic cleaning is to dislodge and remove tenacious debris from instruments with hard-to-reach nooks and crannies.

66. Ultrasonic cleaning is not suitable for lensed instruments, powered instruments, or instruments that are chrome plated or made of plastic or rubber. Consult the instrument manufacturer's IFU to determine whether ultrasonic cleaning is compatible with a specific instrument.

67. High-intensity sound waves generate tiny bubbles that expand until they collapse or implode (cavitation), creating negative pressure that dislodges soil from hard-to-reach crevices. Ultrasonic cleaning is especially beneficial for items with box locks, serrations, lumens, and crevices.

68. Follow both the detergent and the ultrasonic manufacturers' IFU when adding detergent to the water in the ultrasonic cleaner. The IFU will also indicate if and when the water needs to be degassed.

69. Before placing instruments in the ultrasonic washer, ensure that they are free of gross soil.

70. Place instruments in a specially designed instrument basket or tray. Instruments should not rest on the bottom of the unit because that will prevent cavitation on the part of the instrument not in contact with water.

71. Attach adaptors that flush cleaning solution through the lumens of cannulated instruments.

72. Only instruments of the same kind of metal should be placed in the ultrasonic machine at one time. If instruments constructed of dissimilar metals are combined in the ultrasonic cleaner, etching and pitting may occur as a result of ion transfer from one metal to another.

73. To prevent aerosolization of contaminants, the lid on the ultrasonic cleaner should remain closed during use.

74. If an automated rinse phase is not included in the ultrasonic cycle and instruments are not placed in an automated washer using treated water, instruments should be manually rinsed with treated water.

75. The solution in the ultrasonic washer should be changed at least daily or whenever it is visibly soiled. The manufacturer's IFU will have instructions for changing the solution.

76. Most facilities use an ultrasonic cleaner following initial decontamination and prior to manual cleaning. Some facilities use ultrasonic cleaning for most instruments; others use it exclusively for specialty or difficult-to-clean instruments. Some washer-disinfectors/decontaminators include an ultrasonic cycle.

Lubrication

77. Instruments with movable parts should be lubricated according to the device manufacturer's IFU with an antimicrobial, water-soluble lubricant that protects against rusting and staining. Because the lubricant is usually white, it often called *instrument milk*.

78. The lubricant must be water soluble to allow penetration of steam during sterilization. The residue from oil-based lubricants can prevent penetration of the steam.

Section Questions

1. How does OSHA require that contaminated materials be transported to a decontamination site away from the work area? [Refs 37–38]

2. What is the purpose of the negative pressure in the "decontam" area of the SPD? [Ref 40]

3. How many air exchanges per hour are required in the decontamination area? [Ref 40]

4. What PPE is required for personnel in the "decontam" area? [Ref 41]

5. Why is cleaning the most important step in preparing items for sterilization? [Ref 42]

6. Why is it preferable to use a mechanical washer rather than to clean manually? [Ref 43]

7. What items might require manual cleaning? [Ref 44]

8. What supplies and equipment should be readily available wherever items are cleaned? [Ref 45]

9. Why is hot water not used to rinse contaminated instruments? [Ref 46]

10. How can mixing detergents in a higher concentration than recommended interfere with sterilization? [Ref 47]

11. Describe the methods employed to prevent aerosolization from occurring. [Refs 48–49]

12. In what area do items enter the washer, and where do they exit? [Ref 53]

13. What causes TASS and how can it be prevented? [Refs 56–58]

14. What resources should be consulted when preparing to clean endoscopes? [Ref 60–61]

15. Why are robotic instruments difficult to clean? [Refs 63–64]

16. What is the purpose of ultrasonic cleaning? [Ref 65]

17. Explain how cavitation dislodges soil. [Ref 67]

18. What instruments should not be subjected to ultrasonic cleaning? [Refs 66, 72]

19. What determines the amount of detergent to use and the frequency of changing the solution? [Refs 68, 75]

20. What type of lubricant is used for surgical instruments? [Refs 77–78]

Preparation and Packaging

Inspection

79. When instruments arrive in the clean area of the SPD, sometimes called the "prep and pack" area, any remaining moisture should be dried, and instruments should be inspected for cleanliness, integrity, alignment, sharpness of edges, and proper function.

80. It is critical that items that do not function as intended be removed from service and either discarded or sent for repair. At the point of use, there is very limited opportunity to check each instrument for function; therefore, it is

imperative that careful inspection and checking for function occur prior to packaging. An instrument that fails in surgery can be the direct cause of an injury to the patient.

Assembly and Packaging
Selection Criteria for Barrier Protection

81. Packaging materials and systems are intended to maintain the sterility of items until their intended use.

82. Packaging material must be appropriate for both the item and the sterilization process. Not all packaging materials are compatible with every sterilization process; however, all packaging materials must:

    - Provide a barrier to microorganisms.
    - Permit penetration and exit of the sterilant.
    - Allow for adequate air removal.
    - Be intact; resist tears, punctures, and abrasions.
    - Permit complete and secure enclosure of the contents.
    - Be fluid resistant.
    - Be free of toxic ingredients and non-fast dyes.
    - Provide adequate seal integrity.
    - Be large enough to evenly distribute the contained mass.
    - Permit identification of the contents and/or labeling to identify contents.
    - Maintain sterility of items until package is opened.
    - Allow for aseptic delivery of contents to the sterile field.
      (AAMI, 2013, §8.2; AORN, 2015, pp. 652)

83. A wide variety of types of packaging systems is available:

    - Woven fabrics
    - Nonwoven materials
    - Paper
    - "Peel packs" (plastic/paper and plastic/Tyvek pouches)
    - Rigid container systems

Woven Fabric

84. Reusable wrappers constructed of cotton and polyester blend fabrics that have been treated to be water resistant have been largely replaced by disposable, nonwoven fabrics. Woven wrappers:

    - May produce lint.
    - Do not exhibit "memory," a characteristic that causes material edges, when the package is opened, to return to their original folded position.
    - Are compatible with steam and ethylene oxide (EtO) sterilization but may not be used with hydrogen peroxide or ozone.
    - Must be inspected between uses for pinholes and tears. Damaged wrappers must be repaired with heat-sealed patches or discarded.
    - Must be laundered between uses to prevent superheating and deterioration of the fabric. They should be maintained for a minimum of 2 hours at room temperature (i.e., 68–73°F [20–23°C]) and at a relative humidity of 30% to 60% (AAMI, 2013, §8.3.1).
    - Lose their water-resistant properties over time and must be retreated or discarded.
    - Usually require two wrappers (four layers) to protect sterile contents.
    - Packages may be wrapped:
      - Sequentially: Two wrappers are folded one at a time to create a package within a package.
      - Simultaneously: Two wrappers at once: The item is folded into two wrappers at the same to create a single package.
      - Single-layer wrap: Items may be wrapped in a single layer of material when the single-layer wrap meets the same barrier protection requirements as two layers of traditional material.
    - The manufacturer's IFU will describe the number of layers required and the method of folding for each type of wrapping material.
    - The facility's policy for wrapping must be driven by the ability of the wrap available to maintain items in a sterile state.

Nonwoven Materials

85. Nonwoven wrappers are made of a combination of cellulose and/or other synthetic materials.

86. Nonwoven, cellulose-based wrappers are compatible with steam and EtO, but are not

compatible with hydrogen peroxide (H_2O_2) sterilization technologies. Polypropylene wrappers are designed for items to be sterilized with H_2O_2 and with EtO and steam. The manufacturer's IFU will determine the compatibility of each wrapper with each sterilization technology.

87. Nonwoven wrappers are single use, disposable, almost entirely lint free, and tear resistant; they provide excellent barrier protection against dust, airborne microorganisms, and moisture.

88. Items wrapped in nonwoven material are wrapped according to the manufacturer's IFU. Some nonwoven wraps require two layers; others require only a single wrap that is equivalent to a sequential double wrap.

89. Nonwoven wrappers eliminate the need for washing, inspecting, and patching. Quality is consistent because wrappers are used only once and then discarded.

90. Nonwoven wrappers may display undesirable memory, because wrapper edges try to return to their original fold when packages are opened. This creates the potential for contamination of package contents when a wrapper edge that has been handled folds back into the package and contaminates the sterile contents.

91. Some nonwoven packaging products may require a longer sterilization time than woven packaging materials. This information must be supplied by the manufacturer.

92. Packages are secured with pressure-sensitive tape that also serves as a process indicator. Select process indicator tape that is specific to the intended sterilization method. (See Ref 133.)

Pouches: Plastic/Paper, Plastic/Tyvek

93. Pouches (also called "peel packs") constructed from plastic and paper or plastic and Tyvek (a material made from high-density polyethylene fibers) may be used for packaging items for sterilization. The plastic/paper combination is appropriate for steam or EtO sterilization. Tyvek/plastic combinations contain no cellulose and are compatible with H_2O_2 and EtO sterilization, but not with steam.

94. The plastic film is fused to the paper or Tyvek so that one side is clear and the other opaque. The sterilant penetrates the opaque paper or Tyvek portion of the pouch, while the plastic portion permits visualization of the item inside.

95. Advantages of peel packs:
    - Inexpensive
    - Permit visualization of the contents
    - Lint free
    - Provide an effective barrier against airborne microorganisms
    - Suitable for packaging multiple small items and individual lightweight items

96. Disadvantages of peel packs:
    - Provide little resistance to punctures
    - Tendency to display memory
    - Limited to packaging items that can be delivered aseptically to the sterile field

97. Items can be packaged in a single pouch; or the sealed pouch containing the item can be placed within another pouch (double pouched). Double pouching is only permissible if the manufacturer's IFU indicate that the pouch has been validated for that option.

98. When double pouching, the inner pouch should fit inside the outer pouch without being folded (AAMI, 2013; see **Figure 3-2**), and the pouches should be oriented in the same direction (plastic faces plastic, and paper faces paper; AAMI, 2013, p. 73). The contents of the inner pouch will be visible.

99. Pouch material is available in many sizes, and pouches are manufactured as individual pouches or on a continuous roll that can be cut into desired lengths.

100. Pouches are either self-sealing or can be fused with a heat sealer. Self-sealing often provides the most secure seal. When heat sealers are used, consult the manufacturer's IFU to establish the appropriate temperature setting. Sealing at the incorrect temperature may result in a weak or incomplete seal.

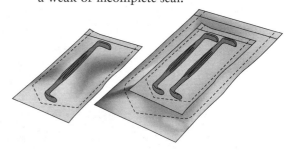

Figure 3-2 Single and double-packaging with paper/plastic pouches.
Reprinted from ANSI/AAMI ST79:2010 & A1: 2010 & A2:2011 with permission of Association for the Advancement of Medical Instrumentation, Inc. © 2011 AAMI www.aami.org. All rights reserved. Further reproduction or distribution prohibited.

101. Remove as much air as possible from the pouch before sealing. Air expands when it is heated and can burst the pouch seams during sterilization.

102. Once a pouch has been opened, the item may not be resealed without being reprocessed. The package seal must not permit resealing once the pouch has been opened.

103. Pouches should be positioned for sterilization on edge (vertically) and all facing in the same direction to promote penetration and evacuation of sterilant. Occasionally, racks are used to facilitate proper positioning.

104. Peel packs should never be placed inside instrument sets because they cannot be maintained in a vertical position (AAMI, 2013, p. 73). Paper bags, foam pouches, and other supplies have been validated for use within sets to contain multiple small items and protect delicate instruments (**Figure 3-3**).

Rigid Container Systems

105. Rigid container systems are packaging receptacles that have an outer case (often called a *casket*) constructed of aluminum, stainless

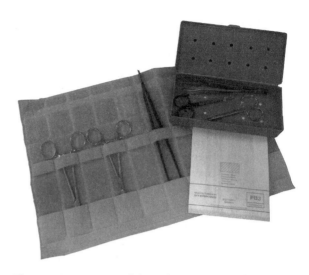

Figure 3-3 Arrange small items in sets in paper bags, foam, and small containers validated for that purpose.
Courtesy of Medical City Dallas, Dallas, TX.

steel, heat-resistant plastic, or a combination of materials. Each system has one or more wire mesh baskets that fit inside to hold instruments (**Figure 3-4**).

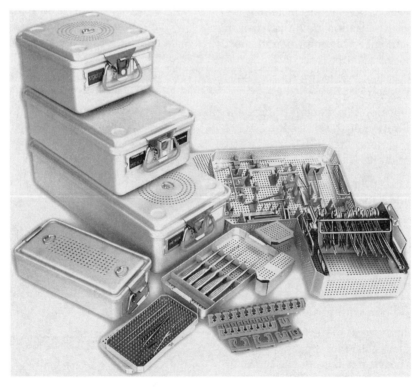

Figure 3-4 Rigid Containers and Accessories.
Courtesy of Case Medical, Inc., South Hackensack, NJ.

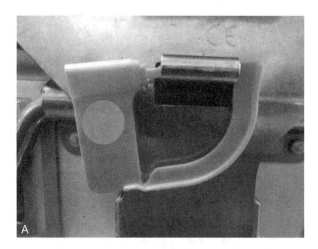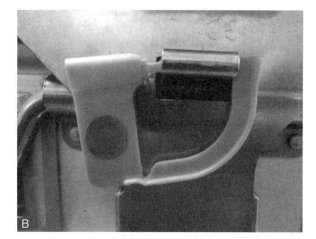

Figure 3-5 Tamper-proof container lock is also a process indicator: (A) Before sterilization and (B) After sterilization. Courtesy of Medical City Dallas, Dallas, TX.

106. Information about compatibility with sterilization technologies and cycles, arrangement of instruments within containers, sealing, labeling, temperature, exposure times, and cleaning instructions must be obtained from the manufacturer's IFU.

107. Container systems have gaskets to promote a secure seal and either a valve or filter system to permit penetration and evacuation of sterilant.

108. After rigid containers have been manually or mechanically cleaned, the gaskets, valves, and filter retainers must be inspected for integrity.

109. Unless the IFU indicates that filters are intended to be used multiple times, a new filter(s) is placed in a container each time one is prepared for use.

110. The lid and base of the container are held together by a latch mechanism.

111. The container is locked with a tamper-evident seal (**Figure 3-5**). Once opened, the contents of the container should be used immediately.

The container cannot be resealed. The seal may also contain a process indicator.

112. Advantages of rigid containers:
   - Durable; provide more protection for instruments than wrapped packages
   - Baskets often have pegs or posts to protect instruments and organize them efficiently
   - Do not require wrapping
   - Can stack for efficient storage

113. Rigid containers can be heavy; an empty container can weigh as much as 10 pounds.

114. If condensation occurs within the container, it is referred to as a "wet pack." When the scrub person opens a container in preparation for surgery and discovers a "wet pack," the instruments are not considered sterile and must not be used. (Note: consult the manufacturer's IFU to see if the container has been FDA cleared to permit moisture while retaining sterility.) An uncleared "wet pack" should be returned intact to the SPD with an explanation of the problem.

Section Questions

1. What do you look for when inspecting surgical instruments? [Ref 79]
2. Why is it important to inspect instruments before they are processed for use? [Ref 80]
3. What characteristics must all packaging materials have? [Ref 82]
4. Explain the concept of "memory" in relation to wrapping materials. [Ref 84]
5. Differentiate between sequential and simultaneous double wrapping. [Ref 84]

(continues)

Section Questions (continued)

6. What determines the number of layers of wrapping material required and the method of folding? [Ref 84]

7. Describe nonwoven wrappers. [Refs 85–87]

8. What differentiates peel packs appropriate for steam sterilization from those for H_2O_2 sterilization? [Ref 93]

9. Describe advantages and disadvantages of peel packs. [Refs 95–96]

10. When is double pouching permissible? [Ref 97]

11. What is the proper protocol for using two pouches to contain an instrument? [Ref 98]

12. Why is it wise to remove air from the pouch before sealing? [Ref 101]

13. Why are pouches constructed so that they cannot be resealed? [Ref 102]

14. How must pouches be arranged on the sterilizer shelf? [Ref 103]

15. Why can't peel packs be used to organize small instruments within instrument sets? [Ref 104]

16. Identify the components of a container system. [Refs 105, 107]

17. Where are the instructions for appropriate sterilization technology and cleaning? [Ref 106]

18. Describe the purpose of the gaskets, valves, and filters. [Ref 107]

19. What is the purpose of the tamper-evident seal that is part of the container's locking system? [Ref 111]

20. Describe advantages and disadvantages of container systems. [Refs 112–113]

Packaging Items for Steam Sterilization

115. Instruments and other items are arranged in container baskets or a perforated or mesh-bottom tray that permits steam to penetrate and also prevents air from being trapped (**Figure 3-6**).

116. Unless contraindicated by the container manufacturer, a lint-free absorbent towel or tray liner may be placed in the bottom of the tray to help absorb condensate that is formed during sterilization and to help speed the drying process (**Figure 3-7**).

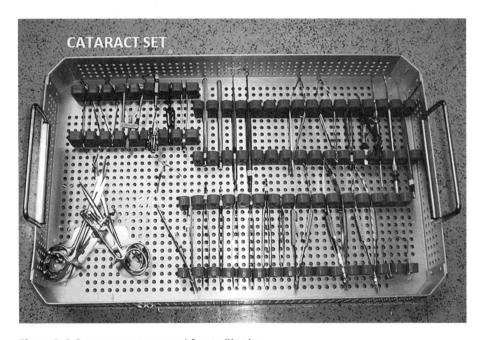

Figure 3-6 Instrument set arranged for sterilization.
Courtesy of Case Medical, Inc., South Hackensack, NJ.

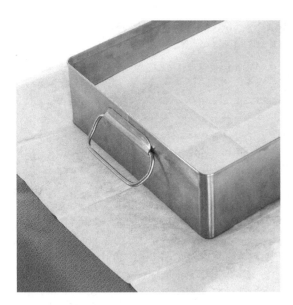

Figure 3-7 Tray liner in instrument tray.
© 2005 Kimberly-Clark Worldwide, Inc. Used with permission.

117. Instruments must be positioned so that every surface of each item will be exposed to the sterilant (**Figure 3-8**).

118. Joints and hinges of instruments must be opened and detachable parts disassembled unless the manufacturer provides validated instructions for sterilization when the device is assembled (AORN, 2015, p. 654). Racks, pins, or stringers may assist in organizing instruments and securing them in an open position.

119. To prevent damage, heavy instruments are placed on the bottom of the tray, and delicate instruments are placed on top. If a container has two baskets, heavier items go into the bottom tray, lighter items in the top.

120. The combined weight of an instrument set, including the container, tray, and/or wrapper, should not exceed 25 pounds (AAMI, 2013, §8.4.2). Sets heavier than 25 pounds should be divided into two sets. In addition to employee safety concerns, instrument sets that are too heavy may concentrate too much metal mass and compromise drying.

121. Basins, bowls, and cups can be nested one inside the other if they are separated with gauze or an absorbent towel. The porous material permits entry of the sterilant, sterilant contact with all surfaces, and exit of the sterilant, and it facilitates the drying process.

122. Basins, bowls, and cups should be positioned vertically in the steam sterilizer to prevent water from pooling in them and to prevent wet packs.

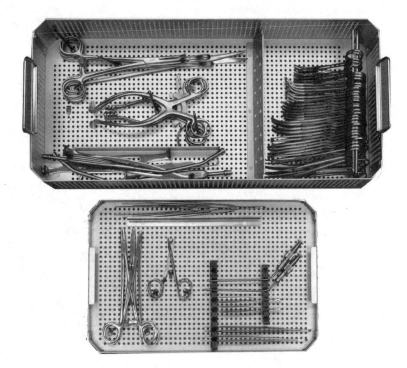

Figure 3-8 Instrument set arranged for sterilization. Note that ringed instruments are held open on a stringer, pins hold larger instruments in place. Heavy instruments are in the larger bottom tray; more delicate instruments are arranged in a separate tray that fits on top.
Courtesy of Case Medical, Inc., South Hackensack, NJ.

123. Nested items should be placed facing in the same direction to prevent air pockets, allow circulation of the steam, and permit condensate to drain out.

124. Rubber sheeting (e.g., Esmarch bandage) or other impervious material cannot be folded on itself or wrapped tightly in a roll for sterilization. The resulting density of the item prevents adequate circulation of the sterilant. (Note: Multiple alternate spellings of *Esmarch* are frequently used, including Eschmark and Esmark. The term is from the German surgeon Johann F. A. von Esmarch.)

125. Open the item and cover with a porous material (e.g., gauze) of the same size, roll or fold loosely, then wrap. This approach promotes sterilant contact with the entire surface of the rubber or other impervious material. Esmarch that is supplied sterile by the manufacturer is preferred.

126. Lumened items, such as cannulas and ventricular and irrigation needles, must be cleaned, rinsed, and dried thoroughly before packaging for sterilization.

Packaging Items for Low-Temperature Sterilization

127. For H_2O_2 or H_2O_2/ozone sterilization systems:
    - All items must be thoroughly dry; lumens should be blown dry with compressed air.
    - If any moisture is present on the objects, the sterilizer cannot achieve a vacuum and the cycle aborts (CDC, 2008).
    - Appropriate packaging includes polypropylene wrap or rigid container systems validated for this sterilization method. The sterilizer manufacturer's and device manufacturer's IFU must be followed when selecting trays and containers.
    - Cellulose-based materials (e.g., paper, gauze, linen, or towels) absorb hydrogen peroxide and cannot be included within the load.

128. For EtO sterilization:
    - Materials used to package items for steam sterilization are also appropriate for EtO sterilization.

129. Items prepared for gas sterilization must be thoroughly dry. Lumens should be blown dry with compressed air. EtO in contact with water forms ethylene glycol, a toxic residue.
    - Oil-based lubricants may not be used, because ethylene oxide cannot penetrate the film left by these lubricants.

Monitoring: Chemical Indicators and Integrators

130. Parameters of the sterilization process are conditions that must be met in order for sterilization to occur:
    - Steam sterilization: time, temperature, and steam quality
    - EtO sterilization: time, temperature, gas concentration, and relative humidity
    - H_2O_2 sterilization systems: H_2O_2 concentration, pressure, time, and temperature

131. Chemical indicators demonstrate a visible change when exposed to parameters of sterilization; indicators differ in the parameter(s) to which they are sensitive.

132. Process, or Class 1, indicators demonstrate only that items have been exposed to the physical conditions within the chamber that are monitored by the indicator.

133. Process indicators include heat-sensitive tape, labels, or strips that are placed on the outside of a package to distinguish between processed and unprocessed units (**Figure 3-9**).

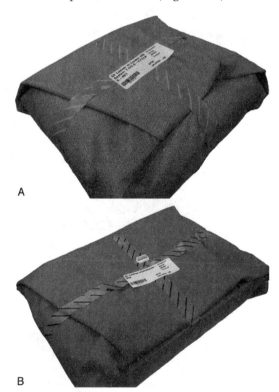

A

B

Figure 3-9 Process indicators change color when exposed to the sterilization process: (A) wrapped item waiting to be sterilized; process indicator stripes are white (B) item that has been removed from the sterilizer; process indicator stripes are black.
Courtesy of Medical City Dallas, Dallas, TX.

Packaging materials such as peel packs and rigid container locking devices often have an integrated process indicator.

134. When there is no visible indicator, the package must be considered contaminated.

135. In addition to the process indicator on the outside of each item, one or more chemical indicators should be placed inside of each package or set (AORN, 2015, p. 655).

136. The manufacturer's IFU will identify the most challenging location(s) within a set or container to determine the most effective placement of the internal indicator. An indicator should be placed in each layer of multilevel sets.

137. Single-variable indicators (Class 3) and multivariable indicators (Class 4) respond to one or more of the critical parameters of sterilization. Class 3 and Class 4 indicators are rarely used in the surgical setting.

138. Integrators (Class 5) react to all critical parameters of the sterilization process. This is the most common internal indicator used in the healthcare setting (**Figure 3-10**).

139. Emulators (Class 6) also react to all critical parameters of the sterilization process and are cycle specific; each steam sterilization cycle has a specific emulator; emulators are not interchangeable (**Figure 3-11**).

140. Chemical indicators are designed specifically for either high-temperature or low-temperature sterilization and are not interchangeable. It is important to select the proper indicator for the sterilization technology being used.

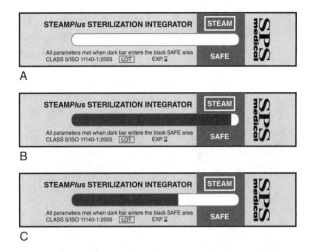

Figure 3-10 Class V integrators change color when exposed to all of the critical parameters of sterilization: (A) unexposed (B) Pass (C) Fail.
Courtesy of SPSmedical, Rush, NY.

Labeling

141. Items packaged for sterilization should be clearly labeled with the contents and initials of the package assembler (**Figure 3-12**).

142. Indelible, nonbleeding, and nontoxic markers may be used to mark packages. Marking on peel packs should be on the plastic side of the pouch (AORN, 2015, p. 658).

143. Before being placed into the sterilizer, a lot control sticker is placed on each package (**Figure 3-13**).

    The lot control number indicates the sterilization date, sterilizer used, and cycle or load

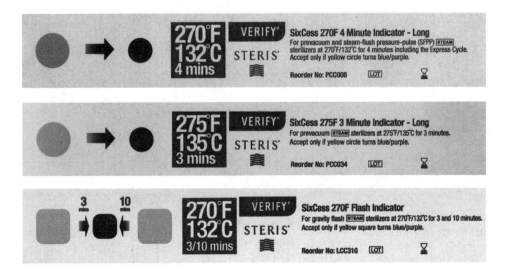

Figure 3-11 Class Six emulating indicators are designed for specific steam sterilization cycles: (A) 270°F/132°C 4 minute cycle (B) 275°F/135°C 3 minute cycle (C) IUSS 3 and 10 minute cycles.
Courtesy of Steris Corporation, Mentor, OH.

number. Lot control numbers, in conjunction with computerized instrument tracking systems, facilitate inventory control, stock rotation, and retrieval of items in the event of sterilization or sterilizer failure.

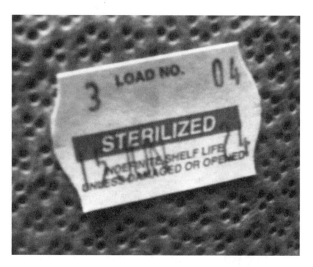

Figure 3-13 Lot control sticker.
Courtesy of Medical City Dallas, Dallas, TX.

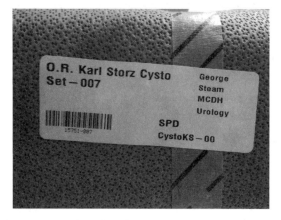

Figure 3-12 Each package is clearly labeled with the contents and identifies the individual who assembled the package.
Courtesy of Medical City Dallas, Dallas, TX.

Section Questions

1. Why do trays that hold instruments for sterilization have perforated bottoms? [Ref 115]

2. What purpose(s) does a towel in the bottom of an instrument tray serve? [Ref 116]

3. How must instruments be positioned in the tray for sterilization? [Refs 117–119]

4. What is the maximum recommended weight of an instrument set? [Ref 120]

5. How are hollow items such as basins and bowls positioned to prevent the accumulation of condensation? [Refs 121–123]

6. Describe preparation of an Esmarch bandage for sterilization. [Refs 124–125]

7. What effect will instruments that have not been thoroughly dried have on an H_2O_2 sterilization cycle? [Ref 127]

8. What packaging materials are appropriate for H_2O_2 sterilization? [Ref 127]

9. Identify the parameters associated with steam, EtO, and H_2O_2 sterilization technologies. [Ref 130]

10. How does a chemical indicator work? [Ref 131]

11. What is the purpose of a Class 1 chemical indicator? [Refs 132–134]

12. How do we determine where to put the chemical integrators inside of an instrument set? [Ref 136]

13. Explain the difference between a chemical integrator and an emulator. [Refs 138–139]

14. What information should be visible on every sterile package? [Refs 141, 143]

15. What is the purpose of a lot control number or lot control sticker? [Ref 143]

Sterilization and Disinfection

144. Sterilization and disinfection processes destroy microorganisms and are among the cornerstones of infection prevention. Protecting the patient from surgical site infection requires the perioperative nurse to understand and apply the principles and practices of sterilization and disinfection.

145. Advances in surgical techniques and technology have created a proliferation of complex, sophisticated, and expensive surgical instrumentation, including endoscopic, fiberoptic, and robotic instruments that require special handling.

146. The appropriate method of cleaning, disinfecting, and sterilizing an item is determined by its composition and configuration, and its compatibility with the sterilization and disinfection methods available within the healthcare facility. It is wise to consult the manufacturers' IFU for processing of instruments and devices when purchasing and processing decisions are made.

147. Whether an item is disinfected or sterilized depends on its intended use. The Spaulding classification of devices, developed in 1968 by Earle Spaulding and adopted by the CDC, categorizes devices as critical, semicritical, or noncritical and determines whether an item must be sterilized or if disinfection is sufficient (**Exhibit 3-1**).

Sterility Assurance Level (SAL)

148. The process of sterilization provides the greatest assurance that items are sterile (i.e., free of known and unsuspected microorganisms).

149. Critical items used in surgery must be sterilized with a sterility assurance level (SAL) of 10^{-6}. This mathematical expression means that there is equal to, or less than, one chance in 1 million that any viable microorganism will be present on an item after sterilization. This is a very high SAL compared to industries where an SAL of 10^{-3} (one chance in 1,000) might be acceptable.

150. In addition to the high level of sterility assurance, a sterilizer must be capable of killing 1 million spores in half the time for which the sterilizer is programmed for hospital use (Favero & Bond, 2001, pp. 885–886). For example, if the exposure phase in the sterilization cycle is 4 minutes, the sterilizer manufacturer must demonstrate that 1 million spores are killed in 2 minutes.

151. Certain pathogenic bacteria such as *Clostridium tetani* (that produces tetanus), *Clostridium peridens* (that causes gas gangrene), and *Clostridium difficile* (that causes serious infections) are capable of developing spores. Spores are the hardiest form of a bacterium; they are more resistant to heat, drying, and chemicals, and can remain alive for many years. When conditions are favorable for growth, such as when the spore gains entry into the body, the spore will germinate to produce a vegetative cell.

152. Disinfection kills all living microorganisms, with the exception of high numbers of bacterial spores. Disinfection does not provide the margin of safety associated with sterilization. Disinfectants vary in their ability to destroy microorganisms and are classified according

Exhibit 3-1 Spaulding Classification System.

Minimum preparation of items is determined by the risk of infection involved with use

Critical Item
- Device enters normally sterile tissue or the vascular system
- Device should be sterilized to destroy all microbial life.
- Examples: surgical instruments, cardiac and urinary catheters, implants, and ultrasound probes used in sterile body cavities

Semicritical Item
- A device that contacts intact mucous membranes and does not ordinarily penetrate sterile tissue.
- Minimum level of processing is high-level disinfection to destroy all vegetative microorganisms, mycobacterium, small or nonlipid viruses, medium or lipid viruses, fungal spores, and some bacterial spores.
- Examples: respiratory therapy and anesthesia equipment, some endoscopes, laryngoscope blades,[24] esophageal manometry probes, cystoscopes

Noncritical
- A devices that does not ordinarily touch the patient or touches only intact skin.
- Such devices should be low-level disinfected.
- Examples: blood pressure cuffs, OR bed safety strap, positioning equipment, computers, environmental surfaces

---

Data from Centers for Disease Control and Prevention. Guideline for Disinfection and Sterilization in Healthcare Facilities, 2008. Last updated December 29, 2009. http://www.cdc.gov/hicpac/Disinfection_Sterilization/2_approach.html

to their cidal activity (i.e., their ability to kill microorganisms).

153. Only sterilization can render an item free of all microorganisms, including spores.

Methods of Sterilization

154. The choice among methods of sterilizing an item depends on its compatibility with the sterilization technology, the configuration of the item, packaging of the item, available technologies, length of time of the sterilization process, and safety factors.

155. Steam is a high-temperature technology that is the least expensive and most common sterilization modality available in hospitals.

156. Two other accepted methods of sterilization, dry heat and ionizing radiation, are not found in U.S. healthcare facilities.

157. Equipment, safety, and cost considerations confine ionizing radiation to industrial settings where it is used for bulk sterilization of commercially prepared items.

158. Dry heat is appropriate for powders, oils, and petroleum products that cannot be penetrated by steam or ethylene oxide or other sterilizing agents. Dry heat sterilization is rarely used in hospitals in the United States because most of these products are supplied sterile from the manufacturer.

159. Heat- and moisture-sensitive items require low-temperature sterilization technologies.

160. EtO, approved for medical device sterilization in the late 1950s, was the first low-temperature technology. Because of the toxicity of EtO and the stringent restrictions for installation and use, it has largely been replaced with H_2O_2 sterilization technologies.

161. Hydrogen peroxide gas plasma was introduced in the 1990s; H_2O_2 vapor and H_2O_2 vapor plus ozone were introduced in the early 2000s. Advantages and disadvantages are associated with all sterilization technologies.

High-Temperature Sterilization
Steam Sterilization

162. Moist heat in the form of saturated steam under pressure is an economical, safe, and effective method of sterilization used for the majority of surgical instruments. Sterilization by this method is accomplished in a steam sterilizer, often called an *autoclave*.

163. For an item to be sterilized, steam must penetrate every fiber of the packaging and contact every surface of the item inside. In addition, the critical parameters of moisture, temperature, and time must be met.

164. Saturated steam contains the greatest amount of water vapor possible. Heated to a sufficient temperature, it is capable of destroying all living microorganisms, including spores, within a relatively short period of time.

165. Saturated steam destroys microorganisms through a thermal process that causes denaturation and coagulation of proteins or the enzyme protein system contained within the microorganism's cell.

166. Steam at atmospheric pressure has a temperature of 212°F (100°C), which is inadequate for sterilization. The addition of pressure to increase the temperature of the steam is necessary for the destruction of microorganisms.

167. An increase in pressure of 15 to 17 pounds per square inch will increase steam temperature to 250–254°F (121–123°C). Twenty-seven pounds of pressure per square inch will increase steam temperature to 270°F (132°C).

168. The minimum generally accepted temperature required for sterilization to occur is 250°F (121°C; Perkins, 1969, p. 161). Typical temperatures for the operation of steam sterilizers are in the range of 270–275°F (132–135°C), although 250°F (121°C) is also used (AAMI, 2013, §8). Steam sterilization is a function of time and temperature. Sterilization at 250°F (121°C) requires more time than sterilization at 270°F (132°C).

169. Steam sterilization has many advantages. Steam:
    - Is readily available (most often supplied from the healthcare facility boiler).
    - Is economical.
    - Enables fast sterilization—destruction of most resistant spores occurs quickly.
    - Is compatible with most in-house packaging materials.
    - Leaves no toxic residue and is environmentally safe.
    - Is suitable for a wide range of surgical instrumentation. The majority of items used for surgery are made from stainless steel and can withstand repeated steam sterilization without sustaining damage.

170. Steam sterilization is also associated with several disadvantages, though preset cycles on more modern autoclaves minimize these challenges.

    • A variety of instruments and devices used in surgery cannot withstand high-temperature sterilization.

    • A temperature of 270°F is not appropriate for all items. A reduced temperature of 250°F may be necessary for a specific item being sterilized. A temperature higher than 270° may be needed to comply with the manufacturer's IFU.

    • Timing of the sterilization cycle must be adjusted based on the type of cycle, variances in materials, device configuration, and size of the load.

171. Efficacy of steam sterilization depends on attention to detail. Improper preparation of items or improper placement within the autoclave can interfere with steam circulation, draining of condensate, or proper drying, any of which can cause the process to fail.

172. A steam sterilizer, sometimes called an *autoclave*, generally consists of a rectangular metal chamber and a shell. Between the two is an enclosed space referred to as a *jacket*. When the autoclave is ready to use, steam and heat fill the jacket and are maintained at a constant pressure, keeping the autoclave in a heated, ready state (**Figure 3-14**).

173. Items are placed in the chamber, the door is shut tightly, and the sterilization cycle is initiated. Steam enters the chamber and displaces all the air from both the chamber and the items in the load. As the pressure rises, steam penetrates the packaging and contacts all surfaces of the items within. The steam forces the air out of the chamber through a discharge port outlet at the bottom front of the autoclave.

174. It is essential that all the air in the chamber be displaced by steam. Trapped air will act as an insulator that interferes with heating and prevents steam contact with every surface of every item.

175. Proper loading of the autoclave is critical. Items must be placed so that steam can circulate freely throughout the chamber and can contact all surfaces. Placement of items must also promote drainage of condensate to prevent water from collecting within items. For example, items such as cups or basins must be placed on their side to facilitate drainage.

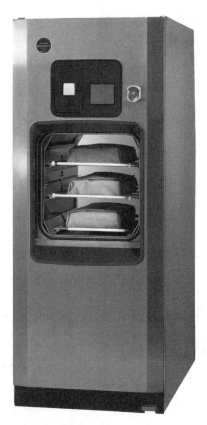

Figure 3-14 Steam Sterilizer.
Courtesy of Steris Corporation, Mentor, OH.

176. The discharge port outlet is the beginning of a filtered waste line. Beneath the filter is a thermometer. This is the coolest part of the autoclave.

177. The actual exposure or sterilization time does not begin until the thermometer senses that the steam has reached the necessary preset temperature.

178. If air is not trapped and the parameters of time, moisture, and temperature have been met, microbial destruction will occur.

179. When the exposure time is complete, the steam is exhausted through the outlet port and a drying cycle follows. A drying cycle is required for wrapped items.

180. Wrapped packages and instrument containers should be allowed to cool on the sterilizer rack. They should not be touched while they are cooling. Rigid containers can be hot enough to burn skin. Grabbing a hot package may result in strikethrough, causing condensate that has not yet evaporated to penetrate the wrapper. The package would then be considered contaminated and would need to be reprocessed.

181. A minimum drying time of 30 minutes is recommended, although some instrument sets may require as much as 2 hours to cool adequately (AAMI, 2013, §8.8.1).

182. Warm packages must not be placed on cool surfaces because condensate will form, causing the package to become damp. Microorganisms are capable of penetrating wet materials; therefore, moist packages that contact an unsterile surface must be considered contaminated.

183. Two types of steam sterilizers or autoclaves are in use today: the older gravity displacement and newer dynamic air removal technologies (high vacuum, prevacuum, and pulse pressure). These autoclaves differ in how air is removed from the chamber during the sterilization process.

184. Sterilizers vary in terms of their design and performance characteristics. Some sterilizers offer both a gravity-displacement and a dynamic air-removal cycle; some offer only one type of cycle.

185. The nature of the items and the container in which they are sterilized determine the necessary time and temperature for sterilization. No single setting is appropriate for all items. The manufacturers' IFU for the items and for the autoclave must be consulted to determine the correct cycle settings.

Section Questions

1. How is the method of cleaning, disinfecting, and sterilizing an item determined? [Ref 146]

2. Differentiate the need for sterilization versus high-level disinfection. [Ref 147]

3. What level of processing is required for crutches, thermometers, and hemostats? [Ref Exhibit 3-1]

4. What is the significance of a sterility assurance level of 10^{-6}? [Ref 149]

5. Why are spores important when determining the efficacy of a sterilizer? [Refs 150–151]

6. Disinfection and sterilization both kill pathogens. How does sterilization differ from disinfection? [Refs 152–153]

7. What factors must be considered when choosing a sterilization technology to process an item? [Ref 154]

8. Why are there both high-temperature and low-temperature sterilization technologies in healthcare? [Refs 155, 159]

9. What must occur inside the autoclave for an item to be sterilized? [Ref 163]

10. Why does an autoclave require steam under pressure to achieve sterilization? [Refs 166–167]

11. List advantages and disadvantages of steam sterilization. [Refs 169–170]

12. Describe how a steam sterilizer works to achieve sterilization. [Refs 172–179]

13. What factors can keep sterilization from occurring? [Ref 178]

14. Describe reasons for allowing packages to cool following sterilization. [Ref 180]

15. How can strikethrough cause a sterilized item to be considered contaminated? [Ref 180]

Gravity Displacement

186. In a gravity-displacement cycle or autoclave, steam replaces the air in the chamber by gravity.

187. As steam enters from a port located near the top and rear of the chamber, it is deflected upward. Air is heavier than steam; thus, by the force of gravity, the air is forced to the bottom while the steam rides on top of the air. The steam rapidly displaces the air under it and forces the air out through the discharge outlet port (**Figure 3-15**).

188. Most gravity-displacement autoclaves are operated at temperatures between 250°F and 274°F (121–134°C) with a 10- to 30-minute exposure time. For example, a wrapped instrument set requiring 30 minutes at 250°F (121°C) might require a 15-minute exposure at 270°F (134°C; AAMI, 2013, §8.6.1).

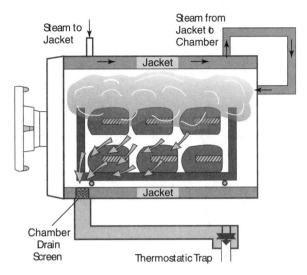

Figure 3-15 Steam sterilizer – Steam entry and air removal.
Courtesy of AMSCO International, Inc.

189. Certain powered equipment may require prolonged exposure times of as much as 55 minutes when sterilized in a gravity displacement sterilizer.

190. Sterilization at a higher temperature requires less time than at a lower temperature. A temperature of 270°F (132°C) will accomplish sterilization more rapidly than a temperature of 250°F (121°C). All recommended cycles achieve an SAL of 10^{-6}.

191. The disadvantages of a gravity-displacement process are the length of time required for sterilization and the dependence on gravity to remove air. A prevacuum or steam–flush–pressure–pulse cycle offers a greater margin of safety with regard to air removal.

192. Gravity-displacement cycles should not be used when a prevacuum or steam–flush–pressure–pulse cycle is available, nor when the item manufacturer's IFU recommend a dynamic air-removal cycle.

193. Gravity-displacement sterilizers are common in dentist and physician offices, clinics, and small surgicenters. Sterilizers that permit only a gravity-displacement cycle can still be found in healthcare facilities; however, most sterilizers sold today for hospitals and large ambulatory surgery centers run dynamic air-removal cycles (though they may also offer gravity-displacement cycles).

194. Some medical devices, because of their design, may require a gravity-displacement cycle. The device manufacturer's IFU will determine the cycle type, time, and temperature.

Dynamic Air Removal (Prevacuum Sterilizer)

195. The prevacuum autoclave is equipped with a vacuum pump that evacuates almost all air from the chamber prior to the injection of steam. The evacuation process, which takes approximately 5 minutes, essentially creates a vacuum within the chamber. When the steam enters the chamber, the force of the vacuum causes instant steam penetration and contact with all surfaces of the contents regardless of the size of the package or load.

196. Following the prevacuum phase, an exposure time of 3 to 4 minutes at 270°F to 275°F (132–135°C) is usually recommended for accomplishing sterilization (AAMI, 2013, §8.6.1). It is imperative that the device manufacturer's instructions for use be consulted before selecting the cycle time and temperature.

197. A dynamic air-removal (prevacuum sterilization) cycle has several advantages:

- Incorrect placement of objects within the chamber will have less effect upon air removal than in a gravity-displacement cycle.

- The entire load will heat rapidly and more uniformly than with a gravity-displacement autoclave; therefore, the exposure time is shorter.

- Loading the autoclave is more efficient, allowing more supplies to be sterilized within a given time.

198. The disadvantage of a dynamic-air-removal (prevacuum) sterilizer is that in the event of a leak, such as in the door seal, an air pocket can form that will inhibit sterilization.

Extended Cycles

199. With proliferation of the number and types of surgical devices, the variety of cycle times has likewise increased. We cannot assume that a 4-minute exposure at 270°F (132°C) is always appropriate.

200. Although a 4-minute exposure time is typical, exposure times of 5, 8, and 15 minutes are not uncommon. These cycles are commonly referred to as *extended cycles*. Temperature requirements vary from 270°F to 275°F (132–135°C). The manufacturer's IFU for sterilization of any instrument will determine the

correct cycle length and temperature. If a device calls for an extended cycle or temperature variation, other devices that require less time should not be included in the load unless they have been validated by the device manufacturer for these extended cycles.

201. An extended cycle of 18 minutes at 270°F (134°C) minutes is also required for instruments exposed to prions (AAMI, 2013, Annex C).

Steam–Flush–Pressure–Pulse Sterilizer

202. Instead of creating a vacuum to remove air from the chamber, a sterilizer may use a repeated sequence of steam, flush, and pressure pulses above atmospheric pressure. Because a vacuum is not drawn, a Bowie-Dick test or daily air-removal test is not required for this type of sterilizer.

203. A variety of cycle times can be selected, based on the nature of the items to be sterilized.

204. The advantage to a steam–flush–pressure–pulse sterilizer is that sterilization is not affected in the event of an air leak into the sterilization chamber.

Immediate-Use Steam Sterilization (IUSS)

(AORN, 2015, pp. 671–673; AAMI, 2013, §8.6.2)

205. IUSS has replaced the term *flash sterilization*, derived from "sterilization in a flash," a quick way to sterilize an unwrapped item.

206. IUSS is appropriate only for processing an item needed urgently and for which there is no sterile replacement immediately available. For instance, IUSS might be used to sterilize a one-of-a-kind item that was contaminated during surgery and is essential to complete the procedure.

207. IUSS should not be used for routine sterilization of instruments and was never intended for sterilizing whole sets of instruments.

208. IUSS should be used only in carefully selected, urgent clinical situations and should not be used to sterilize implantable devices (AORN, 2015, p. 673). Use of IUSS is discouraged by a number of standards-setting organizations.

209. According to the CDC, IUSS is not intended to be used for convenience, as an alternative to purchasing additional instrument sets, or to save time (CDC, 2008).

210. Cleaning is absolutely critical to proper instrument processing, because inadequate cleaning will compromise the sterilization process. At no time is it appropriate to rinse or clean an item in the scrub sink.

211. An item intended for IUSS must be cleaned in the same manner that it would be cleaned in the SPD. In many instances, instruments prepared for IUSS are cleaned and prepared under less-than-ideal conditions. Many operating rooms do not have the processes and resources in place that are available in the SPD. In addition, a separate decontamination area for cleaning instruments may not exist in the operating room.

212. Regardless of where instruments are cleaned, the cleaning process should be consistent and in compliance with accepted standards. Appropriate PPE is required for personnel, regardless of what is being cleaned or where cleaning is done. A scrub sink is not appropriate for cleaning instruments.

213. Items subject to IUSS should be sterilized in containers specifically validated for IUSS. These containers facilitate aseptic delivery of the item to personnel at the sterile field. Some containers used for IUSS have also been cleared by the FDA, for terminal sterilization that allows storage of sterilized items for later use. There are some new rigid containers designed specifically for IUSS that allow for an item to be stored for a short period of time. Rigid containers *not* intended specifically for IUSS should not be used for this process.

214. Although it is recommended that items sterilized via IUSS be placed in a dedicated container, a single wrapper may be used for certain types of instruments if the sterilizer IFU indicate this is appropriate.

215. IUSS may be done in a gravity-displacement or a dynamic air-removal (prevacuum or steam–flush–pressure–pulse) sterilizer. The cycles for IUSS are preset by the sterilizer manufacturer.

216. Exposure times for IUSS can vary by more than 30 minutes and are determined by factors such as the nature and configuration of the item, the type of sterilizer, and whether a dedicated container is available. For example, at 270°F (134°C), a 3-minute exposure is appropriate in both a gravity-displacement and a prevacuum sterilizer for most metal or nonporous or nonlumened items only. However, for metal items with a lumen, a 10-minute cycle in a gravity-displacement sterilizer is required. In a prevacuum sterilizer, metal items with a lumen might

require only 4 minutes. If a dedicated IUSS container system is used, the exposure time and temperatures may vary further. For this reason, it is critical that sterilizer, container, and device manufacturer guidelines be followed.

217. Because there is little or no dry time with an IUSS cycle, items may be wet or moist at the end of the process. IUSS cannot be used to terminally sterilize wrapped or containerized items intended for storage.

218. When a device manufacturer does not provide instructions for IUSS, the item should not be sterilized in this manner. Perioperative nurses should always refer to the manufacturer's IFU when selecting the cycle type, time, and temperature. Inconsistencies between the device manufacturer's and the sterilizer manufacturer's IFU should be resolved before sterilization.

219. If IFU are not available within the operating room, the perioperative nurse should consult with personnel from the SPD. In the absence of instructions, IUSS should not be used to sterilize the item. It is important to refer to the most recent manufacturer's IFU, because instructions for sterilization continue to evolve.

220. Another disadvantage of IUSS is that, following sterilization, aseptic transfer of the item from the autoclave to the sterile field may be challenging. Sterilizers are often located at a distance from the operating room, increasing the risk of contamination during transport.

221. Using the special containers designed for use with IUSS reduces the risk of contamination during transfer from the autoclave to the sterile field.

222. Ideally, a sterilizer used for IUSS would open directly into the operating room. This configuration facilitates transport without contamination.

Section Questions

1. What is the relationship between time and temperature for steam sterilization cycles? [Ref 190]

2. What are the disadvantages of gravity-displacement steam technology? [Ref 191]

3. What is the typical exposure time and temperature for a dynamic air-removal sterilizer? [Ref 196]

4. List some advantages of a dynamic air-removal sterilizer over a gravity-displacement sterilizer. [Ref 197]

5. What determines when an extended cycle might be necessary? [Refs 200–201]

6. What advantage does steam–flush–pressure–pulse technology have over the prevacuum autoclave? [Ref 202]

7. What differentiates an IUSS cycle from a regular steam sterilization cycle? [Ref 205]

8. For what circumstance is IUSS intended? [Ref 206]

9. What are some identified situations for which IUSS should *not* be used? [Refs 207–209]

10. Under what circumstances is it acceptable to clean instruments in the scrub sink? [Ref 210]

11. Why is cleaning an instrument prior to IUSS difficult in the operating room? [Refs 211–212]

12. In what type of autoclave can IUSS be done? [Ref 215]

13. What is the length of time associated with an IUSS sterilization cycle? [Ref 216]

14. When can an item *not* be sterilized in an IUSS cycle? [Refs 218–219]

15. Why is the location of the sterilizer a factor in safe IUSS sterilization? [Refs 220–222]

Low-Temperature Sterilization Technologies
Hydrogen Peroxide Plasma

223. Plasma is a state of matter that is produced through the action of a strong electric or magnetic field. In low-temperature hydrogen peroxide plasma sterilization, a plasma state is created by the action of radiofrequency or electrical energy on hydrogen peroxide vapor within a vacuum (**Figure 3-16**).

224. Items to be sterilized are placed in a sterilizing chamber, a vacuum is established, and liquid

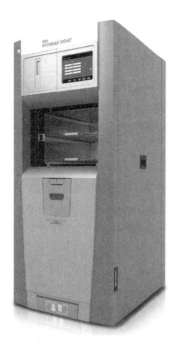

Figure 3-16 Hydrogen peroxide plasma sterilizer – Sterrad 100NX.
Courtesy of Advanced Sterilization Products, division of Ethicon, Inc.

hydrogen peroxide is injected into a cap and enters the chamber in a vaporized or gas form. Hydrogen peroxide vapor is effective in killing microorganisms. The hydrogen peroxide gas is charged with radiofrequency energy that creates plasma. The levels of residual hydrogen peroxide are removed, and at the end of the cycle the reactive species recombine to form oxygen and water vapor. The water vapor is in the form of humidity and cannot be felt.

225. Monitoring includes a special chemical indicator designed to change color in the presence of H_2O_2 and a biological indicator containing the spore *Geobacillus stearothermophilus*.

226. Packages are dry at the end of the cycle and may be used immediately or stored for future use.

227. Advantages of low-temperature hydrogen peroxide gas plasma sterilization include:

   • Gas plasma offers an efficient alternative to EtO sterilization, no toxic chemicals are retained, and no aeration is required. Because there are no toxic byproducts, PPE or monitoring of the environment is not required.

   • The sterilization cycle is short (approximately 30 minutes to more than 1 hour depending up the sterilizer model).

   • The sterilant is compatible with most metals and plastics.

   • The sterilizer is simple to operate. Cycle times are preset and temperature does not require adjustment.

   • There is no plumbing, no drain, nor other fixed requirements. Because the sterilizer connects to an electrical outlet, it can easily be relocated if the need arises.

228. Disadvantages of low-temperature hydrogen peroxide gas plasma include:

   • Hydrogen peroxide gas plasma is not compatible with powders, liquids, textiles, and other cellulose-containing items such as linen, gauze, and paper.

   • Packaging materials are limited to nonwoven polypropylene wraps, Tyvek and Mylar pouches, and specific container systems.

   • In some hydrogen peroxide gas plasma sterilizer models, lumen restrictions may prevent long, narrow-lumened devices, such as ureteroscopes, from being processed by this method.

Vapor-Phase Hydrogen Peroxide

229. In a vapor-phase hydrogen peroxide sterilizer, H_2O_2 is added to the sterilization chamber through a vaporizer under low pressure, creating a vapor that fills the sterilization chamber. As the H_2O_2 diffuses and contacts surfaces, an oxidative process inactivates microorganisms. Byproducts of the process are oxygen and water vapor in the form of humidity, so no additional aeration is required.

230. Programmed cycles address specific parameters for sterilizing instruments of different types: instruments with and without lumens and instruments with diffusion-restricted spaces (e.g., hinges, ratchets, box locks) and single- or dual-channel flexible endoscopes or other features.

231. For both vapor and plasma H_2O_2, all items to be sterilized must be thoroughly cleaned, rinsed, and dried before being packaged and loaded into the chamber.

232. Items should be arranged in a single layer with minimal overlap to ensure proper diffusion of sterilant vapor throughout the load.

233. Cycle phases include:

   • Conditioning: Sterilant fills the reservoir and a vacuum pulse removes air and moisture from the chamber, filtered dry air is introduced, and the load is tested electronically for acceptable moisture content.

- Sterilization: A series of four pulses creates a vacuum and introduces sterilant vapor and filtered air into the chamber.

- Aeration: The sterilant vapor is evacuated from the chamber. When the aeration phase is complete, the chamber pressure is brought to atmospheric level and the chamber door unlocks.

234. Monitoring includes a special chemical indicator designed to change color in the presence of H_2O_2 and a biological indicator containing the spore *Geobacillus stearothermophilus*.

235. Advantages of low-temperature hydrogen peroxide vapor sterilization include:

- Vaporized H_2O_2 offers an efficient alternative to EtO sterilization; there are no toxic byproducts, only water vapor and oxygen.

- The sterilant is compatible with most metals and plastics, glass, and silicone.

- The sterilizer is simple to operate. Cycle times are preset and temperature does not require adjustment.

- There is no plumbing, no drain, nor other fixed requirements. The sterilizer connects to an electrical outlet and can be relocated easily if necessary.

236. Disadvantages of vaporized hydrogen peroxide include:

- Hydrogen peroxide vapor is not compatible with liquids, linens, powders, and cellulose materials such as linen, gauze, and paper.

- Packaging materials are limited to nonwoven polypropylene wraps, Tyvek and Mylar pouches, or specific container systems.

Ethylene Oxide Gas (EtO)

237. EtO is a toxic gas used to sterilize items that cannot tolerate the temperature and moisture of steam sterilization. Ethylene oxide achieves sterilization by interfering with protein metabolism and cell reproduction.

238. Because OSHA (2012b) identifies EtO as a human carcinogen, the sterilizers must be housed in a location that is closely monitored and vented.

239. OSHA requires specific training, PPE, exposure monitoring, and warning signs. Exposure to EtO can cause eye irritation, nausea, dizziness, vomiting, nasal and throat irritation, shortness of breath, tissue burns, and hemolysis.

Insufficiently aerated items may cause patient or personnel injury (OSHA, 2012b, 29CFR 1910.1047 (j)(2)(i)(A)).

240. Because of safety issues and prolonged aeration time, most healthcare facilities have significantly reduced or eliminated the use of EtO, replacing it with newer low-temperature sterilization technologies that do not have the same safety issues, lengthy process, and aeration time.

241. Because EtO is toxic and a variety of materials can absorb EtO, items must be thoroughly aerated following sterilization to remove vestiges of the chemical from the packaging and the sterile items.

Liquid Chemical Sterilant Processing System

242. Peracetic acid is acetic acid (vinegar) plus hydrogen peroxide that provides an extra oxygen atom. Peracetic acid disrupts protein bonds and the extra oxygen atom inactivates cell systems and causes immediate cell death.

243. Liquid peracetic acid is a low-temperature, nonterminal process that can be used to prepare reusable heat-sensitive devices such as endoscopes and their accessories that cannot be processed using steam.

244. The items to be processed are placed in a dedicated container, then placed into the tabletop unit (**Figure 3-17**). The sterilant circulates through the container and tray, contacting all surfaces of the items. Items are then rinsed with filtered and UV-treated water.

245. Items with internal lumens are connected to irrigator adapters to ensure sterilant contact within the lumens. It is important to ensure that devices with lumens are fitted with the appropriate irrigator adaptors prior to processing.

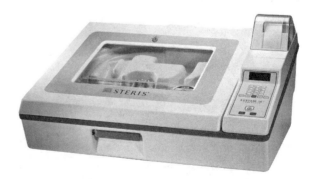

Figure 3-17 Steris Liquid Chemical Serilant Processing System 1E.
Courtesy of Steris Corporation, Mentor, OH.

The manufacturer of each device should be consulted to determine if the device is validated for processing in a liquid peracetic acid processing system. Both the device manufacturer's and the liquid chemical sterilant processor manufacturer's IFU should be consulted to determine the appropriate irrigator adaptor(s).

246. Contact time is standardized at 6 minutes at a temperature of 45.5°C to 60°C (113.0–140°F). A rinse period follows the contact period; the rinse time depends on the water temperature and fill time. An entire cycle takes less than 30 minutes.

247. Following processing, the circulating nurse opens the lid, retrieves the tray, transports it to the operating room, and opens it. The sterile scrub person removes the items (which are wet) from the tray and places them on the sterile field.

248. Processing using liquid chemical peracetic acid is a "just in time" process. Processed items must be used immediately; they cannot be packaged and stored for later use. Processed items that are not delivered to the sterile field are hand dried and returned to storage for future processing; these stored items are not considered sterile.

249. The system uses microprocessors to ensure that the required parameters are met.

250. Monitoring includes a special chemical indicator designed to change color in the presence of peracetic acid. Biological monitoring is performed with a spore strip containing *Geobacillus stearothermophilus*.

251. Advantages of liquid chemical peracetic acid processing include:
    • The cycle is less than 30 minutes and offers quick turnaround time.
    • Peracetic acid is combined with anticorrosive and buffering agents that prevent corrosion of instruments and render the sterilant nontoxic to personnel and the environment.
    • Liquid chemical peracetic acid processing is compatible with many materials that cannot withstand high-temperature sterilization.

252. Disadvantages of liquid chemical peracetic acid processing include:
    • The size of the tray used for processing does not permit large loads to be processed. Only one flexible scope can be processed at a time.
    • Only immersible items that fit within the dedicated tray may be processed.
    • Items are wet at the end of the cycle.
    • Processed items must be used immediately. The nature of the process permits point-of-use processing but not storage. Processed items must be used immediately or dried and returned to storage for later processing; they cannot be left in the system to be used at a later time.

Vaporized Hydrogen Peroxide and Ozone

253. Combined vaporized hydrogen peroxide and ozone sterilization have recently been introduced to the market. Ozone is an emerging low-temperature technology.

254. Manufacturer's IFU should be consulted to determine the appropriate application of this technology.

Section Questions

1. What are the end products of H_2O_2 plasma sterilization? [Ref 224]
2. What are the advantages and disadvantages of H_2O_2 sterilization compared to EtO and steam technologies? [Refs 227–228, 235–236]
3. How should items be arranged in the sterilizer to promote successful sterilization? [Ref 232]
4. Why has EtO sterilization been largely replaced with other low-temperature technologies? [Refs 237–240]
5. Why is aeration of items sterilized with EtO so important? [Ref 241]
6. What items are appropriate for processing with peracetic acid? [Ref 243]
7. Why is peracetic acid considered a nonterminal process? [Ref 248]
8. How are chemical and biological monitoring done with peracetic acid?
9. Describe the advantages and disadvantages of a liquid chemical sterilant processing system. [Refs 251–252]
10. What additional low-temperature processes have been introduced to the market? [Ref 253]

Sterilization Monitoring: Quality Control

255. Items that have been sterilized for patient use cannot, themselves, be tested for sterility; the packages would have to be opened for testing and the items would no longer be available for patient use. Hence, we must assume that if a sterilizer is performing properly, it is, in fact, sterilizing the contents of each load. We assume the sterility of the contents if we can demonstrate that the sterilizer has performed properly.

256. Assumption of sterility is based on the following:

    • Chemical and mechanical process indicators insure that all of the required parameters of sterilization have been met.

    • Biological indicators provide proof that microorganisms that are the most difficult to kill have, in fact, been destroyed.

257. Depending upon where sterilizer monitoring is done, the circulating nurse, the scrub person, and SPD personnel all share responsibility for checking these monitors.

Physical Monitors

258. Physical monitors include temperature and pressure recorders, digital printouts, and gauges that record activities within the chamber during the sterilization cycle.

259. A digital printout record correlates the exact times, temperatures, and pressures achieved during the conditioning, exposure, and exhaust phases of the sterilization cycle. The operator who opens the sterilizer at the end of the load should verify that the cycle was complete and correct. The printout includes space for the operator to initial and include the load identification (**Figure 3-18**).

260. Gauges on the autoclave may register pressure and temperature within the jacket and the chamber. Gauges on the EtO sterilizer may register temperature, gas concentration, and humidity.

261. With liquid peracetic acid, a diagnostic cycle is run to check electricity supply, filters, temperature, pressure, and system integrity at the beginning of each day, and a printout of the results is filed. A microprocessor system will abort the cycle if parameters are not met.

Chemical Indicators

262. A Class 2 chemical indicator, the Bowie-Dick or daily air-removal test (DART), is run each day before the first processed load to

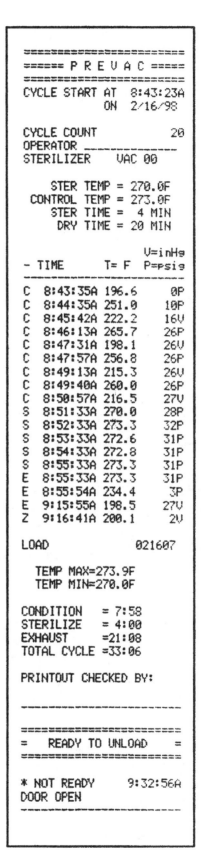

Figure 3-18 Steam sterilizer cycle printout. Courtesy of Steris Corporation, Mentor, OH.

demonstrate that air is being eliminated from the chamber of each dynamic air-removal autoclave effectively enough to achieve steam penetration of a standard load (AAMI, 2013).

263. The Class 2 indicator contains a commercially prepared sheet of paper with various patterns of heat-sensitive ink that is contained in a commercially prepared package or placed in a specially constructed pack of towels. The Bowie-Dick or DART is placed over the drain in an otherwise empty autoclave.

264. Following the cycle, a uniform color change indicates that the air-removal process was successful (**Figure 3-19**).

Biological Monitors

265. Biological monitoring determines whether or not microorganisms have been destroyed and is, therefore, the most accurate method of ensuring that the conditions necessary for sterilization have been achieved.

266. Biological indicators (BI) are available as capsules that contain a known, living, and highly resistant spore population; spore strips; and ampoules with spores suspended in the culture medium (**Figures 3-20** and **3-21**).

267. *Geobacillus stearothermophilus* spores are used to test steam autoclaves and hydrogen peroxide sterilizers. Ethylene oxide sterilizers are tested with *Bacillus atrophaeus* spores. Both types of spores are highly resistant nonpathogenic microorganisms.

268. A BI should be run in each steam sterilizer at least weekly and preferably every day that the sterilizer is in use (AAMI, 2013, §10.5.3.2).

269. A BI should be run in every sterilizer load containing an implant. In some facilities, a BI is run with each sterilizer load (AAMI, 2013, §10.5.3.2).

270. Implants should not be released for implantation until the results of biological monitoring are known to be negative for growth.

271. EtO sterilizers should be tested with every load (AORN, 2015, p. 674).

272. Hydrogen peroxide sterilizers should be tested daily and preferably with every load (AORN, 2015, p. 676).

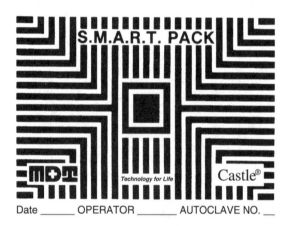

SATISFACTORY TEST

TYPICAL TEST FAILURE

Figure 3-19 Air removal test.
Courtesy of MDT Biologic Company, Rochester, NY.

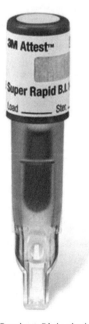

Figure 3-20 Rapid Readout Biological Monitor.
Courtesy of 3M, St. Paul, MN. The image is reproduced herein with permission. © 3M, 2013. All rights reserved.

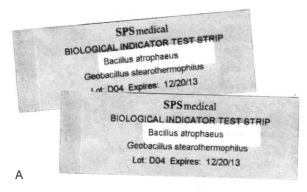

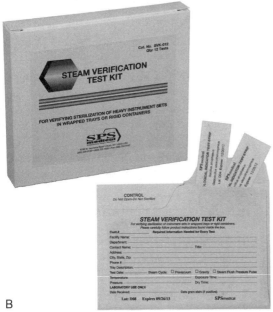

A

B

Figure 3-21 Biological indicator spore strips - dual (steam, EtO, dry heat, and chemical vapor): (A) Hospitals sometimes send spore strips to an outside validation lab for third party verification; (B) Clinics and office-based surgery often use a biological indicator mailing system.
Courtesy of SPSmedical, Rush, NY.

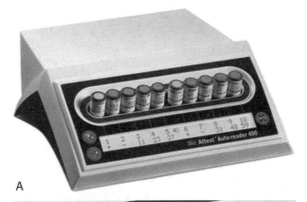

A

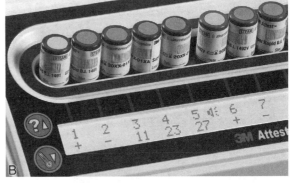

B

Figure 3-22 Rapid readout biological indicator incubation system (A) Incubator and (B) The + sign in well #1 indicates growth (the spores in the ampoule have not been killed); the − sign in well #2 indicates that there has been no growth after incubation for the required time (the spores in the ampoule have been killed); the 11, 23, and 27 in wells #3, 4, and 5 indicate the number of minutes left before incubation time is reached. At the end of that time, the numbers will be replaced by a + or a − sign.

273. To routinely test the ability of the sterilizer to operate effectively, one or two strips, ampoules, or capsules containing the spores are placed at a specific location within the chamber (determined by the manufacturers' IFU), and a sterilizer cycle is run.

274. For cycles used for terminal sterilization, the biological monitor should be contained within a process challenge device (PCD). A PCD represents a defined challenge to the sterilization process. Most PCDs used are commercially prepared, but a PCD may be assembled by the user. Commercially prepared PCDs are equivalent in performance to an AAMI BI test pack (**Figure 3-13**).

275. For IUSS cycles, the biological monitor is placed directly in the tray/container to be used, because the tray/container is considered to be the PCD.

276. Rapid-readout BIs whose growth is visible in 3 hours, 1 hour, or as little as 30 minutes, have largely replaced the traditional BI that took 24–48 hours before bacterial growth was visible (**Figure 3-22**).

277. It is essential to select the biological monitor specific to each sterilizer technology and cycle.

278. The traditional biological indicator must be incubated before results can be read. Before the BI is placed in the incubator, it is crushed in order to expose the spores to the growth medium in the capsule. A control BI (one that has *not* been through a sterilization cycle) must be incubated at the same time. The

microorganisms in the control BI are alive and will grow when they are exposed to the growth medium. As the bacteria grow, the medium exhibits a distinct color change. Microorganisms in the BI from the sterilizer should be destroyed and therefore will not grow when exposed to the growth medium and no color change will occur. At the end of the incubation period, a distinct difference in color between the control and the test BI indicates a "negative BI" and successful sterilization.

279. Rapid-readout BIs must also be incubated. However, they detect the presence of *Geobacillus stearothermophilus* by recognizing the activity of alpha-glucosidase, an enzyme present within the organism. The presence of the enzyme is detected by reading fluorescence produced by the enzymatic breakdown of a nonfluorescent substrate. This creates a fluorescence change, which is detected by the auto-reader. A fluorescence change indicates a steam sterilization process failure.

280. A positive BI reading (demonstrating bacterial growth) indicates that sterilizing conditions have not been met, indicating a "failed load."

281. A positive BI should be reported immediately to the appropriate supervisor, the load quarantined, and the sterilizer taken out of service until the cause is determined.

282. With rapid-readout BIs, the length of time between sterilization and available BI results is short enough that items in the "failed load" will most likely not have been used for patient care.

283. In addition to sterilizer malfunction, a positive reading can indicate incorrect packaging, an incorrect cycle, items incompatible with the process, or incorrect placement of items within the sterilizer.

284. When the cause of the sterilizer failure can be immediately identified and the failure is confined to one load or one item within the load, corrective action is taken, the sterilizer is returned to service, and the load is reprocessed.

285. When the cause of failure is unknown, all items from the failed load must be recalled, as well as any items processed between that load and the last load with a negative BI.

286. The sterilizer is returned to service after repair and subsequent BI testing is negative.

287. If a traditional BI is used, the incubation time may be lengthy and sterilized items might be sent to the operating room before the results of the biological testing are available, and a portion of the contents of the sterilizer may have been used.

288. Identification of items to recall is made from the load list/lot number. The SPD advises the operating room staff if any items to be recalled have been delivered to the operating room.

289. It is essential that all of the items from the sterilizer be accounted for. When items have been opened for procedures and patient exposure is known, facility policy determines the notification process that usually involves infection prevention staff and the operating surgeon.

Sterilization: Documentation

290. The following records for each sterilizer should be filed daily and kept as a permanent record (**Figure 3-23**):
    - Results of Bowie-Dick/DART
    - Results of biological monitoring
    - For each sterilizer load:
        - List of all contents of the load
        - Load lot control sticker (sterilizer number, sterilizer load, date)
        - Chemical monitor included in load
        - Biological monitor results if implant included in load
        - Sterilizer printout, initialed by the operator for verification of cycle parameters (if one person puts in a load and another removes it, both persons should initial the document)
    - Sterilizer failure results (if applicable)

291. IUSS records should be fully traceable to the patient on whom the sterilized item was used.

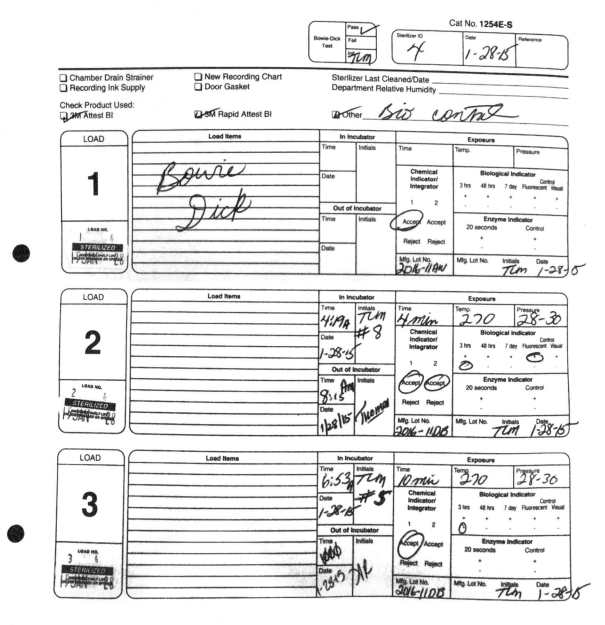

A

Figure 3-23 Daily documentation for each steam autoclave: (A) Each sterilizer has an envelope that contains all of the monitoring documentation for a 24-hour period.
Courtesy of Medical City Dallas, Dallas, TX.

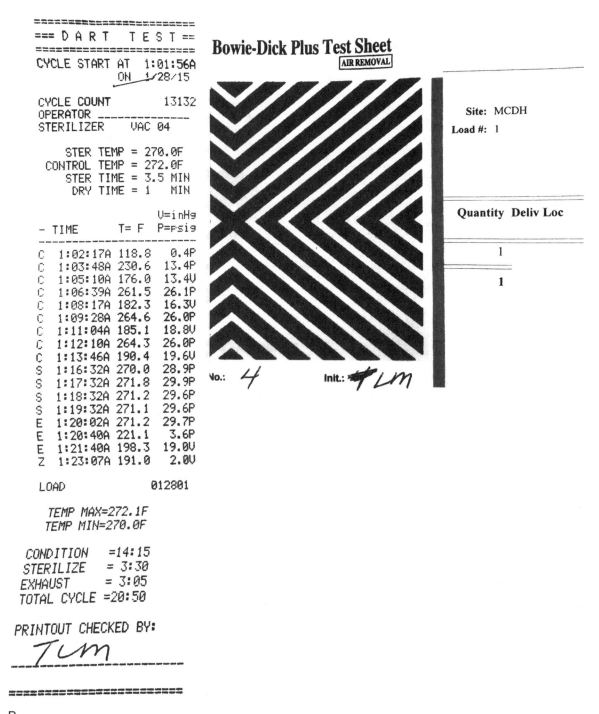

```
===========================
=== D A R T   T E S T ==
===========================
CYCLE START AT  1:01:56A
            ON  1/28/15

CYCLE COUNT         13132
OPERATOR ---------------
STERILIZER    VAC 04

    STER TEMP = 270.0F
 CONTROL TEMP = 272.0F
    STER TIME = 3.5 MIN
     DRY TIME = 1   MIN

                   V=inHg
- TIME      T= F  P=Psig
-------------------------
C  1:02:17A 118.8   0.4P
C  1:03:48A 230.6  13.4P
C  1:05:10A 176.0  13.4V
C  1:06:39A 261.5  26.1P
C  1:08:17A 182.3  16.3V
C  1:09:28A 264.6  26.0P
C  1:11:04A 185.1  18.8V
C  1:12:10A 264.3  26.0P
C  1:13:46A 190.4  19.6V
S  1:16:32A 270.0  28.9P
S  1:17:32A 271.8  29.9P
S  1:18:32A 271.2  29.6P
S  1:19:32A 271.1  29.6P
E  1:20:02A 271.2  29.7P
E  1:20:40A 221.1   3.6P
E  1:21:40A 198.3  19.0V
Z  1:23:07A 191.0   2.0V

LOAD            012801

  TEMP MAX=272.1F
  TEMP MIN=270.0F

CONDITION  =14:15
STERILIZE  = 3:30
EXHAUST    = 3:05
TOTAL CYCLE =20:50

PRINTOUT CHECKED BY:
   TLM
  --------------------

===========================
```

B

Bowie-Dick Plus Test Sheet
AIR REMOVAL

Site: MCDH
Load #: 1

Quantity   Deliv Loc

1

1

No.: 4   Init.: TLM

Figure 3-23 (B) Bowie Dick test documentation; note that the Bowie Dick test is listed on the envelope as the first load of the day.

Courtesy of Medical City Dallas, Dallas, TX.

Sterilizer Load Contents

Sterilizer: Stm04
Time Opened: Wed 28-Jan-2015 2:17:57 pm
Cycle: Cycle 2 PV 270.6.36
Employee: Thomas Thomas
Comments:

Site: MCDH
Load #: 6

Set Type	Index Unique ID	Site	Quantity Deliv Loc
Biological Indicator	000	MCDH	1
ENT NSR Set	002	MCDH	1
ENT Tympanoplasty Set	001	MCDH	1
General Laparoscopy Instruments	015	MCDH	1
Neuro Midas Electric Drill	005	MCDH	1
New Ortho Lami Retractor Pan	002	MCDH	1
New Ortho Lami Set	001	MCDH	1
Ortho De Mayo Knee Positioner - Base	004	MCDH	1
Ortho De Mayo Knee Positioner - Boot	004	MCDH	1
Pediatric Set	005	MCDH	1
PL Debridement Set	004	MCDH	1
Plastic Minor Set	001	MCDH	1
PN Irrigating Bipolars	001	MCDH	1
PP Ortho	000	MCDH	1
Robot Camera Pan	000	MCDH	1
Robot Camera Pan	002	MCDH	1
Robot Camera Pan	004	MCDH	1
Robot Camera Pan	008	MCDH	1

18

```
============================
===== P R E V A C =====
============================
CYCLE START AT   2:18:09P
           ON  1/28/15

CYCLE COUNT        13137
OPERATOR _____
STERILIZER    VAC 04

     STER TEMP = 270.0F
  CONTROL TEMP = 272.0F
     STER TIME =  6 MIN
     DRY TIME = 36 MIN

                      V=inHg
  - TIME       T= F   P=Psig
---------------------------
C  2:18:30P 112.4    0.2P
C  2:20:01P 217.5    7.7P
C  2:21:18P 180.0   10.1V
C  2:23:44P 263.7   26.0P
C  2:25:42P 202.7   10.0V
C  2:27:27P 264.8   26.1P
C  2:29:27P 205.2   10.1V
C  2:31:07P 264.8   26.1P
C  2:33:06P 207.4   10.4V
S  2:36:46P 270.0   29.2P
S  2:37:46P 271.9   30.5P
S  2:38:46P 271.5   30.1P
S  2:39:46P 271.0   29.8P
S  2:40:46P 271.1   29.9P
S  2:41:46P 271.2   29.9P
E  2:42:46P 271.2   29.9P
E  2:43:52P 217.9    3.7P
E  3:19:53P 163.8   27.6V
Z  3:22:02P 126.9    2.0V

LOAD            012806

  TEMP MAX=272.1F
  TEMP MIN=270.0F

CONDITION   = 0:18:15
STERILIZE   = 0:06:00
EXHAUST     = 0:39:16
TOTAL CYCLE = 1:03:31

PRINTOUT CHECKED BY:


=  READY TO UNLOAD  =
============================

* NOT READY      3:22:33P
DOOR OPEN
```

3M Comply™ SteriGage™
Class 5 Steam
Chemical
1243 Integrator   REJECT   ACCEPT

Figure 3-23 (C) Documentation for each load includes a load list, chemical indicator, lot number, and sterilizer load printout.
Courtesy of Medical City Dallas, Dallas, TX.

Section Questions

1. Explain why items sterilized for patient use cannot be tested to insure their sterilit. [Ref 255]

2. On what methods do we base our assumption of sterility of the contents of a sterilizer? [Ref 256]

3. Describe the physical monitors used to assess the performance of sterilizers. [Refs 258–260]

4. What is the purpose of a Bowie-Dick test or DART? [Ref 262]

5. When is the Bowie-Dick test (or DART) run and how is the package placed in the autoclave? [Ref 262–263]

6. How do we determine that the Bowie-Dick test or DART has either passed or failed? [Ref 264]

7. What is the purpose of a biological monitor? [Ref 265]

8. What spores are used to test each type of sterilization technology? [Ref 267]

9. When should BIs be run? [Refs 268–279]

10. At what point are implants released after sterilization? [Ref 270]

11. How frequently are H₂O₂ sterilizers tested with a BI? [Ref 272]

12. Why is the BI contained within a PCD? [Ref 274]

13. How do rapid-readout BIs compare to traditional BIs? [Ref 276]

14. Describe the process of incubating a BI. [Ref 278]

15. Explain the purpose of using a control when incubating a BI. [Ref 278]

16. How can you tell if an incubated BI is positive or negative? [Refs 278–279]

17. What reasons might there be for a failed BI? [Ref 283]

18. What process must follow a failed BI? [Refs 284–285]

19. What documentation should be captured for every sterilizer load? [Ref 290]

20. What additional documentation is required for IUSS? [Ref 291]

Disinfection

292. Disinfection is a process that destroys pathogenic microorganisms through the use of a liquid chemical germicide.

293. A disinfectant is an agent that destroys vegetative forms of harmful microorganisms. Some disinfectants kill some spores; however, disinfectants do not kill high numbers of spores.

294. Liquid chemical disinfectants are used to destroy pathogens on inanimate objects such as walls, tables, small equipment, and surgical instruments.

295. Disinfectants must be selected according to their intended use. Disinfectants suitable for housekeeping purposes such as cleaning walls and surfaces are not suitable for disinfection of surgical instruments. Likewise, the most appropriate disinfecting agent for surgical instruments is not the most suitable for housekeeping.

296. Examples of disinfectants include alcohol, chlorine and chlorine compounds, formaldehyde, glutaraldehyde, hydrogen peroxide, iodophors, *ortho*-phthalaldehyde, phenolics, and quaternary ammonium compounds.

297. Disinfectants vary in their ability to destroy microorganisms, and they are not interchangeable. Disinfectants are categorized as high level, intermediate level, and low level.

298. Factors that influence the efficacy of a disinfectant include the type of chemical, concentration and temperature of the chemical, amount and types of microorganisms present, configuration of the item to be disinfected, adequacy of prior cleaning, and exposure time.

299. High-level disinfectants kill all microorganisms, including vegetative bacteria forms, the tubercle bacilli, viruses, and fungi. They do not kill large numbers of spores, although some high-level disinfectants can achieve sterilization after prolonged exposure of 8 hours or

more. Because waiting for such a long period of time is impractical, high-level disinfectants are not used for sterilizing instruments. Disinfectants used for disinfecting instruments and medical devices are not used on environmental surfaces.

300. Intermediate- and low-level disinfectants are formulated to be used on environmental surfaces and are never to be used on instruments and medical devices.

301. Intermediate-level disinfectants inactivate most vegetative bacteria, the tubercle bacillus, fungi, and viruses, but not necessarily bacterial spores.

302. Low-level disinfectants kill most vegetative bacteria, some fungi, and some viruses; they do not kill the tubercle bacillus.

303. For instrument disinfection, only high-level disinfection is appropriate. The most frequently used high-level disinfectants are solutions of 2% to 3.2% alkaline glutaraldehyde or 0.55% *ortho*-phthalaldehyde.

304. Following exposure to the solution, the device must be thoroughly rinsed, preferably in sterile water. It is important to refer to the manufacturer's IFU, because some disinfectant products require as many as three separate rinses.

305. To avoid dilution of the disinfectant and compromising the disinfection process, all items to be disinfected should be thoroughly cleaned, rinsed, and dried prior to immersion.

Glutaraldehyde

306. Glutaraldehyde is a commonly used high-level disinfectant. High-level disinfection is achieved in minutes, although the exact number of minutes varies with the concentration and temperature of the solution. The manufacturer's IFU and institutional policy describe the exact required immersion time.

307. Glutaraldehyde is irritating to mucous membranes and can irritate skin, eyes, throat, and nasal passages. It should be mixed in a well-ventilated room with a minimum of 10 air exchanges per hour. Local exhaust ventilation located at the level of the point of discharge is the preferred method of preventing vapor from escaping. Self-contained workstations with a fume hood should be installed where glutaraldehyde is used. Glutaraldehyde should always be stored in a closed container.

308. Protective eyewear, nitrile gloves or a double set of latex gloves, a mask, and a repellent gown should be worn during use of glutaraldehyde. Exposure varies with the activity. Mixing and discarding the solution and immersing and retrieving items from the solution are the activities that pose the greatest risk of exposure.

309. Like all disinfectants, glutaraldehyde must be mixed and used strictly according to the manufacturer's IFU and standards of practice. Information regarding mixing instructions, temperature, use, immersion time, toxicity, and length of effectiveness can be found on the product's label.

310. The current OSHA ceiling threshold limit value for exposure to glutaraldehyde is 0.5 part glutaraldehyde to 1 million parts air during any part of the work day. Monitoring of the work area and employee exposure is not required by OSHA; however, monitoring should be employed when high levels of exposure are suspected (OSHA, 2015).

311. Glutaraldehyde that is heated will achieve microbial killing faster than glutaraldehyde at room temperature. Some automated systems are programmed to heat glutaraldehyde. However, when glutaraldehyde is heated, the vapor pressure is raised, which in turn increases the amount of vapor released into the air.

Ortho-phthalaldehyde

312. *Ortho*-phthalaldehyde (OPA) is a nonglutaraldehyde disinfectant used in operating rooms and endoscopy suites. Because it achieves disinfection faster than glutaraldehyde and does not release any irritating odors, OPA has replaced glutaraldehyde in many facilities.

313. *Ortho*-phthalaldehyde has a very low vapor pressure; as a result, it is rarely irritating to staff. Although there are no OSHA requirements and no monitoring requirements for OPA, high-level disinfectant monitoring systems are available.

314. *Ortho*-phthalaldehyde will stain protein and items that are not thoroughly cleaned and rinsed prior to immersion. It will stain gray in spots where there are protein residuals.

Quality Control

315. Disinfectant solutions have an expiration date that represents the length of anticipated

effectiveness, as indicated on the label. Date of mixing and expiration date should be indicated on the container in which the disinfectant is stored.

316. Some disinfectant solution instructions for use call for a specific quality control test prior to initial use to ensure that the required effective concentration is present. In addition to an initial quality control test, concentration testing should be conducted before each use. A disinfectant can lose its minimum effective concentration (MEC) before the expiration date. The number of times the solution is used, the amount of debris introduced into the solution, and any dilution that occurs when items are washed, rinsed, and not dried before immersion can all affect the MEC and cause a solution to fail.

317. One should never rely entirely on the label for proof of the expiration of the solution. The MEC of disinfectant solutions should be monitored before each use with indicators designed for this purpose, usually supplied as paper or plastic strips that are dipped into the solution and then observed for appropriate color change as indicated on the label. Indicators are not interchangeable, and only those supplied with a particular product should be used to test that product.

318. Chemical properties and appropriate hazard warnings should be posted.

Documentation

319. When liquid chemical germicides are used for high-level disinfection, the following should be documented:
    - Results of quality control testing—performed according to the manufacturer's instructions
    - Results of testing for minimum effective concentration
    - Date solution is mixed/activated/opened/prepared
    - Expiration date—should be visible on the container
    - Person responsible for mixing
    - Item disinfected
    - Patient for whom the disinfected item was used

Section Questions

1. Describe disinfection. [Ref 292]
2. What is the difference between sterilization and disinfection in relation to spores? [Ref 293]
3. How are disinfectants selected? [Ref 295]
4. Identify some disinfectant chemicals. [Ref 296]
5. Explain the factors that influence the efficacy of disinfection. [Ref 298]
6. Differentiate among high-, intermediate-, and low-level disinfection. [Refs 299–302, Exhibit 3-1]
7. Which level of disinfection is used for surgical instruments? [Ref 303]
8. What are the most commonly used high-level disinfectants for instrument disinfection? [Ref 303]
9. How is a high-level disinfected instrument prepared for patient use? [Ref 304]
10. What is the effect of not thoroughly rinsing and drying instruments on the disinfectant? [Ref 305]
11. Which factors affect the length of time it takes to disinfect an item with glutaraldehyde? [Ref 309]
12. Describe the responsibilities associated with using glutaraldehyde. [Refs 308–310]
13. What is the impact of heat on glutaraldehyde? [Ref 311]
14. Describe the characteristics of OPA. [Refs 312–314]
15. How does the MEC correlate with the expiration date of a disinfectant solution? [Ref 316]

Reuse of Single-Use Devices

320. Under current FDA (2000) regulations, any hospital that chooses to reprocess single-use Class 3 devices (devices that carry a significant risk in the event of failure) that have been opened and used will be held to the same standard as the original manufacturer of that item. The requirements for the original manufacturer are extremely stringent and virtually impossible for a hospital to replicate.

321. The perioperative nurse in the operating room should never attempt to reprocess a single-use device. When a question arises about whether a single-use device will be reprocessed, a group including infection preventionists and risk management should refer to the FDA's (2000) "Guidance Document: Enforcement Priorities for Single-Use Devices Reprocessed by Third Parties and Hospitals" to determine the facility policy.

Storage of Sterile Items

322. Sterilized items should be stored in a well-ventilated, limited-access area, with controlled temperature and humidity, at least four air exchanges per hour, and that is clean and dust free.

323. To reduce dust accumulation, wire mesh shelving is preferable to closed shelving. The bottom shelf should be solid or items on the bottoms shelf should be stored in bins.

324. Cabinets and shelves should permit adequate cleaning and air circulation.

325. Closed cabinets are best for items that are used infrequently.

326. Storage cabinets and shelves should be far enough away from floors, ceiling fixtures, vents, sprinklers, and lights to prevent contamination. Shelves should be at least 18 inches below the ceiling or level of a sprinkler head, 2 inches from outside walls, and 8 to 10 inches above the floor (AAMI, 2013, §8.9).

327. Sterile items should be stored separately from clean items. If sterile and clean items are stored on the same cart, sterile items should be on the uppermost shelves and clean items on lower shelves.

328. Sterile items should not be stored under or next to sinks or other areas where they might become wet.

329. Wrapped packages should not be bent, crushed, crammed, or stacked.

330. No outside shipping containers or corrugated cartons should be brought into the sterile storage area.

Shelf Life

331. Shelf life is the amount of time following sterilization that an item may be considered sterile.

332. Event-related sterility: Theoretically, if an item is not contaminated during transport and storage, it will remain sterile indefinitely. Shelf life is related to the events that can occur that will cause an item to become contaminated. A package remains sterile until it is opened or an event occurs that renders the package unsterile.

333. Proper packaging, handling, and storage can prevent contamination. Poor quality wrappers, poor storage conditions, and improper handling of sterile items increase the potential for contamination.

334. A small percentage of institutions have policies requiring that an expiration date be placed on stored items. Most institutions have eliminated the use of expiration dates.

335. Before any package is opened for surgery, it must be visually inspected to determine whether the package may have been compromised. Stains, pinholes, and tears are obvious examples of potential contamination that would preclude using the item in surgery.

336. Shelf life is determined by many factors:

   - Type and configuration of packaging material: Items packaged in rigid container systems may have a longer shelf life than items packaged with woven and nonwoven materials, which are more readily contaminated.

   - Use of dust covers: Plastic pouches specifically designed to prolong the shelf life of sterilized items by protecting them from moisture and dust can extend shelf life.

   - Conditions of storage: Dust, temperature, humidity, and traffic can affect shelf life.

   - Number of times a package is handled before use: The more the package is handled, the greater the risk for contamination.

337. Expiration dates on commercially prepared items may indicate that the integrity of the device or material will be compromised (material degradation) after the indicated date, and the item should not be used once this date has been reached.

Section Questions

1. What is the FDA requirement for reprocessing Class 3 devices? [Ref 320]

2. Describe the type of shelving best suited for storing sterile items. [Ref 322]

3. What are the required distances from walls, floor, and ceiling for stored items? [Ref 326]

4. When sterile items are stored with clean items, how should they be arranged in relation to one another? [Ref 327]

5. What should be done with outside shipping containers and corrugated cartons? [Ref 330]

6. Explain event-related sterility. [Ref 332]

7. What factors lead to potential contamination of sterile packages? [Ref 333]

8. What is the responsibility of the perioperative nurse prior to opening a sterile package? [Ref 335]

9. What factors impact the shelf life of sterile packages? [Ref 336]

10. What is the significance of the expiration date on commercially sterilized packages? [Ref 337]

References

Al-Ghoul, A., Charukamnoetkanok, P., Dhaliwal, D., Allinson, R., Law, S., Charles, A.,& Brown, L. (2014). Toxic anterior segment syndrome. Retrieved from http://emedicine.medscape.com/article/1190343-clinical#showall

American National Standards Institute (ANSI), & Association for the Advancement of Medical Instrumentation (AAMI). (2001). *Processing CJD: Contaminated patient care equipment and environmental surfaces* (ST79: 2013 & A1:2010 & A2:2011 Annex C). Washington, DC: Author.

ANSI/AAMI (2001). Comprehensive guide to steam sterilization and sterility assurance in health care facilities. ST79: 2010 & A1:2010 & A2:2011. Washington, DC: ANSI/AAMI.

Association for the Advancement of Medical Instrumentation (AAMI). (2013). *Comprehensive guide to steam sterilization and sterility assurance in health care facilities* (ST79:2010/A4:2013). Arlington, VA: Author.

Association of periOperative Registered Nurses (AORN). (2015). *Guidelines for perioperative practice.* Denver, CO: Author.

Center for Biofilm Engineering at Montana University. (2011). BIOFILMS: *The hypertexbook.* V4.3. Retrieved from http://www.hypertextbookshop.com/biofilmbook/v004/r003/

Centers for Disease Control and Prevention (CDC). (2008). *Guideline for disinfection and sterilization in healthcare facilities.* Retrieved from http://www.cdc.gov/hicpac/Disinfection_Sterilization/13_0Sterilization.html

Centers for Disease Control and Prevention (CDC). (2015a). *CDC statement: Los Angeles County/UCLA investigation of CRE transmission and duodenoscopes.* Retrieved from http://www.cdc.gov/hai/outbreaks/cdcstatement-LA-CRE.html

Centers for Disease Control and Prevention (CDC). (2015b). *Interim protocol for healthcare facilities regarding surveillance for bacterial contamination of duodenoscopes after reprocessing.* Retrieved from http://www.cdc.gov/hai/organisms/cre/cre-duodenoscope-surveillance-protocol.html

Centers for Disease Control and Prevention (CDC). (2015c). *Procedure-associated events: Surgical site infection (SSI) event.* Retrieved from http://www.cdc.gov/nhsn/PDFs/pscManual/9pscSSIcurrent.pdf

Dancer, S. J., Stewart, M., Coulombe, C., Gregori, A., & Verdi, M. (2012). Surgical site infections linked to contaminated surgical instruments. *Journal of Hospital Infection,* 81(4), 231–238.

Facility Guidelines Institute. (2014). *Guidelines for design and construction of hospitals and outpatient facilities.* Chicago, IL: American Hospital Association.

Favero, M.,& Bond, W. (2001). Chemical disinfection of medical and surgical materials. In S. S. Block(Ed.), *Disinfection, sterilization, and preservation* (5th ed., pp. 881–915). Philadelphia, PA: Lippincott Williams & Wilkins.

Henning, C. (Ed.). (2011). *Care and handling of ophthalmic microsurgical instruments* (3rd ed.). San Francisco, CA: American Society of Ophthalmic Registered Nurses.

Occupational Safety and Health Administration (OSHA). (2012a). *Toxic and hazardous substances: Bloodborne pathogens.* Retrieved from http://www.osha.gov/pls/oshaweb/owadisp.show_document?p_table=STANDARDS&p_id=10051

Occupational Safety and Health Administration (OSHA). (2012b). *Toxic and hazardous substances: Ethylene oxide.* Retrieved from https://www.osha.gov/pls/oshaweb/owadisp.show_document?p_table=standards&p_id=10070

Perkins, J. J. (1969). *Principles and methods of sterilization.* Springfield, IL: Charles C. Thomas.

Petersen, B., Chennat, J., Cohen, J., Cotton, P. B., Greenwald, D. A., Kowalski, T. E., . . . Rutala, W. A. (2011). Multisociety guideline on reprocessing flexible GI endoscopes. *Infection Control and Hospital Epidemiology, 32*(6), 527–537.

Rutala, W., & Weber, D. (2010). Guideline for disinfection and sterilization of prion-contaminated medical instruments. *Infection Control and Hospital Epidemiology, 31*(2), 107–117. Retrieved from http://www.shea-online.org/Assets/files/other_papers/Prion.pdf

Saito, Y., Kobayashi, H., Uetera, Y., Yasuhara, H., Kajiura, T., & Okubo, T. (2013). Microbial contamination of surgical instruments used for laparotomy. *American Journal of Infection Control, 42,* 43–47.

Retrieved from http://www.ajicjournal.org/article/S0196-6553%2813%2901102-4/pdf

Society of Gastroenterology Nurses and Associates (SGNA). (2013). *Guideline for use of high level disinfectants & sterilants for reprocessing flexible gastrointestinal endoscopes.* Retrieved from http://www.sgna.org/Portals/0/Issues/PDF/Infection-Prevention/6_HLDGuideline_2013.pdf

U.S. Department of Health and Human Services (HHS). (2013). *National action plan to prevent health care-associated infections: Roadmap to elimination.* Retrieved from http://www.health.gov/hcq/prevent_hai.asp#hai

U.S. Food and Drug Administration (FDA). (2000). *Guidance document: Enforcement priorities for single-use devices reprocessed by third parties and hospitals.* Retrieved from http://www.fda.gov/regulatoryinformation/guidances/ucm107164.htm

World Health Organization (WHO). (2003). *WHO manual for surveillance of human transmissible spongiform encephalopathies including variant Creutzfeldt-Jakob disease.* Retrieved from http://www.who.int/bloodproducts/TSE-manual2003.pdf

Post-Test

Read each question carefully. A question may have more than one correct answer.

1. Disinfection differs from sterilization in what way?
    a. High-level disinfection and sterilization are the same.
    b. Sterilization kills all spores; disinfection does not.
    c. High-level disinfection kills vegetative bacteria; sterilization does not.
    d. Disinfection and sterilization both kill microorganisms, but only disinfection kills high numbers of spores.

2. Which of the following definitions is correct?
    a. Bioburden represents the population of viable organisms on an item.
    b. A Bowie-Dick test demonstrates that air and noncondensable gases are adequately removed from the chamber of any steam sterilizer.
    c. An autoclave is another term for any sterilizer.
    d. A chemical indicator is a sterilization monitor with a known population of resistant spores.

3. Which of the following statements is/are true?
    a. Surgical-site infections are responsible for increased length of stay and increased healthcare costs.
    b. Contaminated surgical instruments are a known source of infection.
    c. Perioperative diagnoses include increased risk for infection.
    d. Sterilization and disinfection are cornerstones of infection prevention.

4. Which of the following is the most valid reason for the perioperative nurse to have a comprehensive knowledge of instrument processing?
    a. Perioperative nurses rotate through the SPD and need to be prepared.
    b. Perioperative nurses must have a frame of reference when they are complaining to the SPD about instruments.
    c. The perioperative nurse is a partner in instrument processing and assumes varying degrees of responsibility for the care and preparation of instruments.
    d. There is an instrument-processing department in most operating rooms.

5. Critical items
    a. contact sterile tissue and the vascular system.
    b. must undergo high-level disinfection.
    c. do not penetrate mucous membranes.
    d. include thermometers, crutches, and blood pressure cuffs.

6. Semicritical items include
    a. surgical instruments.
    b. cystoscopes and laryngoscopes.
    c. blood pressure cuffs and crutches.
    d. warming blankets and sequential compression devices.

7. The sterility assurance level is
    a. the number of organisms killed during sterilization.
    b. the amount of time it takes to kill 1 million organisms.
    c. a mathematical expression of the time, temperature, and pressure needed to kill microorganisms.
    d. a mathematical expression of the probability of a viable microorganism being present on an item after sterilization.

8. Spores are used to test for sterility because they are
    a. more resistant than any other bacteria to heat, drying, and chemicals.
    b. easier to process, incubate, and analyze.
    c. larger than bacteria and easier to see.
    d. a form of bacteria that is also representative of viruses and fungi.

9. The choice of sterilization technology for an item depends first on
    a. what is most convenient for the facility.
    b. what is least expensive and readily available.
    c. the compatibility of the item with the sterilization process.
    d. the type of wrapping that must be used for sterilization.

10. For an item to be successfully steam sterilized
    a. it must be sequentially wrapped and placed upright in the sterilizer.
    b. steam must penetrate the packaging completely and the intended parameters of moisture, temperature, and time must be met.
    c. it must be subjected to unsaturated steam for the appropriate amount of time and under the correct amount of pressure.
    d. the temperature must remain at 250°F at atmospheric pressure for the proper amount of time.

11. Which statement(s) is/are true about steam sterilization?
    a. Moist heat under pressure is economical.
    b. Steam sterilization denatures and coagulates protein.
    c. Steam sterilization occurs at atmospheric pressure.
    d. Parameters of steam sterilization include time and temperature.

12. What are some advantages of steam sterilization?
    a. One cycle time is appropriate for all items.
    b. Cycles are preprogrammed to prevent operator error.
    c. It is economical and sterilization is achieved quickly.
    d. It is suitable for all surgical instruments.

13. Which statement(s) is/are true about autoclaves?
    a. Air trapped in the chamber will interfere with sterilization.
    b. Sterilization begins only when the correct temperature has been reached.
    c. Cups and basins must be placed so that water will collect in them and form steam.
    d. Wrapped packages should be removed from the sterilizer immediately and allowed to cool for at least 2 hours.

14. How might trapping of air in a steam autoclave interfere with sterilization?
    a. The presence of air forces the temperature above the target range.
    b. Air in the chamber prevents the sterilizer from reaching the target pressure.
    c. Air interferes with the humidity level in the chamber.
    d. Trapped air acts as an insulator that interferes with heating and prevents contact of steam with every surface of every item.

15. Which statement(s) is/are true about steam sterilizers?

    a. A Bowie-Dick test is done once each day in all gravity-displacement sterilizers.

    b. Exposure time in a prevacuum sterilizer is longer because it takes a while to create the vacuum.

    c. Prevacuum sterilizers are used for liquids.

    d. Prevacuum sterilizers are less affected by incorrect arrangement of objects in the chamber.

16. Which statement(s) is/are true about immediate-use steam sterilization?

    a. IUSS is not intended for sterilizing sets of instruments.

    b. IUSS is intended for urgent situations in which there is no sterile replacement for an item that has been contaminated.

    c. Drying time is the same in IUSS as with regular sterilization.

    d. In an emergency, items can be rinsed in the scrub sink and sterilized with IUSS.

17. Which statement(s) is/are true about immediate-use steam sterilization?

    a. IUSS is perfect for implants that arrive immediately before a procedure.

    b. IUSS is not an alternative to purchasing an adequate supply of instruments.

    c. IUSS is appropriate when there is only one specialty set of instruments.

    d. IUSS can be done only in a prevacuum sterilizer.

18. Which statement(s) is/are true about immediate-use steam sterilization?

    a. Only devices with manufacturer's IFU for IUSS should be sterilized in this manner.

    b. Proper cleaning is critical to effective sterilization with IUSS.

    c. OSHA validates specific rigid containers for IUSS.

    d. Any rigid container can be used for IUSS.

19. The two most challenging factors involved with processing items using IUSS are that

    a. most device manufacturers don't validate their items for IUSS.

    b. aseptic transfer of the sterilized item to the sterile field may require traversing an unsterile area.

    c. many operating rooms don't have a cleaning process equivalent to the sterile processing department.

    d. the IUSS sterilizer is small and it takes too long to process trays of instruments between procedures.

20. What are some advantages of H_2O_2 sterilization?

    a. Items to be sterilized can be wrapped in any material.

    b. There is a single cycle for all items.

    c. There are no toxic residues remaining following the cycle.

    d. Cycle times are preset and the sterilizer is easy to operate.

21. The spore used to monitor H_2O_2 sterilization is

    a. *Bacillus atrophaeus.*

    b. *Geobacillus atrophaeus.*

    c. *Geobacillus stearothermophilus.*

    d. *Bacillus subtilis.*

22. Which packaging materials can be used for H_2O_2 sterilization?

    a. Muslin wrappers

    b. Tyvek pouches

    c. Polypropylene wraps

    d. Paper pouches

23. Which statement(s) is/are true about ethylene oxidesterilization?

    a. EtO is a toxic gas that must be closely monitored and vented.

    b. EtO is appropriate for items that cannot tolerate the temperature and moisture of steam sterilization.

    c. EtO provides a rapid cycle and is the sterilization option of choice when heat- and moisture-sensitive items are required quickly.

    d. Aeration must be done for all loads sterilized using EtO.

24. Which statement(s) is/are true about liquid chemical processing?

    a. It is a low-temperature, nonterminal process.

    b. Items must be used immediately following processing; they cannot be packaged or stored for later use.

    c. Only one flexible endoscope can be processed at a time.

    d. Peracetic acid disrupts protein bonds and inactivates cell systems, causing immediate cell death.

25. Which statement(s) is/are true about liquid chemical processing?

    a. The unit has connectors to insure circulation of sterilant through lumens.

    b. The units must be vented and therefore are not very portable.

    c. The process is lengthy, taking nearly an hour to complete a cycle.

    d. There is no biological monitor appropriate for monitoring peracetic acid.

26. Which statement(s) is/are true about sterilization monitoring?

    a. Physical monitors record activities within the sterilizer chamber.

    b. Chemical indicators exhibit a visual change when sterilization has been achieved.

    c. A chemical indicator should be placed both on the inside and on the outside of each package.

    d. The nurse relies on the outside indicator to determine whether the contents of a sterilized package are sterile.

27. A Class 5 indicator is a(n)

    a. process indicator that demonstrates an item has been exposed to the sterilization process.

    b. single-parameter indicator designed to react to one of the critical parameters of the sterilization process.

    c. integrator that reacts to all of the critical parameters of the sterilization process.

    d. emulator that reacts to all parameters of the sterilization process and is cycle specific.

28. Which statement(s) is/are true about biological indicators?

    a. A biological indicator is the most accurate method of establishing that items within the load have been sterilized.

    b. A biological indicator contains a known quantity of a highly resistant virus.

    c. A biological indicator must be incubated before it can be read.

    d. A biological indicator should be contained within a process challenge device (PCD) for cycles used for terminal sterilization.

29. Which statement(s) is/are true about a "failed load"?

    a. It should be reported immediately, the load quarantined, and the cause of failure researched.

    b. Failure can be caused by incorrect packaging, incorrect cycle, items incompatible with the process, or incorrect placement within the sterilizer.

    c. When the cause of failure is unknown, all items from the failed load must be located and recalled for reprocessing.

    d. Items from a failed load that have already been used in or for a patient must be reported to The Joint Commission.

30. Documentation of sterilization should include
    a. a supervisor's signature for every sterilizer load.
    b. a list of each item included in the sterilizer load.
    c. indication that biological tests were run in every sterilizer twice a day.
    d. Bowie-Dick test results for gravity-displacement sterilizers.

31. A biofilm
    a. consists of microorganisms living within a polysaccharide matrix that adheres to a surface.
    b. prevents sterilant from reaching the microorganisms incorporated within the glycocalyx.
    c. prevents antibiotics from reaching cells.
    d. is readily dissolved by disinfectants.

32. Which statement(s) is/are true?
    a. In the operating room, any item that is not sterile is considered contaminated.
    b. Following surgery, items on the sterile field that have not come in contact with the patient are processed separately from the ones that were used.
    c. Decontamination is a process that renders a contaminated item safe for handling.
    d. Decontamination is an automated process.

33. Which statement(s) is/are true about nursing responsibilities?
    a. Cleaning, packaging, and storing of sterile supplies requires judgment and an understanding of scientific principles.
    b. The SPD processes instruments and supplies and makes the final determination of what is sterile and what is not.
    c. The perioperative nurse may assume primary responsibility for high-level disinfection and IUSS.
    d. Assuming responsibility for ensuring that all instruments and supplies delivered to the sterile field are, in fact, sterile is part of the perioperative nurse's commitment to advocating for patient safety.

34. Sterilization is required for
    a. all semicritical items.
    b. all instruments that contact mucous membranes.
    c. all instruments that penetrate mucous membranes.
    d. anything used in the operating room.

35. The first and most important step in instrument decontamination is
    a. disinfecting with an enzyme soak.
    b. cleaning
    c. decontamination.
    d. sterilization.

36. How should instruments be managed after a surgical procedure?
    a. Separate the used from the unused instruments.
    b. Close all clamps and scissors to protect the tips and blades.
    c. Use enzymatic spray or gel to prevent debris from drying.
    d. Store contaminated instruments in a safe place before returning them to the SPD at the end of the day.

37. What should be used to keep instruments clean on the sterile field?

    a. Soak them in a basin of normal saline.

    b. Wipe them with a moist sponge.

    c. Spray them with an enzymatic detergent.

    d. Wipe or flush them with sterile water.

38. Which statement(s) is/are true about instrument cleaning?

    a. An instrument can be clean, but not sterile.

    b. An instrument can be sterile, but not clean.

    c. Instruments opened for a procedure should be cleaned immediately following the procedure, whether they were used or not.

    d. Instruments should be kept as clean as possible on the sterile field.

39. Which statement(s) is/are true about postoperative cleaning?

    a. Used instruments from a set should be returned to the set before returning them to the SPD.

    b. Blood and debris allowed to dry on instruments can cause rusting and pitting.

    c. Instruments for IUSS can be washed in the scrub sink.

    d. Instruments can remain in water safely for an unlimited period of time.

40. Before instruments are sent to the SPD

    a. remove disposable sharps and discard them in a sharps container.

    b. reusable drill bits should be wiped clean.

    c. heavy instruments should be placed on the bottom of the tray, with lighter instruments on the top.

    d. scissors and clamps should be closed to protect blades and tips.

41. Which statement(s) is/are true about manual cleaning?

    a. It should be done where required supplies and equipment are available.

    b. A higher concentration of detergent is necessary to remove heavy debris.

    c. Brushes, syringes, and compressed air should be available.

    d. Instruments should first be washed in hot water.

42. Immersible items should be cleaned below the surface of the water

    a. to be sure that all surfaces are wet.

    b. to drown microorganisms.

    c. to prevent aerosolization of debris.

    d. to avoid wasting water.

43. Which statement(s) is/are true about TASS?

    a. TASS is caused by foreign matter that is not removed from instruments during cleaning and sterilization.

    b. TASS is a noninfectious inflammation of the anterior segment of the eye.

    c. TASS can result in permanent visual impairment.

    d. Endotoxins from bacteria in ultrasonic cleaners have been associated with TASS.

44. Which statement(s) is/are true about prions?

    a. A prion is an infectious protein particle.

    b. Creutzfeldt-Jakob disease, a prion disease of the central nervous system, is always fatal.

    c. Prions can be managed by routine sterilization and disinfection routines.

    d. Brain, spinal cord, and dura mater are considered high-risk tissues for transmission of prion disease.

45. Instruments that are exposed to tissue at high risk for prions should be
    a. kept dry until cleaned or contaminated.
    b. kept separate from instruments not exposed to high-risk tissue.
    c. cleaned with all other instruments as soon as possible following the procedure.
    d. soaked overnight in a phenolic solution.

46. Which statement(s) is/are true about ultrasonic cleaning?
    a. Ultrasonic cleaning is used to flush all ports and articulations of robotic instruments.
    b. Ultrasonic cleaning removes tenacious debris through cavitation.
    c. Cavitation is the implosion of bubbles generated by sound waves.
    d. Ultrasonic cleaning is especially well suited to removing debris from lensed and powered instruments.

47. Which statement(s) is/are true about ultrasonic cleaning?
    a. Only instruments of the same type of metal should be processed at one time.
    b. It is especially useful for difficult-to-clean instruments.
    c. Instruments do not need to be free of gross soil before immersion in the ultrasonic cleaner.
    d. Instruments that rest on the bottom of the ultrasonic cleaner are subject to the strongest cavitation.

48. Which statement(s) is/are true about lubrication and inspection?
    a. Oil-based lubricants are most protective and extend instrument life.
    b. Water-soluble lubricants permit penetration of sterilant.
    c. Items that are defective should be tagged before being placed in sets.
    d. Defective instruments can result in injury to the patient.

49. Which statement(s) is/are true about packaging materials?
    a. Packaging materials must be compatible with the method of sterilization.
    b. The purpose of packaging material is to maintain sterility of the package contents until their intended use.
    c. Packaging materials must be able to maintain an adequate seal.
    d. Packaging materials must allow for aseptic delivery to the field.

50. Which statement(s) is/are true about nonwoven wrappers?
    a. They are virtually lint free, are tear resistant, and provide excellent barrier protection.
    b. They are disposable and synthetic.
    c. They can display memory, creating a potential for contamination when packages are opened.
    d. The same synthetic wrapper can be used for all sterilization technologies.

51. Which statement(s) is/are true about pouches?
    a. The same pouch cannot be used for both steam and hydrogen peroxide sterilization.
    b. Pouches are inexpensive and permit visualization of the contents.
    c. One side of a pouch is clear and the other side is opaque.
    d. Plastic/paper and plastic/Tyvek pouches display memory and provide little resistance to puncture.

52. Which statement(s) is/are true about pouches?
    a. They can hold multiple small items in a sealed inner pouch contained within an outer pouch.
    b. The inner pouch should be positioned within the outer pouch so that the contents of the inner pouch are visible.
    c. Pouches should be stacked loosely on top of one another in the autoclave to provide maximum penetration of the sterilant.
    d. Pouches can be used to contain small items within instrument trays.

53. Which statement(s) is/are true about rigid containers?
    a. There may be a valve system to permit entry and exit of sterilant.
    b. Rigid containers are durable and protect instruments from damage.
    c. They are lightweight; an empty container weighs no more than 5 pounds.
    d. Cleaning before placing instruments inside a rigid container involves checking gaskets, valves, or filters.

54. Which statement(s) is/are true about packaging for steam sterilization?
    a. Placing a towel in the instrument set creates condensate and delays drying.
    b. The surfaces of all instruments must be exposed to the sterilant.
    c. Scissors and clamps must be open to allow contact of sterilant with inner surfaces.
    d. Instruments with multiple parts may be assembled to prevent loss or misplacement of the individual pieces.

55. Which statement(s) is/are true about packaging for steam sterilization?
    a. The combined weight of the tray and instrument cannot exceed 15 pounds.
    b. Peel packs are used to contain small items within instrument sets.
    c. Pouches used within instrument sets should not be sealed.
    d. Basins and bowls should be positioned vertically to prevent pooling of water.

56. Which statement(s) is/are true about low-temperature H_2O_2 sterilization?
    a. Items must be thoroughly dried before being placed in the sterilizer.
    b. Cellulose wrappers cannot be used with H_2O_2 sterilizers.
    c. The end products of the sterilization process are oxygen and water vapor.
    d. The system is flexible; it has no plumbing or drain and can be plugged in anywhere.

57. Which statement(s) is/are true about low-temperature EtO sterilization?
    a. EtO sterilizers are not usually located in the operating room because EtO is a human carcinogen and must be closely monitored and vented.
    b. Aeration is required so materials can absorb EtO during the sterilization process.
    c. Exposure times are relatively short, ranging from 30 to 90 minutes.
    d. Proximity to EtO requires monitoring PPE because exposure is irritating.

58. Which statement(s) is/are true about process indicators?
    a. A process indicator shows that a package has been exposed to the sterilization process.
    b. A process indicator is placed at the very center of the package or instrument set.
    c. Pouches sometimes have a built-in process indicator.
    d. Pouches with a built-in process indicator do not need a second chemical indicator.

59. What are the parameters of steam sterilization?
    a. Steam concentration, time, pressure
    b. Relative humidity, time, temperature
    c. Steam concentration, relative humidity, time
    d. Time, temperature, steam quality

60. What are the parameters for H_2O_2 sterilization?
    a. Relative humidity, H_2O_2 concentration, time
    b. H_2O_2 concentration, time, pressure
    c. Time, pressure, temperature
    d. H_2O_2 concentration, pressure, time, temperature

61. Which statement(s) is/are true about indicators?

    a. One or more chemical indicators should be placed inside of each sterile package.

    b. There should be an indicator on each layer of a sterile multilevel set.

    c. An indicator that functions properly will ensure that the set is sterile.

    d. If the indicator is questionable or the internal indicator is missing, the set can be used if the process indicator on the outside of the pack demonstrates that the set has been exposed to the parameters of sterilization.

62. Which statement(s) is/are true?

    a. A pouch that has been opened but not used can be resealed if the type of seal permits it.

    b. The assembler must label the package clearly with the contents and initials of the assembler.

    c. Lot control numbers can be used to track packaged items from a "failed load."

    d. Packages should be marked on the paper side of the pouch.

63. Which statement(s) is/are true about shelf life?

    a. Solid steel shelving is preferable to mesh shelving because it is durable and supports heavy sets.

    b. Shelves should be 8 to 10 inches above the floor and at least 18 inches from the ceiling or sprinkler head.

    c. Shipping cartons should be placed on lower shelves to avoid contaminating sterile items.

    d. Expiration dates on commercial packages indicate that the contents' integrity may degrade and should not be used after the expiration date has been reached.

64. Which statement(s) is/are true about shelf life?

    a. When clean and sterile items are stored in the same unit, clean items should be on the uppermost shelves.

    b. Shelf life is the amount of time following sterilization that an item can be considered sterile.

    c. Poor-quality wrappers, poor storage conditions, and inappropriate handling of sterile items can increase the likelihood of contamination.

    d. Event-related sterility is based on the theory that an item remains sterile until something contaminates it.

65. Which statement(s) is/are true about reuse of single-use devices?

    a. The FDA holds facilities that choose to reprocess single-use devices to the same standards as the original manufacturer of the item.

    b. Perioperative nurses should choose single-use items carefully for resterilization, inspecting them carefully for contamination.

    c. Items opened but not delivered to the field are not considered contaminated and can be resterilized.

    d. The facility's infection preventionist can determine which single-use items can be resterilized.

Competency Checklist: Instrument Processing

Under "Observer's Initials," enter initials upon successful achievement of competency. Enter N/A if competency is not appropriate for institution.

Name _____

	Observer's Initials	Date

Point of Use

1. Items are rinsed/wiped/irrigated during the procedure.   _____ _____
2. Disposable sharps and trash are discarded appropriately.   _____ _____
3. All instruments are returned to proper sets for return to SPD.   _____ _____
4. Enzymatic soak solution, spray, or gel is applied before transport to the decontamination area.   _____ _____
5. Contaminated instruments are contained during transportation to the decontamination area.   _____ _____

Cleaning

6. Personal protective equipment is worn during cleaning.   _____ _____
7. Items requiring cleaning by hand are separated from those going to the washer/disinfector.   _____ _____
8. Manual cleaning:
   a. Detergent is prepared according to IFU.   _____ _____
   b. Spray nozzle is held close to instruments in sink to avoid splashing.   _____ _____
   c. Manual cleaning is performed under the surface of the water to avoid aerosolization.   _____ _____
   d. Proper approach is selected for decontamination of equipment according to IFU.   _____ _____
9. Washer/disinfector is properly used.   _____ _____
   a. Appropriate items are selected for washer/disinfector.   _____ _____
   b. Machine is loaded properly.   _____ _____
10. Ultrasonic cleaner is loaded properly (single layer; same type of metal).   _____ _____
11. Appropriate instruments are lubricated.   _____ _____
12. Instruments are inspected for cleanliness and good condition; all components are present.   _____ _____

Packaging

13. Rigid containers are inspected and assembled appropriately:
    a. Caskets and inner baskets are thoroughly cleaned between uses.   _____ _____
    b. Gaskets, valves, and filters are checked prior to placement of instruments.   _____ _____
    c. Following assembly, the lock is placed and contents are identified.   _____ _____
14. Instrument sets are assembled properly.   _____ _____
    a. Items are placed in a tray/container compatible with the sterilization method.   _____ _____
    b. Multi-part instruments are disassembled.   _____ _____
    c. Hinged instruments are opened.   _____ _____
    d. Small, multi-part, and delicate instruments are organized in appropriate containers (no peel packs).   _____ _____
    e. Heavy items are on bottom; more delicate on top.   _____ _____
    f. Items with broad surfaces are placed on edge.   _____ _____
    g. Nested items are separated with porous material and placed facing the same direction.   _____ _____
15. Appropriate chemical indicator(s) are in place.   _____ _____
16. Set is wrapped properly in packaging material appropriate to the method of sterilization.   _____ _____
17. Package is sealed with the appropriate process indicator.   _____ _____
18. Package is labeled with contents and initials.   _____ _____

Sterilization

19. Appropriate method of sterilization is identified for each item.   _____   _____

20. Appropriate process indicator is confirmed on outside of package.   _____   _____

21. Load lot sticker is placed on each item in the load.   _____   _____

22. Chamber is loaded properly so that sterilant can contact surfaces of all items.   _____   _____
    a. Heavy trays lie flat in a single layer.   _____   _____
    b. Small wrapped packages are loosely stacked.   _____   _____
    c. Peel packs are placed on edge and all facing in the same direction.   _____   _____
    d. Basins (anything that can trap moisture) are placed on edge to promote draining.   _____   _____

23. Appropriate sterilization cycle is chosen.   _____   _____

24. Sterilizer is operated according to the manufacturer's instructions.   _____   _____

25. When sterilization is complete:
    a. Printout/to is reviewed to insure all parameters achieved.   _____   _____
    b. Package is allowed to cool before it is removed from autoclave and distributed.   _____   _____

Immediate-Use Steam Sterilization (IUSS)

26. Items are cleaned properly (IFU) before sterilization.   _____   _____

27. Appropriate container is selected for sterilization.   _____   _____

28. Correct sterilization cycle is chosen for item.   _____   _____

29. Inspection of printout:
    a. Patient information is included.   _____   _____
    b. Printout is signed or initialed.   _____   _____

30. Sterile item is transported aseptically to sterile field.   _____   _____

Sterilization Monitoring

31. Demonstrates or verbalizes the process for running a Bowie-Dick/DART sterilization   _____   _____
    monitor:
    a. Correct autoclave (dynamic air removal)   _____   _____
    b. Correct monitor   _____   _____
    c. Correct placement of monitor (IFU)   _____   _____
    d. No other items in autoclave during test run   _____   _____
    e. Documentation correct   _____   _____

32. Demonstrates or verbalizes the process for running a biological monitor:
    a. Appropriate monitor   _____   _____
    b. Correct placement of monitor (IFU)   _____   _____
    c. Prepares ampule and incubates monitor correctly   _____   _____
    d. Documents results correctly   _____   _____
    e. Verbalizes the process following a failed monitor   _____   _____

33. Demonstrate or verbalizes the documentation process for each sterilizer load:
    a. Envelope for each sterilizer to contain sterilization documentation for a 24-hour   _____   _____
       period
    b. Results of Bowie-Dick testing   _____   _____
    c. Results of biological monitoring   _____   _____
    d. Documentation of each load   _____   _____
       i. Sterilizer printout for each load   _____   _____
       ii. Load lot sticker   _____   _____
       iii. Load list   _____   _____
       iv. Chemical indicator (if run in load)   _____   _____
       v. Biological indicator (if run in load)   _____   _____

High-Level Disinfection

34. Demonstrates or verbalizes the process for high-level disinfection.   _____   _____

35. Appropriate items are identified for high-level disinfection.   _____   _____

36. Appropriate personal protective equipment (PPE) is donned during preparation and   _____   _____
    use of disinfectant.

37. Disinfectant is properly prepared (IFU).   _____   _____

38. The minimum effective concentration (MEC) test is performed and results are documented.   _____ _____
39. Items are disinfected properly: _____ _____
    a. Appropriately washed and dried before being disinfected   _____ _____
    b. Rinsed after being disinfected and before use   _____ _____
    c. Handled so as to prevent contamination   _____ _____
40. Documentation is appropriate.   _____ _____

Storage

41. The fire safety/AAMI criteria for locating shelving in sterile storage is verbalized.   _____ _____
42. Sterile items are protected from being compressed, dropped, ripped, or getting wet.   _____ _____
43. Sterile items are shelved so that those sterilized first are first in line for use.   _____ _____
44. Heavy sets are placed on center shelves; stacking heavy packages is avoided.   _____ _____
45. Peel packs are stored in a container to protect and organize them.   _____ _____

Observer's Signature   Initials   Date

_____

Orientee's Signature

_____

Aseptic Practices: Preparing the Sterile Field and the Patient for Surgery

LEARNER OBJECTIVES

1. Describe categories of surgical site infection.
2. Explain the relationship of aseptic practice to the prevention of infection.
3. Identify the perioperative nurse's responsibility for aseptic practice.
4. Identify four sources of infection.
5. Describe the precautions for contact, airborne, and droplet-transmitted infections.
6. Describe the purpose and technique of a surgical prep.
7. List the desired characteristics of topical antimicrobial agents.
8. Describe two processes for surgical hand antisepsis.
9. Describe open-gloving and closed-gloving techniques.
10. Identify restricted, semi-restricted, and unrestricted areas of the operating room.
11. Describe appropriate attire within the restricted, semi-restricted, and unrestricted areas of the operating room.
12. Discuss the term *surgical conscience*.
13. Discuss six guidelines for draping.
14. List the desired characteristics of surgical gowns and drapes.
15. Discuss four techniques to help maintain a sterile field.
16. Identify the recommended number of air exchanges per hour, temperature, and humidity in the operating room.
17. Describe the process for cleanup of small and large spills.
18. Discuss protocols for cleaning in the operating room.
19. Describe appropriate traffic patterns relative to movement around a sterile field.
20. Identify one nursing diagnosis related to a surgical incision.

LESSON OUTLINE

Nursing Diagnosis: Desired Patient Outcomes

1. The links in the chain of infection are the components that must be present for infection to occur: (a) presence of an infectious agent in a sufficient amount and virulence, (b) a mode of transmission, (c) a portal of entry for the microorganisms, (d) and a susceptible host.

2. Pathogenic microorganisms are ubiquitous, and a surgical incision creates the perfect portal of entry to a susceptible host. Based on this scenario, one common nursing diagnosis for the patient undergoing surgical intervention is high risk for surgical site infection.

3. Activities in the operating room (e.g., hand hygiene, patient prep, creating a sterile field) focus on breaking the chain of infection by reducing the presence of microorganisms.

4. Evidence of infection includes fever, erythema, tenderness, induration, cellulitis, purulent drainage, abscess, or dehiscence. The desired patient outcome is for the patient to exhibit none of the signs or symptoms of infection. Although the exact incidence of surgical site infection (SSI) is unknown, it is one of the most frequently reported healthcare-acquired infections. SSIs are usually diagnosed after discharge.

5. Surgical site infections are defined as superficial incisional, deep incisional, or organ/space:

   • Superficial incisional infection involves only the skin or subcutaneous tissue. It is the most common SSI, and the usual treatment is removal of sutures or staples and drainage of the area.

   • Deep incisional infection involves deep soft tissue (e.g., fascia and/or muscle). Deep incisional SSIs occur less frequently than superficial incisional SSIs, usually follow more extensive surgeries, and are usually diagnosed prior to discharge. Prolonged hospitalization or rehospitalization is common for deep incisional infections.

   • Organ/space infection involves the visceral cavity or anatomic structures not opened during the procedure. These infections are the most severe and require extended hospitalization, often with multiple reoperations. Organ/space SSI is associated with long-term morbidity and death.

6. The Centers for Disease Control and Prevention (CDC, 2015b) reported that SSIs are the most common healthcare-associated infection (HAI), accounting for 31% of all HAIs among hospitalized patients. There is a 3% mortality rate among patients who experience an SSI, and 75% of the deaths are directly attributable to the SSI (Magill et al., 2014).

7. Many states require hospitals to publish their infection rates. They believe that mandatory reporting of risk-adjusted infection rates will permit better gathering of statistics, create an increased awareness of the problem of infection, and champion efforts to reduce the incidence of HAIs.

Nursing Responsibilities

8. There are many extrinsic (environmental) and intrinsic (patient-related) variables that contribute to the development of SSI. Asepsis refers to the absence of pathogenic organisms. Aseptic technique involves practices that prevent contamination with microorganisms, thereby breaking the chain of infection by minimizing the presence of infectious agents in the operating room. Aseptic practices differentiate the operating room from other patient care areas.

9. The perioperative nurse is responsible for implementing aseptic practice and monitoring the aseptic technique of the entire surgical team. Aseptic practices include attire, environmental sanitation, scrubbing, gowning, gloving, setup and maintenance of the sterile field, prepping and draping of the patient, and protection of the sterile field until the patient's procedure is completed.

10. Everyone working in the perioperative environment shares the responsibility for reducing the number of microorganisms in the operating room to the lowest level possible. As the coordinator of activities in the operating room, the perioperative nurse assumes responsibility for providing each patient with an aseptic environment where the risk for SSI is reduced to its lowest potential. The perioperative nurse continuously monitors all aspects of the operating room environment to ensure adherence to aseptic principles and compliance with aseptic practice.

Section Questions

1. What are the four links in the chain of infection? [Ref 1]

2. Why is a surgical site considered a high risk for infection? [Ref 2]

3. What is the focus of activities in the operating room? [Ref 3]

4. Identify some of the symptoms of an infection. [Ref 4]

5. Differentiate among the three types of surgical site infection: superficial incisional, deep incisional, organ/space. [Ref 5]

6. How do surgical site infections rank among hospital-acquired infections? [Ref 6]

7. What are some of the ramifications of a surgical site infection? [Ref 6]

8. What good do states feel results from mandatory reporting of HAIs? [Ref 7]

9. What is aseptic technique? [Ref 8]

10. What is the perioperative nurse's responsibility in the operation room? [Refs 9–10]

Pathogenic Microorganisms

11. Pathogenic microorganisms are microorganisms that cause disease. The pathogens most commonly associated with SSIs are *Staphylococcus aureus*, *Staphylococcus epidermidis*, coagulase-negative staphylococci, and *Enterococcus* species. An increasing proportion of SSIs are caused by microorganisms resistant to antibiotics. These infections are difficult—and sometimes impossible—to resolve.

12. The more virulent the microorganism, the greater the potential for infection. More virulent strains of bacteria or bacteria with an endotoxin in their outer cell membrane require a smaller inoculum to cause an infection than less virulent strains. An endotoxin is part of the outer wall of gram-negative bacteria such as *Escherichia coli* and *Pseudomonas*. Endotoxins are released when the bacteria cell is destroyed.

13. Multidrug-resistant organisms (MDROs) are microorganisms, predominantly bacteria, that

are resistant to one or more classes of antimicrobial agents. Although the names of certain MDROs describe resistance to only one agent (e.g., methicillin-resistant *Staphylococcus aureus* [MRSA], vancomycin-resistant enterococci [VRE]), these pathogens are frequently resistant to most available antimicrobial agents. Control of MDROs has significant implications for antibiotic stewardship and the appropriate prescribing of antibiotics.

14. MDROs are of significant concern because options for treating patients with these infections are often extremely limited, and MDRO infections are associated with increased lengths of stay, costs, and mortality (CDC, 2015a).

Sources of Infection (Endogenous)

15. Endogenous sources of infection are those that are related directly to the large number of microorganisms found on the skin, in mucous membranes, and in hollow viscera of the patient himself. In fact, the majority of SSIs are caused by the patient's own flora. However, if these microorganisms remain in their normal environment, and if their numbers are not altered by external factors, they will not cause infection.

16. The skin is our primary defense against the entry of microorganisms into the body. Incising the skin exposes the patient to the risk of infection by creating a portal of entry for pathogenic microorganisms.

17. The risk of infection increases with the length of exposure of internal tissues to the environment (surgical time), the presence of implants, and the amount of ischemic tissue present.

18. In addition, certain factors such as extremes of age, poor nutritional status, obesity, compromised immune system, preexisting disease (especially diabetes), preexisting infection, burns, and use of nicotine may significantly increase a patient's risk for developing an SSI.

19. Smoking decreases the delivery of oxygen to the tissues, which delays wound healing and increases the risk for developing an SSI.

20. Geriatric and neonatal patients are at higher risk for postoperative surgical site infection. Impaired healing in older adults is often related to inadequate circulation due to atherosclerosis or the presence of coexisting disease. Delayed healing increases the potential for surgical site infection. The premature infant's immature globulin synthesis increases susceptibility to infection, antibody formation, and cellular defense. The smaller the neonate, the less resistance to infection the child has. Invasive procedures increase the risk of infection.

21. Poor nutritional status frequently accompanies drug or alcohol addiction or is attributable. Treatment for disease can delay wound healing and increase risk for infection.

22. Obesity is a risk factor because fatty tissue is not well vascularized, and avascular tissue is susceptible to infection.

23. Defense mechanisms are impaired in immunocompromised patients—for example, patients receiving radiation therapy, chemotherapy, or corticosteroids; those on immune-suppressive drugs; and those who have acquired immune deficiency syndrome (AIDS).

24. Additional stress is placed on the immune system of patients with chronic conditions such as diabetes, cancer, and cardiac and respiratory diseases.

25. The presence of infection anywhere in the body significantly increases the risk of an SSI and is always a contraindication for elective surgery. Whenever possible, surgery should be postponed until any preexisting infection is resolved.

26. When skin integrity is destroyed, such as with a burn, the patient becomes susceptible to infection.

27. Although necessary, catheters and drains can increase the risk of infection because they provide a pathway for pathogenic microorganism migration. The longer catheters and drains are left in place, the greater the risk for infection.

Sources of Infection (Exogenous)

28. Exogenous sources of infection come from the environment and other people.

29. Exogenous factors include length of surgery, type of procedure, surgical technique, and an extended preoperative hospital stay.

30. Colonization of the patient with healthcare-associated microbes is especially likely when the patient has an extensive preoperative or postoperative hospitalization.

31. Personnel are a major source of microorganisms in the operating room. The greater the

number of personnel in the operating room, the greater the number of microorganisms present.

32. A colonized individual is one who carries the organism but is not infected. Colonized personnel can be transmission sources of microorganisms that can subsequently cause an infection. It is not unusual to discover personnel in the operating who are colonized with MRSA.

33. While the skin is our first line of defense against microbial invasion, the skin itself is covered with microorganisms. Cells and microorganisms are constantly being shed from the skin. Certain body areas, such as the head, neck, axilla, hands, groin, legs, and feet, harbor an especially large number of microorganisms. Hair is a major source of *Staphylococcus*. The number of microorganisms present in hair is related to its length and cleanliness. For this reason, surgical attire should cover and contain microorganisms.

34. Talking, coughing, laughing—even breathing—release organisms into the environment.

35. Chipped fingernail polish can harbor pathogens in large numbers and should be removed prior to entry into the operating room environment (Association of periOperative Registered Nurses [AORN], 2015, p. 32). Because it is impractical to continually monitor the state of fingernail polish, facility policies usually state that fingernail polish should not be worn in the perioperative environment.

36. A 2009 World Health Organization (WHO) study found higher bacterial counts on the hands of nurses with fingernails longer than ¼ inch, whether natural or artificial.

37. Research studies continue to demonstrate that artificial nails may contribute to the transmission of healthcare-associated infection. Artificial nails are more likely to harbor gram-negative pathogens both before and after hand washing, and the longer the artificial fingernails are worn, the greater the number of microorganisms are present. Healthcare personnel who wear artificial nails may also limit hand hygiene and surgical hand scrub practices to protect their manicures (AORN, 2015, p. 32).

38. Jewelry has also been shown to harbor microorganisms. AORN (2015, p. 32) recommends that jewelry not be worn in the operating room. Any jewelry worn should be completely covered by surgical attire.

39. The Joint Commission's National Patient Safety Goals (since 2007), the AORN, the CDC, and the WHO all recommend against artificial nails for members of the surgical team.

Environment

40. The operating room itself is not sterile. Organisms are present in the air, on dust particles, and on dirt in the environment.

41. Dust particles settle on the walls, floors, overhead lights, light tracks, cabinets, door handles, and other stationary fixtures in the operating room that may harbor microorganisms and, therefore, are potential sources of infection. For this reason, the first thing the perioperative nurse must do when "opening" a room is to wipe all horizontal surfaces with a damp cloth.

42. All supplies and equipment that come in contact with personnel become potential sources for infection, because personnel transfer organisms to and from whatever they touch.

Section Questions

1. Define the term *pathogenic microorganism*. [Ref 11]
2. Which types of bacteria require a smaller inoculum to cause an infection? [Ref 12]
3. Describe an endotoxin. [Ref 12]
4. Identify two bacteria that have an endotoxin. [Ref 12]
5. What challenge is associated with an MDRO? [Ref 13]

(continues)

Section Questions (continued)

6. What practices have a significant impact on MDROs? [Ref 13]

7. Define "endogenous source of infection". [Ref 15]

8. How does a surgical procedure itself expose the patient to the risk of infection? [Ref 16]

9. Describe endogenous factors that increase a patient's risk for developing an infection. [Ref 18]

10. How does smoking increase the risk for SSI? [Ref 19]

11. Describe the increased risk for SSI in the geriatric and neonate populations. [Ref 20]

12. How does nutrition influence the risk for SSI? [Ref 21]

13. Describe one risk of obese patients for developing an SSI. [Ref 22]

14. Why might surgery be canceled if a patient is found to have an existing infection? [Ref 25]

15. Why might catheters and drains increase the risk of developing an SSI? [Ref 27]

16. Describe exogenous factors that influence the patient's risk for an infection? [Refs 28–29]

17. Which body areas harbor especially large numbers of microorganisms? [Ref 33]

18. Explain why AORN's recommended practices expect that the perioperative nurse will remove jewelry and avoid wearing nail polish and artificial nails? [Refs 35–38]

19. Which other organizations recommend against artificial nails for surgical team members? [Ref 39]

20. What is the rationale for damp dusting horizontal surfaces before every procedure in the operating room? [Ref 41]

Standard and Transmission-Based Precautions

43. Universal precautions were defined by the CDC in 1987. They comprised a set of precautions for handling blood and body fluids of infected patients designed to prevent the transmission of human immunodeficiency virus (HIV), hepatitis B virus (HBV), and other bloodborne pathogens.

44. Universal precautions evolved into standard and transmission-based precautions in 1996. Standard precautions consider that the blood and body fluid of *all* patients be considered-potentially infectious and that the same safety precautions be taken whether or not the patient is known to have a bloodborne infectious disease.

45. The practice of standard precautions is a method of infection control that protects both the patient and operating room personnel. Standard precautions apply to blood, all body fluids, secretions, and excretions except sweat, regardless of whether they contain visible blood (Siegel, Rhinehart, Jackson, & Chiarello, 2007, p. 66).

46. Standard and transmission-based precautions are methods of infection control that can prevent the transmission of pathogens and protect both the patient and the healthcare worker from exposure.

47. Standard precautions include the use of personal protective equipment (PPE) and prompt and frequent hand washing. PPE includes using gloves when touching blood, body fluids, secretions, excretions, and contaminated items, and wearing masks, eye protection, and gowns during procedures with the potential to generate splashes of blood, body fluids, secretions, and excretions. Shoe and leg coverings may also be used as needed.

48. Hands should be washed after touching blood, body fluids, secretions, excretions, and contaminated items, whether or not gloves are worn (Siegel et al., 2007, p. 66). Also, wash hands after removing gloves and before and after eating.

49. Transmission-based precautions are used in addition to standard precautions for patients who are known or suspected to be infected or colonized with infectious agents that require

additional measures to effectively prevent their transmission (Siegel et al., 2007, p. 66).

50. There are three types of transmission-based precautions: airborne, droplet, and contact.

51. Airborne precautions are appropriate against pathogens that are 5 microns or smaller and are spread by airborne transmission. Rubeola, tuberculosis, and varicella require airborne precautions. The patient is often required to wear a mask during transport.

52. Airborne precautions include respiratory protection (e.g., an N95 mask approved by the National Institute of Occupational Safety and Health [NIOSH], and special air handling and ventilation). Persons susceptible to airborne pathogens should wear respiratory protection, and infected patients should wear a mask during transport.

53. Elective surgery should be postponed for patients who are on airborne precautions. If surgery cannot be postponed, the procedure should be scheduled when the fewest personnel are present. In addition, only personnel required for the surgery should be allowed to enter the room. Following surgery, the room should remain vacant and closed until the air in the room has been completely exchanged. The time required for a complete exchange will depend on the rate of air exchange in that operating room, typically 28 minutes based on 15 air exchanges with an efficiency removal effectiveness of 99.9% (Petersen, 2006, p. 648).

54. Droplet precautions are appropriate for protection against pathogens that are transmitted through droplets (particles 5 microns or larger), such as influenza and mumps. Droplet precautions require wearing a mask within 3 feet of an infected patient and positioning other patients at least 3 feet away from infected patients. Droplets are transmitted by sneezing, talking, and coughing. Infected patients should wear a mask during transport.

55. Contact precautions are used when caring for patients who are known or suspected to be infected or colonized with microorganisms transmitted by direct or indirect contact. Contact precautions include wearing gloves and gowns when anticipating contact with microorganisms, wearing a mask if contact with aerosolized infectious organisms is possible, and cleaning and disinfecting patient equipment.

56. In 1992, the Occupational Safety and Health Administration (OSHA) established mandatory universal precautions practice standards. The three critical components of universal precaution standards are (1) use of personal protective barriers, (2) proper hand washing, and (3) precautions in handling sharps.

57. The standards include the following provisions:

- Employers must list job classifications, tasks, and procedures in which employees have occupational exposure to blood or other potentially infectious body fluids. PPE is selected based on the potential for exposure to blood and body fluids.

- Gloves must be worn when direct contact with blood or other potentially infectious body fluids is expected to occur.

- Masks with face shields or protective eyewear with side shields must be worn when splashes, splattering, or aerosolization of blood and body fluids is anticipated.

- Gowns, appropriate to the procedure being performed, must be worn when aerosolization or splattering of blood or other body fluids is anticipated. Gowns must not permit passage of blood or body fluids.

- PPE (e.g., gloves, masks, face shields, gowns) must be provided by the employer at no cost to the employee.

- Hands and other skin surfaces must be washed as soon as feasible if contaminated with blood or body fluids.

- Contaminated needles are not recapped or removed unless required by a specific procedure. If recapping or removal is required, it must be accomplished with a mechanical device.

- Sharps are deposited in rigid, leak-proof, puncture-resistant containers that must be readily accessible.

- A written schedule of cleaning and appropriate disinfection of equipment and the environment must be implemented and maintained.

- Contaminated laundry is placed in labeled or color-coded laundry bags that prevent leakage.

- Infectious waste containers must be closable, prevent leakage, and be labeled or color coded as potentially infectious.

- The employer must provide a hepatitis B vaccination and a postexposure follow-up program. A preexposure vaccine must be offered free of charge.

- Training and education programs must be made available to all employees who may be exposed to blood or other body fluids that are potentially contaminated with HBV or HIV.

58. In addition, OSHA revised the Bloodborne Pathogens Standard (CFR 29 1910.1030) to require employers to identify, evaluate, and implement safer medical devices. The revision also requires that nonmanagerial healthcare workers be involved in evaluating and choosing safer needle devices. The standard also requires maintaining a sharps injury log (OSHA, 2011).

Section Questions

1. How do standard precautions differ from universal precautions? [Ref 44]

2. What are the two major components of standard precautions? [Ref 44]

3. Which body fluids do standard precautions include? [Ref 45]

4. Describe PPE. [Ref 47]

5. Which patients require transmission-based precautions? [Ref 49]

6. Describe the three types of transmission-based precautions. [Ref 50]

7. A microorganism of what size particle determines the need for airborne precautions? [Ref 51]

8. Which type of protection is required for airborne precautions? [Ref 52]

9. If surgery must be performed on a patient on airborne precautions, which special interventions should be considered? [Ref 53]

10. How many air exchanges in which period of time result in 99.9% air removal effectiveness? [Ref 53]

11. What are some diseases spread by droplet transmission? [Ref 54]

12. A mask is required within how many feet of a patient on droplet precautions? [Ref 54]

13. Which precaution should be taken when transporting a patient on droplet precautions? [Ref 54]

14. Describe the PPE required when managing patients with contact precautions. [Ref 55]

15. What are the three critical components of the universal precautions established by OSHA? [Ref 56]

16. What does OSHA say about the wearing of eye protection? [Ref 57]

17. How does OSHA say contaminated needles/sharps should be handled? [Ref 57]

18. According to OSHA, what are the requirements for containers of infectious waste? [Ref 57]

19. What does OSHA require of the employer in reference to hepatitis B vaccination? [Ref 57]

20. How does OSHA include the perioperative nurse in managing sharps safety? [Ref 58]

Control of Sources of Infection

59. Aseptic practices designed to prevent infection distinguish the operating room from other clinical areas. The perioperative nurse's primary responsibility is to implement and monitor aseptic practices:

- Surgical attire
- Sterilization of instruments and equipment
- Hand hygiene
- Patient skin preparation
- Creation and maintenance of a sterile field
- Environmental hygiene

60. Some aseptic practices, such as PPE, are mandated by regulatory bodies such as OSHA. Others are derived from standards-setting bodies such as AORN and the Association for the Advancement of Medical Instrumentation (AAMI).

61. Regardless of the source of the aseptic practices, they are only as good as the surgical conscience of the individual practitioner. A *surgical conscience* is a personal commitment to adhere

strictly to aseptic practice, to report any break in aseptic practice, and to correct any violation. Like *integrity,* a surgical conscience is what you do *"when no one is looking"*.

62. The sterile environment created for a surgical procedure is intended to isolate the operative site from contamination from the surrounding area.

63. AORN's (2015) *Guidelines for Perioperative Practice* address all aspects of care of the patient in surgery, providing evidence to support best practices.

Control of Patient Sources of Infection: Skin Prep

64. Efforts to reduce patient sources of infection are aimed at lowering the number of bacteria on the skin prior to surgery and reducing potential bacterial contamination from within the patient during surgery. Although the skin cannot be sterilized, the incision site and surrounding area should be as free of microorganisms as possible prior to surgery.

65. Cruse and Foord (1980, pp. 27–40) performed the landmark study demonstrating that hair removal is associated with increased risk of surgical site infection. Hair at the incision site should be removed only when its presence interferes with the intended procedure. If required, hair removal should be done as close to the time of surgery as possible, and in a location outside the operating room (AORN, 2015. p. 48).

66. Before hair is removed from the surgical site, the patient's skin should be assessed for the presence of rashes, moles, warts, or other conditions. Trauma to these lesions can provide an opportunity for the colonization of pathogenic microorganisms.

67. Hair should be removed with single-use clippers or clippers with a reusable head that can be disinfected between patients—never a razor (AORN, 2015, p. 48). Clippers decrease the potential for nicks in the skin that can provide a portal of entry for microorganisms.

68. Hair removal may also be done with a depilatory cream. Depilatory creams are used infrequently because of potential irritation to the skin. They also tend to be messy and time consuming.

69. To prevent airborne dispersal of hair and possible contamination of the sterile field, hair removal should be performed outside the room where surgery will be performed.

70. The operative site and the immediate surrounding area are cleaned, and an antiseptic is used to prep the patient's skin prior to surgery. The objective of skin cleansing is to remove dirt and skin oils, to reduce the number of microorganisms on the skin to a minimum, and to prevent further microbial growth throughout the procedure.

71. The patient should be instructed to shower or bathe the night before surgery and/or just prior to surgery to lower the microbial count on the skin.

72. Traditionally, the use of chlorhexidine gluconate (CHG) was recommended, but seven recent trials involving more than 10,000 patients showed no clear evidence that the use of CHG was better than other wash products at preventing SSIs (Webster & Osborne, 2015).

73. Skin antisepsis immediately before surgery needs to start with the patient's skin being clean. It may be necessary to remove adhesive residue, oils from skin, or other debris prior to the skin prep. The choice of antiseptic agent for the preoperative skin prep depends on the condition of the patient's skin, patient allergies, the incision site, and surgeon and hospital preference.

74. Antiseptic products should:
    - Clean effectively
    - Reduce microbial count rapidly
    - Have a broad spectrum of activity
    - Be easy to apply
    - Be nonirritating and nontoxic
    - Provide residual protection

75. There is no conclusive data to support better patient outcomes with the use of sterile gloves and a sterile prep kit over clean gloves and a clean prep kit. Facility policy and surgeon preference will determine the approach.

76. Prep solutions:
    - The most commonly used antimicrobial agents include CHG, iodophors, and alcohol preparations in concentrations of 60–90%.
    - Antiseptic solutions containing CHG should not be used near the eyes due to the danger of corneal ulcerations. CHG can cause deafness if it comes in contact with the inner ear. CHG is not recommended for prepping mucous membranes (AORN, 2015, p. 51).
    - Alcohol-based prep solutions should not be used near eyes or on mucous membranes.

- Prep solutions based on new technologies are being introduced to overcome these challenges.
- Some prep agents include a soap preparation for cleansing and an antiseptic solution to be applied after cleansing (often referred to as "scrub and paint").

77. Follow the manufacturer's instructions for use (IFU) for amount of prep to be used, duration of the prep, any specific application technique, and dry time if necessary. Antiseptic contact time is an important consideration. Some solutions must dry in order to be effective.

78. Alcohol-based antiseptics must be allowed to dry completely before draping is done. Draping before the alcohol has completely evaporated traps the flammable fumes beneath the drapes and creates a significant fire hazard.

79. Selection of skin-prep agent must take into consideration any patient allergies or sensitivities.

80. The area prepped should include the incision site and area surrounding it to allow for enlarging the incision, anticipated additional incision sites, and the insertion of drains. (**Figures** 4-1, 4-2, 4-3, 4-4, 4-5, 4-6, and 4-7).

81. If the patient is awake, provide an explanation of the prep. Avoid unnecessary exposure; expose only the area to be prepped to maintain the patient's dignity and prevent unnecessary heat loss.

82. Prevent prep solutions from pooling beneath the patient, soaking tourniquet cuff padding, or contacting the electrosurgical dispersive electrode. Pooled prep solutions can cause chemical burns. Place dry towels around the prep site to absorb excess fluid, to prevent saturation of drapes or linens, and to prevent pooling. Be sure to remove the towels after the prep and before draping.

83. Prep progresses from clean to dirty, beginning with the incision site and working to

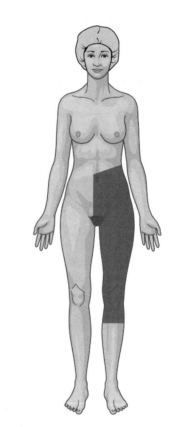

Figure 4-2 Hip prep.

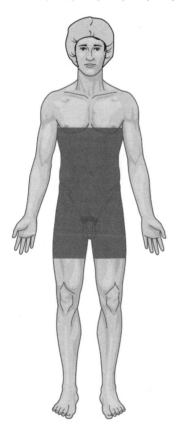

Figure 4-1 Abdominal prep.

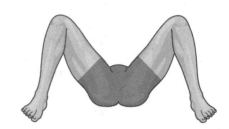

Figure 4-3 Perineum prep.

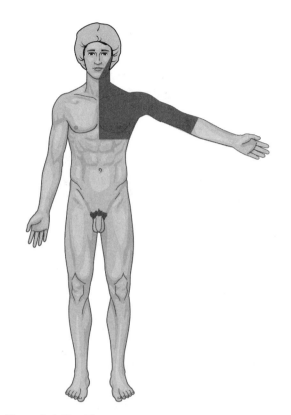

Figure 4-4 Shoulder prep.

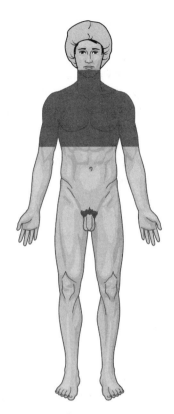

Figure 4-5 Head and neck prep.

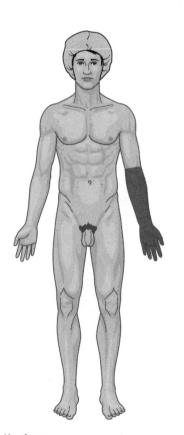

Figure 4-6 Hand prep.

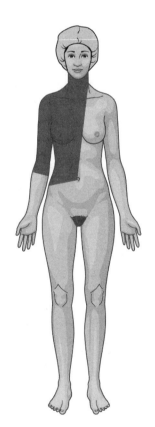

Figure 4-7 Breast prep.

the periphery of the area to be prepped. Once a prep sponge or applicator reaches the periphery, it is considered contaminated and discarded. If the prep is not complete, a clean sponge or applicator should be used.

84. Some preps include parts of the body considered "dirty" because they harbor microorganisms:

    • The umbilicus is cleaned with cotton-tipped applicators before the skin prep begins.

    • A colostomy or stoma is covered until the surrounding area is prepped, and then it is prepped with a separate sponge.

    • In a perineal prep, the vagina and/or anus is prepped last with a separate sponge. In a shoulder prep, the axilla is prepped last.

    • For unusual wounds or incision sites when it may be difficult to know where to begin, use good judgment to determine the approach that will minimize contamination at the incision site.

85. Wash eyes with cotton balls with a nonirritating solution. Begin the prep at the nose and continue outward. Warm sterile water may be used to rinse off the solution. Prevent solution from pooling around the patient's eyes.

86. For traumatic wounds, large amounts of irrigating solution may be used prior to and in addition to the prep to remove dirt and debris.

87. Normal saline should be used to prep burned or denuded skin.

88. When it is necessary to prep a limb, arrange for an additional person or an apparatus to hold the limb securely so the entire circumference can be prepped adequately and safely.

89. A scrub brush or sponge may be useful for cleaning hands and feet prior to the prep. Avoid irritating tender skin or creating scratches that could become a portal of entry for bacteria. Take care to prevent aerosolization of prep solutions and skin debris.

90. Warm prep solutions are preferable. They may help maintain body temperature and are more comfortable for the awake patient. Take care not to overheat the prep solution, because the efficacy of the antiseptic may be compromised at elevated temperatures.

91. Be gentle when prepping fragile skin sites and over pressure-sensitive areas such as the carotid body.

92. Documentation of the skin prep should include the following elements:

    • Assessment of the skin at the operative site

    • Hair removal, if performed, including site, method, time, location, and person who removed hair

    • Patient skin allergies or sensitivities

    • Prep agents or solution

    • Area prepped

    • Name of person performing the prep

    • Skin condition postoperatively/patient response to prep, such as allergic reaction

Section Questions

1. What distinguishes the operating room from other clinical areas? [Ref 59]

2. Provide examples of aseptic practices. [Ref 59]

3. Give three examples of regulatory bodies that mandate aseptic practices. [Ref 60]

4. Define the term *surgical conscience*. [Ref 61]

5. What is the purpose of creating a sterile environment for a surgical procedure? [Ref 62]

6. What is the purpose of AORN's recommended practices? [Ref 63]

7. Discuss criteria involved in considerations for hair removal for a surgical procedure. [Refs 65–69]

8. What is the objective of skin cleansing prior to a surgical procedure? [Ref 70]

9. What factors influence the choice of antiseptic agent for the skin prep prior to the procedure? [Ref 73]

10. Describe the ideal properties of an antiseptic agent for preoperative skin prep. [Ref 74]

11. What determines the duration of the preoperative skin prep and dry time, if any? [Refs 77–78]

(continues)

Control of Environmental Sources of Infection: Traffic Patterns

93. The operating room itself is divided into three areas defined by the activities that occur within each area. These areas are unrestricted, semi-restricted, and restricted (AORN, 2015 p. 267):

    - *Unrestricted area*: An area peripheral to the operating room with a central control point where designated personnel monitor the entrance of patients, personnel, and materials into the semi-restricted area. Surgical attire is not required. The unrestricted area contains the locker rooms/dressing rooms, break room, waiting room, and preoperative areas where patients and family arrive in street clothes. Movement from unrestricted to semi-restricted areas should be through a transition zone such as a locker room, break room, holding area, or office.

    - *Semi-restricted area*: The peripheral support areas of the surgical suite. The area may include storage areas for equipment and clean and sterile supplies; work areas for processing instruments; sterilization processing room(s); scrub sink areas; corridors leading from the unrestricted area to the restricted areas of the surgical suite; and the entrances to locker rooms, preoperative admission area, the postanesthesia care unit (PACU), and sterile processing. This area is entered directly from the unrestricted area past a nurse's station or from other areas. Personnel in the semi-restricted area should wear surgical attire and cover all head and facial hair. Access to the semi-restricted area should be limited to authorized personnel and patients accompanied by authorized personnel.

    - *Restricted area*: A designated space contained within the semi-restricted area and accessible only through a semi-restricted area. The restricted area includes the operating and other rooms in which surgical or other invasive procedures are performed. Personnel in the restricted areas should wear surgical attire and cover head and facial hair. Masks should be worn in the presence of open sterile supplies or persons who are completing or have completed a surgical hand scrub. Only authorized personnel and patients accompanied by authorized personnel should be admitted to this area.

Control of Personnel Sources of Infection: Attire

94. Personnel who work in restricted and semi-restricted areas of the surgical suite are required to wear surgical attire designed to protect both patient and personnel by inhibiting the passage of microorganisms from personnel to the patient and the environment and from patient to personnel.

95. Appropriate surgical attire in the operating-room suite includes hats or hoods, scrub outfits (commonly referred to as "scrubs"), and shoe covers (optional).

96. Scrubs are either a one-piece coverup, such as a dress, or a two-piece shirt and pants set. To prevent shedding, the shirt should fit close to the body or be tucked into the pants. Scrubs may be made of a tightly woven reusable fabric that minimizes shedding, or they may be disposable. Reusable scrubs should be freshly laundered and changed daily.

97. Attire for the restricted and semi-restricted areas is the same, with the exception of a mask

required when sterile supplies are open or personnel are performing a surgical hand scrub.

98. AORN (2015, p. 109) recommends that all individuals who enter the semi-restricted and restricted areas wear scrub attire that has been laundered at a healthcare-accredited laundry facility or disposable scrub attire provided by the facility and intended for use within the perioperative setting.

99. Controversy exists over whether home laundering rather than hospital laundering is acceptable:

    • Proponents of healthcare facility laundering cite the inability of home laundering to provide controlled load mix, appropriate detergent, cycle time, and water temperature as reasons to mandate laundering in the healthcare facility.

    • Recommendations against home laundering are extrapolated from laboratory data. It is impossible to construct well-controlled studies to evaluate the risks associated with home laundering; the number of variables involved in such a study cannot be controlled.

    • Many healthcare facilities do permit home laundering of scrubs with the exception of grossly contaminated scrubs. OSHA (2011) mandates that garments penetrated by blood or other potentially infectious materials be removed immediately or as soon as feasible. In this event, the facility must supply a fresh scrub suit.

100. Scrub attire should contain skin squames and bacteria shed from the body. The top of a two-piece scrub suit should be secured at the waist, tucked into the pants, or fit close to the body (AORN, 2015, p. 102).

101. Personal clothing should be completely contained within scrub attire (AORN, 2015, p. 102).

102. Hats/caps or hoods are worn so that all head and facial hair is completely covered. Hair is a gross contaminant and major source of bacteria. It attracts and sheds bacteria in proportion to its length, oiliness, and curliness.

103. A hat or hood should be worn in areas where supplies are processed and stored as well as in restricted areas where surgery is performed. Hats are frequently disposable (single use). Reusable hats should be covered with a disposable cap, or should be laundered between each wearing. Hats should be removed, and single-use hats or hoods should be deposited

in a designated receptacle before leaving the operating room suite (AORN, 2015, p. 114).

104. Operating rooms are cool, and warm-up jackets serve to keep personnel warm. Warm-up jackets' sleeves should come down to the wrists; jackets should be snapped or buttoned, or zipped closed to prevent the edges from inadvertently contacting and contaminating sterile supplies (AORN, 2015, p. 103). Warm-up jackets may be reusable or disposable and must be made of fabric validated for surgical attire.

105. Hospital policy dictates whether scrubs are to be removed when leaving the operating room suite and fresh ones donned upon reentry, or if cover gowns or lab coats must be worn over scrubs outside the operating room. Changing of scrubs or use of cover gowns has not been shown to influence the risk of SSI (AORN, 2015, p. 104).

106. High-filtration masks are worn in the restricted area in the presence of open sterile supplies. Droplets expelled from the mouth and nasopharynx during talking, sneezing, and coughing are contained within the mask. Whether masks reduce risk of infection when worn by personnel who are not scrubbed and who are in forced ventilation systems is not clear and requires further research. For this reason, policies on wearing of masks may vary.

107. Masks should cover the nose and mouth completely and securely. Most masks contain a small malleable metal strip that should be pinched to conform to the nose to provide a secure, proper fit. The mask should be tied securely at the back of the head in a manner that prevents venting, which can allow unfiltered exhaled air to escape from the sides.

108. Masks with face shields or splash guards, or masks worn with protective eyewear such as goggles or glasses with side shields, are worn whenever splashes, sprays, or aerosols of potentially infectious agents, such as blood, are anticipated (AORN, 2015, p. 106).

109. Masks should be removed and discarded when they become wet and after use. Masks must be either on or off; they should never be left hanging around the neck or be folded and placed in a pocket for future use.

110. When removing a mask, handle it only by the ties. Masks harbor bacteria, and handling of the material portion of the mask after use can transfer microorganisms from the mask to the hands; therefore, only the ties should

be handled. Masks should be disposed of in a designated receptacle (AORN, 2015, p. 106). Wash your hands after removing your mask.

111. There is no evidence that shoe covers contribute to reducing surgical site infection rates. Shoe covers are considered personal protective equipment and, as such, OSHA (2011) requires that they be worn in situations when exposure to copious or potentially infectious fluids is anticipated.

112. Shoe covers should be removed and deposited in a designated receptacle before leaving the operating room suite. Removal of shoe covers can permit transfer of microorganisms from the shoe covers to the hands. Wash your hands after removing shoe covers.

113. Jewelry increases bacterial counts on skin surfaces. Remove any jewelry that cannot be contained or confined within the surgical attire. Removal of watches and bracelets allows for more thorough hand washing (AORN, 2015, p. 107).

114. Nails should be short and clean. Long nails may puncture protective gloves or scratch a patient during transfer. Chipped fingernail polish should be removed and artificial nails should not be worn. Personnel who wear artificial fingernails may limit hand hygiene and surgical hand scrub practices in order to protect their manicure (AORN, 2015, pp. 31, 32).

115. Other attire worn to protect personnel from infectious agents includes gloves, liquid-resistant aprons, and gowns.

116. Personnel who scrub for surgery are referred to as "members of the sterile team" or "scrubbed personnel." In addition to wearing appropriate operating room attire, scrubbed personnel must perform surgical hand antisepsis, commonly referred to as "scrubbing," prior to donning a sterile gown and sterile gloves.

Section Questions

1. Describe the three distinct areas of the operating room. [Ref 93]

2. What is the purpose of requiring surgical attire in the semi-restricted and restricted areas of the operating room? [Ref 94]

3. What is included in "surgical attire"? [Ref 95]

4. Describe "scrubs." [Ref 96]

5. Attire for restricted and semi-restricted areas is the same with what exception? [Ref 97]

6. Explain why there is controversy over requiring facility-provided scrubs versus home laundering of scrubs. [Ref 99]

7. What rationale do those who support facility-provided scrubs give for prohibiting home-laundered scrubs? [Ref 99]

8. Describe proper wearing of scrub attire. [Ref 100]

9. What is AORN's recommendation about wearing personal attire under scrub clothing? [Ref 101]

10. Describe considerations for choosing a hat, cap, or hood to wear. [Refs 102–103]

11. How is the warm-up jacket to be worn? What is the rationale? [Ref 104]

12. What dictates the use of a cover gown or lab coat when leaving the operating room? [Ref 105]

13. What is venting and how does it influence the effectiveness of a surgical mask? [Ref 107]

14. When are face shields or other protective eyewear required? [Ref 108]

15. Why is it important to discard a mask as soon as it is removed? [Ref 109]

16. What is so important about the familiar phrase "masks are either on or off"? [Ref 109]

17. When are shoe covers mandated by OSHA? [Ref 111]

18. Which jewelry is permissible in the operating room? [Ref 113]

19. How do watches, bracelets, and rings affect hand hygiene? [Ref 113]

20. Describe appropriate care of fingernails for the perioperative nurse. [Ref 114]

Scrubbing, Gowning, and Gloving

Definitions

117. *Alcohol-based hand rub:* A product containing alcohol intended for application to the hands for the purpose of reducing the number of microorganisms on the hands. Alcohol-based hand rub products are available as rinses, gels, and foams and are usually formulated to contain 60–95% alcohol.

118. *Alcohol-based surgical hand antiseptics:* A product containing alcohol and another antiseptic agent (such as CHG) that does not require the use of a scrub sponge/brush or sponge.

119. *Antimicrobial soap:* Soap containing an antiseptic agent.

120. *Antimicrobial surgical scrub agent:* A product intended for surgical hand antisepsis.

121. *Antiseptic agent:* An antimicrobial substance applied to the skin to reduce the number of resident and transient microbial flora.

122. *Antiseptic hand wash:* A hand wash performed with a product formulated with an antiseptic agent.

123. *Hand hygiene:* All measures related to hand condition and decontamination (AORN, 2015, p. 31).

124. *Hand washing:* Washing hands with plain soap (soap without an antimicrobial) and water.

125. *Resident microorganisms:* Microorganisms that are permanent residents of the skin.

126. *Surgical hand antisepsis:* Antiseptic hand wash or antiseptic hand rub performed prior to surgery by surgical personnel to eliminate transient microorganisms and reduce resident hand flora. Products cleared for surgical hand antisepsis may be used in place of the traditional brush/sponge and antimicrobial surgical scrub agent.

127. *Surgical hand antiseptic agent:* An antimicrobial product formulated to significantly reduce the number of microorganisms on skin. Surgical hand antiseptic agents are broad-spectrum agents and should exhibit both persistence and cumulative effect that prevents or inhibits proliferation or survival of microorganisms over time.

128. *Transient microorganisms:* Microorganisms found on the skin that are easily removed with a soap and water hand wash or with an antimicrobial hand rub agent.

Hand Hygiene

129. Hand hygiene is often considered the single most important step in preventing infection. Operating room personnel, like all healthcare personnel, should perform hand hygiene before and after patient contact, before donning gloves, and after removing gloves.

130. Hand hygiene, other than in preparation for surgery, requires washing hands with either plain or antimicrobial soap and water or application of an alcohol-based skin rub. When hands are visibly soiled or contaminated with proteinaceous material, hand washing must precede application of an alcohol-based surgical hand preparation.

131. Mechanical washing is the removal of dirt, oils, and microorganisms by means of friction. Antisepsis is the prevention of sepsis by the exclusion, destruction, or inhibition of growth or multiplication of microorganisms from body tissues and fluids.

132. Surgical hand antisepsis is an activity performed immediately prior to gowning and gloving in preparation for surgery. The purpose of surgical hand antisepsis is to remove dirt, skin oils, and transient microorganisms; to reduce the number of resident microorganisms on the nails, hands, and lower arms to as low a level as possible; and to prevent growth of microorganisms for as long as possible. This is accomplished through mechanical washing and chemical antisepsis. Personnel with respiratory infections should not function in the scrub role.

133. The objective of surgical hand antisepsis is to prevent the transfer of microorganisms from personnel to patients and from patients to personnel in the event of glove tears or gown penetration.

134. Prior to performing surgical hand antisepsis, all jewelry must be removed from hands and arms. All other jewelry should also be removed or be completely contained.

135. Hands and arms should be examined for cuts and other lesions that could ooze serum, which is a medium for microbial growth and serves as a potential means of transmission of microorganisms into the patient. Persons with cuts and abrasions should not function in the scrub role.

136. Protective eyewear should be worn when splash or splatter is anticipated. Goggles or face shields are considered appropriate

eyewear protection. Regular eyeglasses do not always adequately protect against splashes or splatter that may occur. In the interest of safety, goggles or face shields should be worn for all invasive procedures.

137. Surgical hand antisepsis, traditionally referred to as "scrubbing," historically required that personnel scrub their hands and arms with a sponge/brush or sponge using an antimicrobial surgical scrub agent while adhering to either an anatomical timed scrub procedure or a counted stroke method procedure whereby each finger, hand, and forearm is visualized as having four sides and each side is scrubbed. This method has largely been supplemented by the use of alcohol-based surgical hand preparations that have been cleared by the U.S. Food and Drug Administration (FDA) for use as surgical hand antiseptics.

138. Antimicrobial scrub agents are detergent-based products containing alcohol, iodine/iodophors, chlorhexidine gluconate, triclosan, or parachlorometaxylenol. Povidone-iodine and chlorhexidine gluconate products are the most commonly used.

139. Alcohol-based products in combination with other products, such as chlorhexidine gluconate and emollients, add persistence and have been shown to be rapid, effective, and gentle to the hands.

140. Each institution should decide whether the traditional scrub procedure; the newer brushless, alcohol-based antiseptics; or a combination of these will be used by the sterile scrub team. Regardless of whether an alcohol-based antiseptic hand rub or a sponge/brush and surgical hand antiseptic hand agent is used, the hands should first be washed. Hands should also be washed after removing gloves (AORN, 2015, p. 35).

141. Surgical hand antiseptic agents should meet the following criteria:
    • Broad spectrum of activity (effective against gram-negative and gram-positive organisms)
    • Rapid acting
    • Nonirritating
    • Not dependent upon a cumulative effect (the first application is as effective as subsequent applications); however, they should demonstrate a cumulative effect
    • Significantly reduces microorganisms on the skin

• Persistent activity—inhibits the rapid growth of microorganisms

142. Surgical hand antisepsis should be performed according to hospital policy, which should specify the agent and the method to be used. The manufacturer's recommendations and supporting literature regarding use of the agent should be incorporated into this policy.

Traditional Surgical Hand Antisepsis (Traditional Scrub Procedure)

143. Historically, scrub policies called for an anatomical scrub or a timed scrub. In either method, the scrub should include cleaning under nails and scrubbing of all surfaces of each finger, hand, and forearm.

144. Anatomical scrubs may indicate the number of strokes to be applied to each area to be scrubbed. The entire surface to be scrubbed is broken into specified areas with a specified number of strokes for each area. For example, each finger has four surfaces, each of which is scrubbed a specified number of times.

145. Timed scrubs specify the length of time a scrub should last and may specify how long the scrub should last on each specified surface. The number of strokes and time may both be incorporated into a scrub policy.

146. Basic steps in the traditional scrub procedure (scrub sponge/brush and antimicrobial surgical scrub agent) include the following:
    • Individually packaged commercially prepared product intended for traditional surgical hand antisepsis is selected. The product usually contains a sponge/brush combination impregnated with antimicrobial surgical scrub agent and a nail-cleaning tool.
    • The faucet is turned on with water set at a comfortable temperature.
    • Take care throughout the procedure not to splash water onto surgical attire. Wet surgical attire can cause the transfer of microorganisms from personnel to the sterile gown worn during surgery.
    • Hands and forearms are washed with soap and running water.
    • The nail cleaner and sponge/brush are removed from the package.
    • The sponge/brush is held in one hand; under running water, the nail cleaner is used to clean nails and subungual spaces on the

other hand; the process is repeated with the opposite hand, and the nail cleaner is discarded.

- The nails and hands are rinsed.
- The sponge/brush, if it is impregnated with antimicrobial agent, is moistened. If it is not impregnated with antimicrobial surgical agent, an antimicrobial agent is added to the hands, usually from a foot-pump dispenser.
- The arms are held in a flexed position with the fingertips pointing upward. Throughout the scrub, the hands are held up and away from the body/surgical attire. The elbows are flexed and the hands held higher than the elbows. Water and cleanser flow from the fingertips (the cleanest area) to the elbow and into the sink.
- Using circular motion and pressure adequate to remove microorganisms but not sufficient to abrade skin, the nails, fingers, hands, and arms are methodically scrubbed, beginning with the fingertips and continuing through the forearms. The scrub sponge/brush is discarded.
- The hands and arms are rinsed, keeping arms flexed with hands above elbows as the scrubbed person enters the operating room.

147. The length of a surgical hand scrub should be determined by the product manufacturer's IFU.

Use of Alcohol-Based Hand Preparations

148. Alcohol-based surgical hand products (either waterless or water aided) are more effective than traditional scrub products in killing microorganisms. They require less time and reduce costs compared to the traditional products, and added emollients make these products gentle to the hands (CDC, 2002; WHO, 2009, p. 41). Nevertheless, all three types—the traditional scrub sponge/brush and antimicrobial surgical scrub agent, the alcohol-based waterless surgical scrub, and the alcohol-based water-aided solution—are considered acceptable by the CDC.

149. Regarding surgical hand preparation, an alcohol-based waterless surgical scrub was shown to have the same efficacy and demonstrated greater acceptability and fewest adverse effects on skin compared with an alcohol-based water-aided solution and a brush-based iodine solution (WHO, 2009, p. 41).

150. Procedures for using an alcohol-based hand rub vary; however, it is critical that the manufacturer's IFU be followed. The scrub procedure should include the following measures:

- Hands and forearms are washed with soap and running water.
- The nails and subungual areas of both hands are cleaned with a disposable nail cleaner at a minimum at the start of the first scrub of the day.
- Hands and forearms are rinsed and thoroughly dried with a clean towel (AORN, 2015, p. 35).

151. Instead of scrubbing according to the traditional scrub, an alcohol-based hand rub product approved by the FDA for use as a surgical hand antiseptic is applied to the hands and forearms.

- The amount of product applied and the procedure for use must be strictly in accordance with the manufacturer's instructions.
- Rub hands thoroughly until completely dry (AORN, 2015. p. 34).

152. Product selection and policies and procedures for surgical hand scrub should be determined in conjunction with the end users, operating room managers, and the healthcare facility infection control practitioner/committee.

Section Questions

1. Define the term *hand hygiene*. [Ref 123]
2. What is often considered the single most important step in the prevention of infection? [Ref 129]
3. Identify times when hand hygiene should be performed. [Ref 129]
4. When is hand washing with soap and water required? [Ref 130]
5. What is the purpose of mechanical hand washing? [Ref 131]
6. What is the objective of the surgical scrub? [Ref 133]
7. What should a scrubbed person do if he or she has a cut or lesion on the hands or arms? [Ref 135]

(continues)

Surgical Gowns

153. Sterile gowns should provide a barrier to the passage of microorganisms from the surgical team to the patient as well as from the patient to the surgical team. The gown manufacturer's data should validate that the materials used in the gown provide meet these criteria.

154. Gowns should be fire resistant, as lint free as possible, free from tears or holes, and fluid resistant or fluid proof. For procedures where little or no exposure to blood or body fluids is anticipated, a gown with minimal barrier protection is acceptable.

155. Fluid-resistant gowns should be worn whenever splashes or spraying of blood or other infectious fluids is anticipated. Where large amounts of fluid are anticipated, fluid-proof gowns should be worn. Fluid-resistant gowns provide an effective barrier and do not readily permit penetration of liquids. Fluid-proof gowns are coated or laminated with an impervious film that does not permit penetration of fluids.

156. Surgical gowns should also have the following desirable characteristics (AORN, 2015, p. 70):

   - Be resistant to penetration by blood and other body fluids

   - Maintain their integrity and be durable—resistant to tears, punctures, and abrasions

   - Be appropriate for the methods of sterilization available to the healthcare facility

   - Resist combustion

   - Be comfortable and contribute to maintaining the wearer's desired body temperature

   - Have a favorable cost–benefit ratio

157. Gown cuffs are made with stockinette and fit tight to the wrist. Gowns may or may not be wraparound style and are held closed with cotton tapes, snaps, or Velcro fasteners.

158. Sterile gloves provide a barrier to prevent passage of microorganisms from the scrubbed person to the patient and from the patient to the scrubbed person.

159. Selection of gloves takes into consideration-strength, durability, and compatibility. Extra-strength specialty gloves are available for procedures such as bone and joint surgeries where there is a high risk of percutaneous blood exposure.

160. Wearing a second pair of gloves over the first is known as double gloving. Double gloving has been shown to reduce skin contact with the patient's blood and/or body fluids during surgery. This practice also greatly reduces the amount of blood on a needle if a puncture does occur. Double gloving is included in the CDC recommendations for managing exposure to pathogens (CDC, 2012).

161. Double gloving is a widely practiced technique that decreases the risk of perforations of the inner glove. Double gloving is usually a personal preference; however, AORN (2015, p. 113) recommends that facility policies and procedures should indicate when double gloving is required.

162. Double gloving with indicator gloves can enhance the ability to recognize when the integrity of a glove has been compromised. The inner, indicator glove is colored and the outer glove is neutral. When a puncture occurs, a

dark-colored patch is visible through the outer glove at the site of perforation.

163. Most people who double glove recommend wearing a half-size larger inner glove, and one's regular glove size for the outer glove to reduce the amount of compression and maximize tactile sensitivity.

164. Latex-free gloves must be used when personnel or the patient has a latex allergy.

165. Hypoallergenic, powder-free gloves should be chosen to minimize sensitization to natural rubber latex and glove chemicals, especially for allergy-prone personnel.

166. Sterile gloves should be powder free. The potential adverse effects for patients from glove powder include an inflammatory response, delayed healing, foreign body reaction, formation of granulomas, and peritoneal adhesion, especially with multiple surgeries.

167. Powder/talc from latex gloves can serve as a carrier for airborne allergenic natural rubber latex proteins, potentially sensitizing patients and personnel. In 1997 & 2011, the FDA issued a report recognizing that "airborne glove powder represents a threat to individuals allergic to natural rubber latex and may represent an important agent for sensitizing non-allergic individuals" (p. 2). If used, powdered sterile gloves should be wiped clean with sterile water or saline prior to participating in the surgical procedure.

Closed Gloving

168. Closed gloving is one method of donning sterile gloves by oneself. Scrubbed hands remain inside the gown sleeve until the glove cuff is secured over the gown cuff.

169. Closed gloving is the preferred method, because it affords less opportunity for contamination.

170. Closed gloving begins with the hands inside the sleeves (**Figure 4-8**):

- Using the right hand that is still inside the right cuff, the scrubbed person grasps the everted cuff of the left glove.

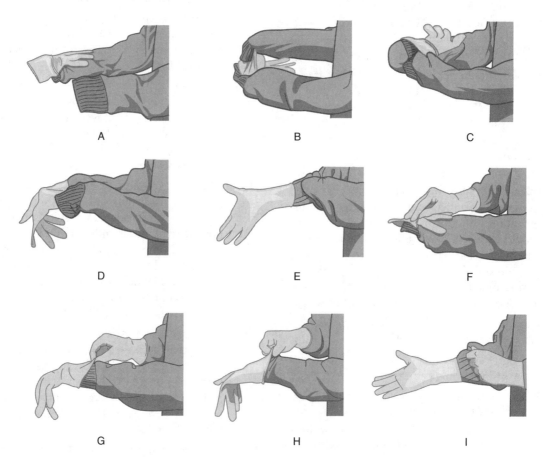

A   B   C

D   E   F

G   H   I

Figure 4-8 Closed gloving.
See Reference #170 for precise instructions.

- The left forearm is extended with the palm facing up and the hand still inside the sleeve. The left glove is then placed palm-side down on the upturned left sleeve, palm to palm, thumb to thumb, with the fingers of the glove pointing toward the scrubbed person's body.

- Using the left thumb and index finger inside the stockinette, grasp the cuff of the glove to hold it in place. The fingers of the left hand must not extend beyond the stockinette cuff.

- Using the sleeve-covered right hand, stretch the cuff of the left glove over the open end of the left sleeve. The glove should totally encompass the stockinette portion of the sleeve. Using the sleeve-covered right hand, pull gently but firmly on the left sleeve of the gown, causing the left hand to slide into the glove.

- To glove the right hand, grasp the right glove with the already gloved left hand and placed on the right sleeve, palm to palm, thumb to thumb, with glove fingers pointing toward the scrubbed person's body.

- Grasp the right glove cuff through the stockinette cuff to hold it in place. The fingers of the right hand must not extend beyond the stockinette cuff.

- Stretch the right glove over the open end of the right sleeve. Using the left hand, pull lightly and evenly on the right sleeve, causing the right hand to slide into the right glove.

Open Gloving

171. With open gloving, the surgically clean hand touches only the inside of the sterile glove and never contacts the exterior of the glove (**Figure 4-9**).

172. Open gloving has greater potential for contamination than closed gloving and it requires significant practice to master the technique.

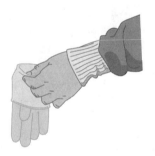

Step 1 – Lift glove touching only the inside (unsterile portion).

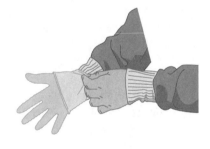

Step 2 – Work other hand into the glove as far as possible, being careful not to touch/contaminate the outside (sterile portion) of the glove.

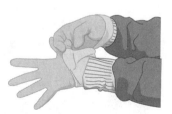

Step 3 – Slip gloved hand under cuff of second glove and work second hand into glove.

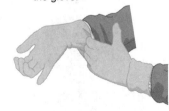

Step 4 – Pull each glove up to cover stockinette of gown, being careful to touch only the outside (sterile portion) of the glove.

Figure 4-9 Open gloving.

173. Open gloving is sometimes used to replace a contaminated glove during a surgical procedure. It is performed as follows:

    • A non-scrubbed person opens a glove package on a clean, dry surface for the scrubbed person replacing gloves.

    • Extend the hands through the stockinette cuff of the gown.

    • The unsterile hand can touch only the inside of the sterile glove.

    • Using the right hand, the scrub person grasps the everted cuff of the left glove and slides the fingers and thumb of the left hand into the glove. The glove cuff remains everted.

    • The scrub person slips the gloved fingers of the left hand under the everted cuff of the right glove and slides the right hand and fingers into the glove.

    • The left hand brings up the right cuff completely enclosing the stockinette cuff of the gown.

    • Using the gloved right hand, the scrub person slips the fingers under the everted cuff of the left glove and completely covers the stockinette cuff of the gown.

    • If the exterior portion of either sterile glove touches skin or stockinette, the glove must be discarded and the process repeated.

Gowning and Gloving

174. A gown package containing a sterile towel and sterile gown is opened on a surface separate from the instrument or back table to prevent contamination of the sterile field. The gown and towel are packaged so that the towel is on top of the gown when the package is opened.

175. Scrub persons who perform a traditional scrub procedure must first dry their hands and arms thoroughly. Wet hands and arms can contaminate the gown by strike-through, and gloves are difficult to pull on.

176. Following are the steps in the gowning procedure (**Figure 4-10**):

    • Grasp the sterile towel and lift it up and away from the folded gown without dripping water on the gown or the sterile field.

    • Step back from the sterile field and allow the towel to unfold without touching anything. If the towel contacts an unsterile surface, the towel is considered contaminated and a new sterile one must be used.

    • Holding the top of the towel with one hand, dry the other hand thoroughly using a rotating, blotting technique beginning at the hand and working down toward the elbow.

    • When the first hand and forearm are dry, grasp the unused lower half of the towel with the dry hand, and dry the opposite hand in the same way. Take care not to return to an area that has already been dried.

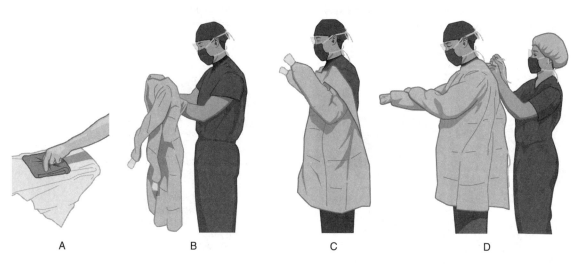

A   B   C   D

Figure 4-10 Gowning.

- The gown is folded so that slots for hands to enter the sleeves are immediately accessible. Lift the gown by reaching into the slots, the inside facing your chest with the neckline at the top.

- Step backward and allow the gown to unfold, being careful that it touches nothing.

- Slide arms into armholes. Do not allow fingers to extend beyond the stockinette. The circulating nurse should be available to assist with fastening the gown at the neck and pulling down at the hem to straighten out folds and wrinkles.

- Using the closed technique to don sterile gloves.

- The last step is wrapping the gown around the body and tying the belt. Extend the cardboard tab attached to one of the gown ties to the circulating nurse. Pivot in the direction that causes the gown to encircle the body. Pull the tie from the cardboard that remains in the circulator's hand and tie the two ends of the belt. A sterile team member can also assist with this final step.

Assisting Others to Gown and Glove

177. The scrub person places a towel over the outstretched hand of the newly scrubbed person, being careful not to touch that person's hands. A towel for drying hands is not necessary if an alcohol-based surgical hand product was used.

178. The scrubbed person then grasps the folded gown at the neck edge, facing in the opposite direction from when gowning oneself. Using the neck and shoulder area of the gown to form a protective cuff over the gloves, the scrubbed person holds the gown firmly while the newly scrubbed team member inserts arms into sleeves (**Figure 4-11**).

179. The circulator should be available to help the individual into the gown, pulling the sleeves from the inside so that the individual's hands pass through the stockinette cuff of the gown. The scrubbed person will then glove the newly scrubbed team member. The sterile glove is grasped under the everted edge, with the thumb of the glove facing the thumb of the person being gloved, and stretching the glove wide so that the person's hand can advance easily into the glove.

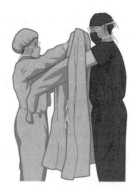

Figure 4-11 Gowning others.

180. Hold the glove steady as the person pushes the hand into the glove. When the hand and stockinette cuff are completely into the glove, gently let go before the person begins to raise his or her hand. If you wait too long to let go, the stockinette will no longer be covered by the glove. Repeat this procedure to glove the other hand.

181. If a team member's glove becomes contaminated, that person steps back from the sterile field and extends the contaminated hand to the circulator who removes the sterile team member's contaminated glove by grasping the outside of the glove approximately 2 inches below the top of the glove and pulling the glove off inside out. The gown cuff must not be pulled down or slip down over the hand because the stockinette is considered contaminated once the original gloves are donned.

182. The scrubbed person may reglove the team member in the same manner as before, or the open-glove technique can be used to reglove without assistance.

183. If a team member's gown becomes contaminated, the circulator unfastens the gown at the neck and waist, grasps it in front at the shoulders, and pulls it forward and off over the scrubbed person's hands, which are still gloved. The gown should come off in an inside-out manner. The contaminated gown should always be removed before the gloves are removed to prevent microorganisms and debris from the gown from being dragged across unprotected, ungloved hands.

184. The circulator removes the sterile team member's gloves, and the scrubbed person regowns and regloves the sterile team member, or the

sterile team member may regown and reglove without assistance.

185. The closed-glove technique is not acceptable for changing a contaminated glove. During initial gowning and gloving, the stockinette cuff is contaminated when the scrubbed, but not sterile, hand passes through it. Using the closed-glove technique, the contaminated cuff would contaminate the new sterile glove.

186. Following the procedure described earlier, gown and gloves are removed. The gown is removed first. Grasp near the neck and sleeve and pull the gown forward over the gloved hands, inverting the gloves you pull your arms from the gown. The gown is folded so the contaminated outside surface is on the inside. It is discarded in a designated linen or waste receptacle.

187. Gloves are removed in a manner that prevents the contaminated external glove from contacting skin. Place the gloved fingers of one hand under the everted glove cuff of the opposite hand and pull the glove off. Grasp the fold on the remaining glove with the bare fingers of the opposite hand and pull the glove off. Perform this technique carefully to prevent bare

skin from contacting the contaminated glove surface. Gloves are discarded in a designated waste receptacle.

188. After gloves are removed, wash your hands or use an antimicrobial product. Hand hygiene lessens the chance of cross-contamination from organisms that might be there as a result of an invisible hole or tear in the glove.

189. Gown and gloves are always discarded before leaving the operating room.

The Sterile Field

Draping

190. Drapes serve as a barrier to prevent the passage of microorganisms between sterile and nonsterile areas. Sterile drapes are used to create a *sterile field* that incorporates the incision site and the area required for sterile supplies and equipment (**Figure 4-12**).

191. The sterile field separates the sterile from the unsterile. Only sterile items are placed on a sterile field.

192. Sterile drapes are positioned over the patient in such a way that only a minimum area of skin around the incision site is exposed.

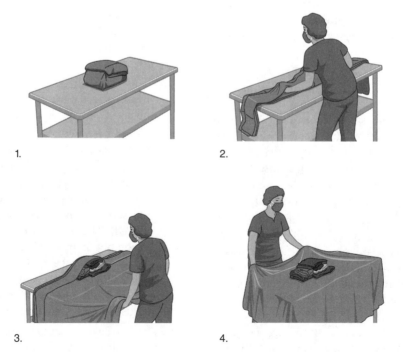

1. 2. 3. 4.

Figure 4-12 Draping a table.

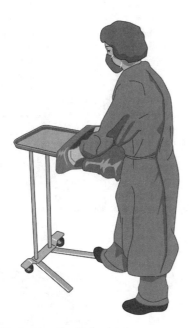

Figure 4-13 Draping the Mayo stand.

193. Furniture draped to be part of the sterile field often includes the instrument table or *back table*, the Mayo (**Figure 4-13**) stands, and ring stands that hold basins.

194. Single-use/disposable drapes are composed of nonwoven synthetic materials and are manufactured with varying degrees of barrier effectiveness. These fabrics include a fluid-proof polyethylene film laminated between the fabric layers at strategic locations of the drape, usually around the drape fenestration. Drapes are available in a variety of configurations and are commercially packaged and sterilized. They are designed for one-time use and must be used or discarded once the package has been opened.

195. Drapes should meet the following criteria:
    - Resistant to blood, body fluids, and liquid penetration and provide an effective barrier to prevent passage of microorganisms from nonsterile to sterile areas
    - Durable—resistant to tears
    - Lint free or low linting to reduce airborne contamination or shedding into the operative site—microorganisms and dust particles may settle on airborne lint and shed into the operative site
    - Flame resistant
    - Memory free—conform easily to body and equipment contours
    - Comfortable

196. As with gowns, drapes may be fluid resistant or fluid proof. Materials have varying degrees of resistance to liquids and should be selected based on the intended procedure and anticipated exposure to fluids.

197. Clear plastic drapes, with an adhesive strip or adhesive backing, are available in various sizes. They may be plain or impregnated with an antimicrobial agent.

198. Plastic drapes with adhesive backing are called *incise drapes* and adhere to the skin at the operative site to aid in preventing migration of microorganisms into the wound. The incision is made through the plastic drape. Incise drapes also adhere to the disposable drapes and can assist in keeping them in place.

199. Some plastic drapes include a pouch to collect fluids that might otherwise accumulate under the drapes where bacteria can proliferate and contaminate the wound.

200. Plastic drapes are useful for draping irregular body areas such as joints, eyes, and ears.

201. Plastic drapes with an adhesive edge may also be used to seal off a contaminated area such as a stoma or to protect a tourniquet from fluids during prepping.

202. Impervious plastic drapes are also available to cover equipment, such as microscopes, portable C arm, and X-ray equipment, that must be close enough to the field to contaminate it without a sterile cover.

Draping Guidelines

203. The following are guidelines for draping (AORN, 2015, pp. 76–78):
    - Only intact sterile drapes can be used for draping. Drapes with defects that compromise barrier protection must be discarded. Whenever the sterility of a drape is in doubt, it is considered contaminated.
    - Drapes should be handled as little as possible.
    - Drapes are carried folded to the operating table; draping begins at the operative site and progresses to the periphery (**Figure 4-14**).
    - Once a drape is placed, it is not moved or repositioned. Repositioning drapes can contaminate the incisional area that has been prepped. Drapes that are placed incorrectly are removed by an unscrubbed person.

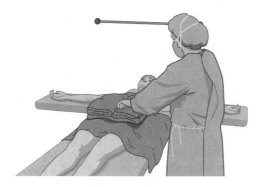

1. Place folded lap sheet over incision site,

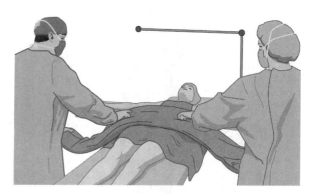

2. and open from side to side, allowing the ends to fall below the table,

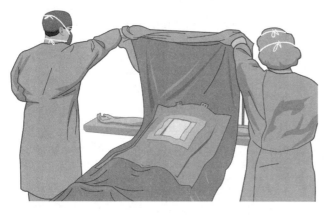

3. then over the top and secured to anesthesia screen or I.V. poles. Arm extensions incorporated into the drape cover the armboards.

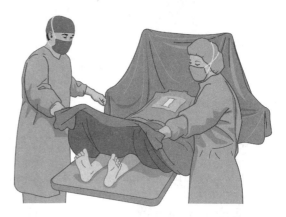

4. Drape lap sheet over the lower portion of patient and table.

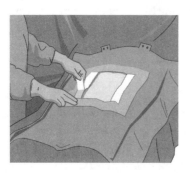

5. Surgeon removes release paper from adhesive strips on both sides of fenestration,

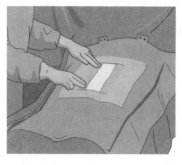

6. and adheres strips to secure the fenestration.

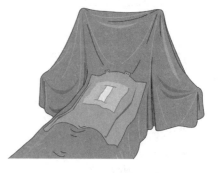

7. The completed laparotomy draping procedure.

Figure 4-14 Draping a patient.

- Drapes are placed gently; they must not be flipped or shaken. Shaking and flipping cause air currents that serve as vehicles for dust, lint, and other particles.

- When draping, a cuff is formed from the drape to protect the sterile gloved hands of the person draping.

- The points of a towel clip that have penetrated a drape are contaminated and must not be removed until the procedure is complete. Use non-penetrating towel clips when possible, because they do not interrupt the integrity of drapes and can be removed and repositioned.

Standard Drapes

204. The number, type, and size of drapes selected for a procedure depend upon the location of the incision, the amount of area around the incision that needs to be included in the sterile field, and the furniture and equipment that will be draped.

205. Standard drapes include the following options:

    - Flat sheets in various sizes
    - Mayo stand covers
    - Towels used to drape the operative site
    - Procedure-specific drapes—drapes with fenestrations of various sizes and configurations to accommodate specific incisions such as laparotomy, chest/breast, thyroid, total hip joint, and extremity. Fenestrations are often reinforced with an impervious barrier. The fenestrated drape is large enough to cover the entire patient and the operating table with sufficient material to extend over the foot of the table, the ether screen (or IV poles) at the head of the table, and the arm boards. If the drape does not cover sufficiently, flat sheets can be used to extend the sterile field.
    - Aperture drape—a small, clear fenestrated plastic drape frequently used in eye and ear procedures
    - Equipment drapes—clear plastic drapes that cover X-ray machines, microscopes, and other equipment
    - Stockinette, with or without an impervious layer, used to drape extremities
    - Leggings—part of the lithotomy drape set
    - Various specialty drapes (e.g., cesarean, craniotomy, cardiac)

Section Questions

1. Describe the desired characteristics of a sterile gown. [Refs 154, 156]

2. Explain the importance of double gloving. [Ref 160]

3. Who determines when two pair of gloves should be worn? [Ref 161]

4. Explain how an indicator glove system can help to identify when the integrity of a glove has been compromised. [Ref 162]

5. What adverse outcomes have been associated with glove powder? [Refs 166–167]

6. Why is the closed method of gloving preferable to the open method? [Ref 169]

7. When is it appropriate to "open glove"? [Ref 173]

8. Why should the scrub person open his or her gown and gloves on a surface away from the back table? [Ref 174]

9. Describe the correct position of the gown when the scrub person holds it before putting it on. [Ref 176]

10. Describe the process of donning gown and gloves. [Ref 176]

11. How does the scrub person wrap the gown around him- or herself and tie it? [Ref 176]

12. How does the circulator assist when the scrub person is gowning another individual? [Ref 179]

13. When gloving another individual, why do you let go of the glove before the other person begins to raise his or her hand? [Ref 180]

14. When a team member requires regloving, what is important about how the circulator removes the contaminated glove? [Ref 181]

15. Why is the contaminated gown always removed before contaminated gloves? [Ref 183]

16. Why is the closed method of gloving not used to change a contaminated glove during a procedure? [Ref 185]

17. How are gown and gloves removed following a procedure? [Refs 186–187]

(continues)

Section Questions (continued)

18. Why must hands be washed (or an antimicrobial product used) after gloves are removed? [Ref 188]

19. What is the purpose of sterile drapes? [Ref 190]

20. Describe a *sterile field* and its purpose. [Refs 190–191]

21. What are some desirable characteristics of sterile drapes? [Refs 194–197]

22. What is the purpose of an incise drape? [Ref 198]

23. Describe some other uses for plastic drapes. [Refs 198–202]

24. How is the sterile field protected when items such as X-ray equipment and microscopes are used? [Ref 202]

25. Which part of the patient is draped first? [Ref 203]

26. Why are drapes not moved once they have been positioned? [Ref 203]

27. Why is flipping or shaking drapes during the draping process prohibited? [Ref 203]

28. What is the purpose of making a cuff of the sterile material when draping? [Ref 203]

29. Why can perforating towel clips not be repositioned? [Ref 203]

30. Describe the variety of drapes available for creating a sterile field. [Ref 205]

Creating and Maintaining a Sterile Field

206. A sterile field should be prepared and maintained for surgical and invasive procedures. Items introduced to a sterile field should be opened, dispensed, and transferred by methods that maintain sterility.

207. Only scrubbed, gowned, and gloved persons can enter the sterile field. Surgical gowns, gloves, and drapes establish a barrier that minimizes the passage of microorganisms between nonsterile and sterile areas.

208. Once donned, the gown is considered sterile in front from the chest to the level of the sterile field. The sleeves are considered sterile from 2 inches above the elbow down to the top edge of the cuff. The neckline, shoulders, axilla, and cuffed portion of the sleeves may become contaminated by perspiration and, therefore, are not considered sterile. The back is considered nonsterile because it cannot be observed by the scrubbed person to ensure that it has not been contaminated. The cuffs are considered contaminated once the hands have passed through them (AORN, 2015, pp. 72–73).

209. Sterile drapes are used to create a sterile field (AORN, 2015, pp. 76–78). Sterile drapes are placed on the patient and on all furniture and equipment that will be part of the sterile field. Sterile drapes serve as a barrier to the passage of microorganisms, isolate the sterile field from the surrounding environment, and minimize passage of microorganisms between sterile and nonsterile areas.

210. Items used within a sterile field must be sterile (AORN, 2015, p. 78). Items for use during surgery are disinfected, packaged, and sterilized prior to surgery.

211. Both the person delivering the item and the person accepting it must ensure sterility of items delivered to the field. The circulating nurse should check the integrity of the wrapper, the expiration date (if there is one), and the color of the process indicator tape.

212. Both the circulator and the scrub person should check the chemical indicator inside the package to ensure that the parameters of sterilization were met during the sterilization process.

213. Only when absolutely necessary can "just in time" sterilization (immediate-use steam sterilization, or IUSS) be used to reprocess an item that is taken directly from the autoclave to the sterile field.

214. If an item is processed with IUSS, the circulating nurse must use proper technique for

cleaning and disinfecting the item, sterilizing it, and transferring it to the sterile field.

215. Wrappers, gowns, gloves, and drapes are all examples of sterile barriers. Whenever the integrity of a sterile barrier is broken, the contents must be considered unsterile. For example, a tear or hole in a wrapper means the contents of the package must be considered contaminated. A glove that has been contaminated must be discarded and replaced.

216. The contents of wet or stained wrappers may have been subject to strike-through, which occurs when liquids soak through a barrier from an unsterile area to a sterile area or vice versa. Strike-through allows for passage of microorganisms through the barrier, so the contents must be considered contaminated.

217. When strike-through occurs, it might not be noticed initially and the wrapper might dry.

Items in a package with a water-stained wrapper should be considered contaminated.

218. If the sterility of any item is in doubt, it is considered contaminated and is discarded. Remember, "*When it doubt, throw it out!*" Contaminated items must not be permitted on the sterile field.

219. Items that remain on the drapes during the procedure, such as suction and electrosurgical pencil, should be secured to prevent them from sliding below the surface of the sterile field. An item that slides below the level of the sterile field is considered contaminated and must be discarded.

220. When delivering an item to the sterile field, the circulator should open the wrapper flap that is farthest away first and the wrapper flap that is closest last. This prevents an unsterile body part from having to reach across a sterile field (**Figure 4-15**).

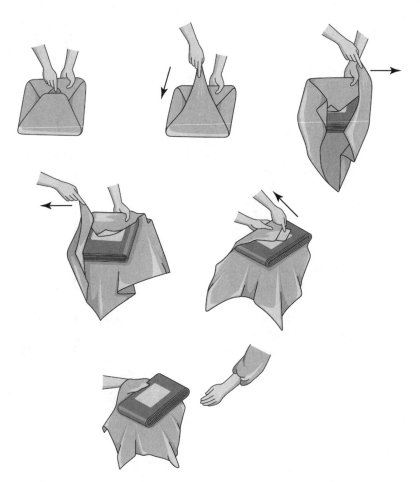

Figure 4-15 Opening a package.

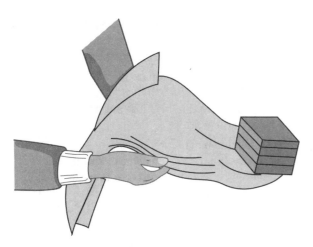

Figure 4-16 Delivering unwrapped item to the sterile field.

221. The circulator should secure all wrapper flaps to prevent accidental contamination of the scrubbed person or sterile field with a wrapper edge.

222. If an item cannot be carefully placed onto the field, the item should be presented directly to the scrubperson or opened on a separate surface.

223. Sterile gowns and drapes and other similar items are placed onto the sterile field, the field is protected from the contaminated hand and arm of the circulator by the sterile drape or wrapper (**Figure 4-16**).

224. Items that are heavy, awkward, or sharp should not be tossed onto the sterile field, because they may roll off the edge, knock other items from the field, or penetrate the sterile barrier. Open these items on a separate surface or deliver them directly to the scrub person (**Figure 4-17**).

225. When delivering solutions to the sterile field, pour the entire contents of bottle into a receptacle placed near the table's edge or held by the scrubbed person. This precludes reaching across the sterile field and decreases the risk of splashing and creating the potential for strike-through.

226. Once removed, the bottle cap should not be replaced. Deliver the entire contents to the field, or discard what is left in the bottle (**Figure 4-18**).

227. Solutions should be verified with the scrubbed person before being delivered to the sterile field. The scrubperson labels the container and verifies the information with the circulating nurse. Use a transfer device such as a sterile vial spike to dispense medications to the sterile field. The stopper of the medicine vial should not be removed, and the medication

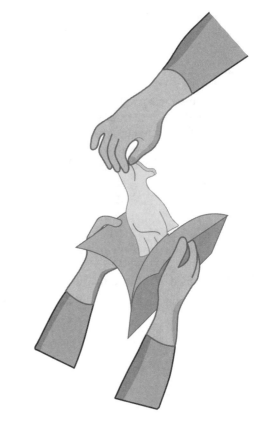

Figure 4-17 Retrieving an item.

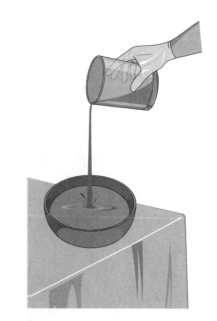

Figure 4-18 Pouring liquid.

should not be poured into a medicine glass on the field (AORN, 2015, p. 307).

228. Open rigid container systems on a separate surface. Verify that the process indicator has

changed color. Ensure the locks are intact to verify that the integrity of the container has not been previously breached.

229. Lift the lid of the container up and toward you to avoid leaning over the sterile contents. Check the filter for integrity and color change of the embedded process indicator.

230. A sterile field should be set up as close to the time of surgery as possible. The longer sterile items are open to the environment, the greater the opportunity for contamination to occur. There is no standard for the length of time a sterile field may remain open before it is considered contaminated. Facility policy may identify a timeframe.

231. Once a sterile field has been created, it should never be left unattended. The field should be monitored at all times for possible contamination (AORN, 2015, p. 83).

232. In the event that a sterile field is created in anticipation of surgery and the surgery is delayed, the sterile field should be under constant visual observation. The nature of the surgical procedure should be considered. If the surgery is emergent and a delay caused by having to set up another sterile field would seriously compromise patient safety, the best decision may be to continue monitoring and preserve the sterile field.

233. Covering a sterile field must be done so that any part of the drape that falls below the level of the field never passes over the field (AORN, 2015, p. 84). This requires two drapes (**Figure 4-19**). A covered field must still be monitored.

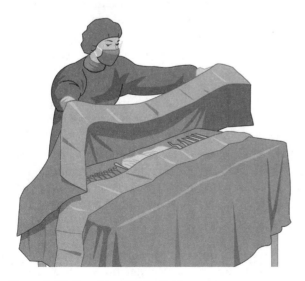

Figure 4-19 Covering a Sterile Field.

234. AORN (2015, p. 86) recommends maintaining a distance of at least 12 inches between the sterile field and unsterile areas and personnel. Some facilities practice the "18-inch rule." Check your facility policy on aseptic technique.

235. Good judgment and keen observation will ensure that only sterile items are introduced to the sterile field.

236. All personnel moving within or around a sterile field should do so in a manner that will maintain the sterility of the field. Scrubbed personnel should remain close to and always face the sterile field (**Figure 4-18**).

237. Unscrubbed personnel should face sterile fields on approach, should not walk between two sterile fields, and should be aware of the need to maintain distance from the sterile field. By establishing traffic patterns around the sterile field and keeping sterile areas in view, accidental contamination can be reduced.

238. Scrubbed personnel should keep their arms and hands above the level of their waists at all times. Hands should remain visible, in front of the body, and above waist level at all times. Contamination may occur when arms and hands are moved below waist level.

239. Arms should not be folded with the hands in the axilla. This area has the potential to become contaminated by perspiration, allowing for strike-through of the gown and, ultimately, contamination of the gloved hands.

240. Scrubbed personnel should avoid changing levels and should be seated only when the entire surgical procedure will be performed at that level. When changing levels, jeopardizing the sterility of the sterile portion of the surgical gown is likely.

241. The patient is the center of the sterile field. All additional sterile equipment is grouped around the patient within view of the scrubbed person.

242. When a break in sterile technique occurs, corrective action should be taken immediately unless the patient's safety is at risk. If the patient's safety is at risk, correct the break in technique as soon as it is safe to do so.

243. When a break in sterile technique occurs and cannot be corrected immediately, it should be reported and recorded, and the wound classification should be adjusted accordingly and documented on the operative record.

Section Questions

1. What are the criteria for entering the sterile field? [Ref 207]

2. Explain why certain parts of a gown are considered sterile and other parts unsterile. [Ref 208]

3. Who is responsible for assuring the sterility of a sterile item—the person delivering the item or the person accepting it? [Ref 211]

4. What steps do the scrub person and circulator take to insure the integrity of sterile items delivered to the sterile field? [Refs 211–212]

5. What is the significance of a water stain on a sterile package? [Refs 216–217]

6. Why is the saying "when in doubt, throw it out" so important in a sterile environment? [Ref 218]

7. What is the purpose of managing the far flap first when opening a sterile package? [Ref 220]

8. How should items that are difficult to manage be delivered to the sterile field? [Ref 222]

9. How is the field protected from contamination when the circulator opens a package and places the contents on the field? [Ref 223]

10. What might happen if heavy, awkward, or sharp instruments are tossed onto the sterile field? [Ref 224]

11. Describe the responsibilities involved in delivering solutions to the sterile field. [Refs 225–227]

12. What responsibilities are associated with opening a rigid container and delivering the contents to the sterile field? [Refs 228, 230]

13. How long can a sterile field remain open in anticipation of a procedure? [Ref 230–231]

14. Describe the proper method for covering a sterile field. [Ref 233, **Figure 4-19**]

15. Why should a scrub person avoid sitting down while waiting for a procedure to begin? [Ref 240]

Operating Room Environment

244. Items that are considered contaminated, soiled, or dirty should not be transported through the same corridors as clean and sterile items. However, when an operating room is accessed by a single corridor, contaminated items leaving the operating room should be secured within a container to protect the environment from contamination.

245. An operating room suite designed with a sterile core surrounded by operating rooms eliminates having to move both sterile and contaminated supplies through the same space. Supplies, sterile storage, equipment, and the elevator from the sterile processing department are contained within the sterile core. Contaminated items leave the operating room into a peripheral hallway that leads to the decontamination area.

246. The operating room is considered a clean environment. The design of the operating room, its location within the healthcare facility, limited access, traffic patterns, and policies and procedures for control and environmental cleaning help to maintain its cleanliness.

247. Items delivered to the operating room from sources outside the healthcare facility should be removed from external shipping cartons before being permitted into the operating room. Outside shipping cartons may harbor insects and dirt collected during transport (AORN, 2015, p. 617).

248. Items and supplies prepared or selected for surgical cases that are delivered to the operating room from departments within the healthcare facility should be transported in closed or covered carts to reduce the potential for contamination.

249. The operating room should have a separate ventilation and air filtration system. All air is filtered through a special filter system. Filters are designed to remove dust and aerosol particles from the air. All airflow is from ceiling to floor.

250. Ventilation systems must comply with local, state, and national regulations. When regulations vary in the requirement for the number

of air exchanges per hour and the number of fresh air exchanges required, the most stringent requirements prevail.

251. To maintain the cleanest air possible, the Facility Guidelines Institute (FGI), U.S. Department of Health and Human Services (HHS), the American Society for Healthcare Engineering (ASHE), and the Centers for Medicare and Medicaid Services (CMS) recommend an airflow rapid enough to change the total volume of air in each operating room a minimum of 20 times per hour with at least 4 exchanges of outside air (CMS, 2011; FGI, HHS, & ASHE, 2014).

252. Air in the operating room is maintained under positive pressure. The air pressure is higher in each operating room than in the hallways so that the more contaminated hallway air cannot enter the room.

253. Special negative-pressure rooms are designed specifically for procedures that produce aerosolized contamination such as bronchoscopy or when the patient has tuberculosis. The negative pressure assures that the air inside the room cannot escape into the less contaminated hallway.

254. To maintain both positive and negative pressures, doors must be kept closed at all times.

255. Some operating rooms have laminar airflow systems for procedures where the risk of infection is high, or when an infection can cause a disastrous patient outcome, such as total joint replacement.

- A laminar airflow system is a unidirectional ventilation system in which filtered, bacteria-free, "ultraclean" air is circulated over the patient from a filtered outlet and returned through a receiving air inlet.
- Air is filtered through high-efficiency particulate air (HEPA) filters that remove all particles equal to or greater than 0.3 micron in size with an efficiency of 99.7%.
- Laminar airflow systems can deliver more than 200 air exchanges per hour.
- Only sterile items are permitted within the area across which the filtered air flows.

256. Temperature in the operating room should be maintained between 68°F and 75°F (20°C and 24°C). This is comfortable enough for the surgical team, yet will inhibit bacterial growth.

257. Relative humidity is maintained at 20% to 60% (AAMI, 2015). Higher humidity can provide an opportunity for mold growth, and lower humidity can result in an excessive amount of dust that can carry bacteria.

Operating Room Sanitation

258. To promote a clean environment, surface materials in the operating room should be nonporous, smooth, washable, and easy to clean. Wall, ceiling, and floor joints are completely sealed. Floor coverings are nonporous.

259. Operating room sanitation practices play a significant role in minimizing the number of microorganisms present. Microorganisms can survive on many environmental surfaces; in fact, the inanimate environment may serve as a reservoir for infectious organisms. MRSA can remain for months, and *Clostridium difficile* can form spores that survive for years on inanimate surfaces. Rigorous cleaning practices are essential to minimize the numbers of pathogens present in the operating room.

260. Although cleaning and housekeeping protocols may vary among healthcare facilities, there are cleaning procedures for implementation prior to the beginning of the day's schedule, during the procedure, between procedures, at the end of the daily schedule, and periodically (e.g., weekly or monthly).

261. Only products registered with the Environmental Protection Agency (EPA) as hospital-grade disinfectants should be used for cleaning inanimate surfaces in the operating room.

262. Persons responsible for cleaning and who, in the course of their work, have the potential to contact contaminated items, blood, or body fluids must wear personal protective attire (e.g., gloves, masks, eyewear, and gowns) that is appropriate to the task performed.

263. Prior to the first procedure of the day, the circulator should visually assess the cleanliness of the room, and if necessary notify housekeeping or environmental services.

264. Damp-dust furniture, equipment, and surgical lights with a lint-free cloth moistened with an EPA-registered hospital-grade disinfectant. Pay particular attention to horizontal surfaces, because dust and lint that transport microorganisms settle on these surfaces. Alcohol and high-level disinfectants used for instrument processing should not be used for operating-room sanitation (AORN, 2015, pp. 12–13).

265. Wipe down equipment from other areas, such as X-ray machines and tourniquet devices that are necessary for the procedure, before they are brought into the room.

266. Video and computer monitors and plasma screens may not be compatible with the germicide used on other surfaces. Consult the manufacturer's IFU to determine the most appropriate cleaning products.

267. If possible, patients known to have a latex allergy should be the first scheduled cases of the day. Latex products used during the day may cause latex particles to remain airborne for a period of time, and damp dusting may not be sufficient to remove all traces of latex protein.

268. Throughout the procedure, confine contamination to as small an area around the patient and sterile field as possible.

269. Clean up spills or splashes of blood and body fluids that occur in the immediate vicinity of the sterile field promptly using a soft disposable cloth and an intermediate-level germicide intended for hospital use. The germicide should be EPA registered and should have a tuberculocidal claim. Amount and dilution should be determined by the manufacturer's IFU.

270. Spill kits should be available for large spills of body fluids and for chemicals such as glutaraldehyde.

271. Persons responsible for cleanup should wear PPE appropriate to the exposure.

272. Disposable items that become contaminated should be discarded into leak-proof and tear-resistant containers to prevent contact with the environment and with personnel who are responsible for handling operating room waste.

273. Sponges are discarded into a plastic-lined bucket or other prepared surface. They are collected in clear, impervious counting bags, counted as soon as possible, and sealed.

274. Blood, body secretions, and other fluids from the sterile field are collected in leak-proof containers.

275. Specimens should be placed in clean, leak-proof containers. Take the specimen from the sterile field, seal the container, and, if necessary, wipe the container with an EPA-registered, hospital-grade germicide. Take care to prevent contamination of specimen documentation and other records.

276. Contaminated reusable items that fall or are removed from the sterile field should be wiped with a germicide and placed in an impervious container. Persons handling contaminated items must wear gloves.

277. All items that are delivered to the sterile field or come in contact with the patient are considered contaminated and, if single use/disposable, should be discarded according to local, state, and national waste regulations that specify what constitutes infectious waste. Disposable items contaminated with infectious waste are deposited in leak-proof containers or bags that are color coded, tagged, or labeled so as to be immediately recognizable as hazardous waste (OSHA, 2011). Examples of such waste include gowns, gloves, sponges, and suture threads.

278. Infectious waste fluids may be poured down a drain connected to a sanitary sewer if regulations permit. Alternatively, the collection container may be sealed and placed in a leak-proof container or bag that is color coded and tagged or labeled so as to be immediately recognizable as hazardous waste. Many institutions use chemical agents to solidify liquid waste to reduce the possibility of spills. Follow local regulations to ensure the safety of the entire community.

279. Noninfectious disposable items are deposited into receptacles not designated for infectious waste; these containers are then sealed and removed from the room.

280. Disposal and treatment of infectious waste is significantly more costly than disposal and treatment of noninfectious waste. It is important to be able to differentiate between infectious and noninfectious waste.

281. Not all items contaminated with blood are defined as infectious waste. Some regulations define infectious waste as items contaminated with blood or other materials that, if compressed, would release blood or other infectious material.

282. Sharp items, such as needles, staples, and scalpel blades, are considered infectious waste. They are deposited in a designated leak-proof, puncture-resistant sharps container identified with a biohazard label (OSHA, 2011). Sharps containers are sealed and replaced by designated personnel.

283. Reusable linen that is identified as infectious is placed in a closeable bag that is color

coded, tagged, or labeled as infectious waste (OSHA, 2011). When contaminated linen is wet, it should be placed in a bag that prevents leak-through. Reusable noninfectious items are transported, cleaned, and disinfected or sterilized according to the healthcare facility's policy.

284. Following the procedure, all instruments opened for the procedure, whether or not they were actually used, are considered contaminated and must be appropriately cleaned and processed. Instruments from sets should be kept together. All items to be returned to the sterile processing department should be placed in designated closed carts, labeled as a biohazard, and transported to a designated area.

285. Following a procedure, the furniture, including operating lights, linen hamper frames, the operating room bed and mattress, suction canisters, and other equipment used during the procedure should be wiped with an EPA-registered, hospital-grade germicidal agent intended for housekeeping purposes. Wipe and reline kick buckets. Wipe down patient transport vehicles, including straps, railings, and other attachments with an EPA-registered hospital-grade germicidal agent. Include items that contact the patient, such as blood pressure cuffs, positioning devices, and tourniquets.

286. Clean any equipment or furniture that is visibly soiled with an EPA-registered, hospital-grade germicide. Wipe down walls, doors, push plates, handles, cabinets, lights, and other areas that are visibly soiled. If visibly soiled, the floor around the operating room table should be cleaned with an EPA-registered, hospital-grade germicidal agent.

287. A clean mop head should be used for each cleanup. The mop should not be dipped back into the solution once it has been used. If the used mop is not dipped into the solution, the solution may be used for subsequent cleanups, provided a clean mop head is also used. A clean mop head should be used for each room/patient procedure. Individual institutional policies for cleaning the floor may vary, and floor cleaning when there is no visible soil may not be necessary after each procedure (AORN, 2015, p. 13).

288. A number of hospitals have switched from string mops to microfiber mops because they are lightweight, require less water for rinsing, attract and retain negatively charged dust and dirt particles and are cost-effective when labor costs are calculated (EPA, 2002).

289. At the conclusion of the day's schedule, operating and procedure rooms, scrub-utility areas, corridors, furnishings, and equipment should be terminally cleaned.

290. Items that should be cleaned daily include the following:

- Surgical lights and tracks
- Equipment towers
- Computer keyboards
- IV poles
- Scrub sinks, including the faucet head and aerator
- Horizontal surfaces such as tables and countertops
- Furniture—particular attention should be given to castors and wheels
- Drawer, door, and cabinet handles
- Push plates
- Ventilation grills
- Cabinet and operating room doors
- Utility carts
- Floors in the operating room, scrub sink area, and corridor (floors in the operating room should be wet-vacuumed)
- Any food left out in the lounge area should be discarded or sealed and/or refrigerated as appropriate

291. Reusable cleaning equipment is disassembled, cleaned, and dried prior to storage.

292. Many items and areas within the operating room are cleaned periodically (e.g., weekly, monthly, or as otherwise indicated in the facility's policies). The facility should have written policies that address cleaning schedules, techniques, and persons responsible for the following:

- Lounges, locker areas, and offices
- Holding areas
- Cabinet shelves
- Walls
- Ceilings
- Air-conditioning vents, grills, and filters
- Ice machines and refrigerators
- Sterilizers
- Restrooms
- Storage areas

293. The anesthesia department is generally responsible for cleaning and caring for its own equipment. The AORN-recommended practices for cleaning, handling, and processing of anesthesia equipment can serve as guidelines for developing institutional policies and procedures.

Additional Considerations: Cleaning and Scheduling

294. Standard precautions consider all surgical patients to be infectious, and the potential for cross-infection exists for all procedures. No special management is required for patients known to be infected with HIV, hepatitis, or other infectious diseases, including scheduling them as the last procedure of the day. Routine cleaning, however, must be adequate and thorough.

295. Patients with airborne- and droplet-transmitted infectious diseases are an exception to this rule. These patients should be scheduled when personnel and patient traffic is minimal so that exposure is reduced. Scheduling as the last case of the day may be appropriate for these patients. A negative-pressure environment is appropriate for these patients.

Special Considerations

Clostridium difficile

296. Although standard and transmission-based precautions are adequate in regard to cleaning of equipment and surfaces contaminated or suspected to be contaminated with resistant microorganisms such as MRSA, there is a heightened awareness of the need for strict adherence to cleaning protocols when organisms are resistant to antibacterial agents and pose an infection risk.

297. *C. difficile* is a spore-forming bacterium that can survive for months on environmental surfaces (CDC, 2015c).

298. When caring for a patient infected with *C. difficile*, alcohol hand rubs are *not* recommended. Alcohol is not effective against *C. difficile*. Hand hygiene should consist of washing hands with antimicrobial soap and water.

299. For surface areas where epidemiology indicates transmission of *C. difficile*, use only cleaning agents that have been validated for the removal of *C. difficile*. Initially, chlorine was the agent of choice but many nonchlorine products are now EPA approved for the removal of *C. difficile* spores.

Creutzfeldt-Jakob Disease

300. Creutzfeldt-Jakob is a prion disease. Prions are abnormal proteins found most often in brain tissue. Though extremely rare—affecting one person per million worldwide (National Institutes of Health [NIH], 2015), prion diseases are usually rapidly progressive and always fatal (CDC, 2015d).

301. While prions (infectious proteins) have been shown to bind tightly to surfaces and to be difficult to remove by cleaning, specific formulations of alkaline and enzymatic detergents can effectively eliminate the infectivity of prions (Rutala & Weber, 2010, p. 108).

302. When preparing for a procedure on a patient with known or suspected prion disease, use as many disposable items (both supplies and instruments) as possible and follow facility policy carefully.

Airborne- and Droplet-Transmitted Infections

303. If possible, surgery should be postponed on patients with airborne- or droplet-transmitted infections. If the patient's condition is such that the surgery cannot be postponed, ideally the procedure should be done in a room with negative pressure. When the pressure in the operating room is lower than the pressure in the surrounding area, microorganisms are contained within the operating room.

304. Some healthcare facilities have a room in which the air pressure can be converted from positive to negative pressure on demand. In these operating rooms, it is critical to check that the airflow has been changed back to positive pressure for patients not on airborne or droplet precautions.

Section Questions

1. How is the clean environment of the operating room protected? [Ref 246]

2. Explain the importance of managing airflow in the operating room. [Ref 249]

3. What rate of air exchange do the CMS, FGI, HHS, and ASHE recommend for the operating room? [Ref 251]

4. Explain the importance of a positive-pressure environment in the operating room. [Ref 252]

5. When is negative pressure an important factor in the operating room? [Refs 253, 303]

6. How is the positive or negative pressure maintained within the operating room? [Ref 254]

7. Describe laminar airflow and explain its application in the operating room. [Ref 255]

8. What are the temperature and humidity recommendations for the operating room? [Refs 256–257]

9. What cleaning procedures does the circulator implement before the first case of the day? [Refs 263–266]

10. What is the rationale for scheduling a latex-allergic patient for the first procedure of the day? [Ref 267]

11. Discuss management of spills during a surgical procedure. [Refs 269–271]

12. What type of container is required for the disposal of contaminated items? [Refs 272, 277]

13. How does the circulator manage specimen containers? [Ref 275]

14. What items delivered to the field are considered sterile and which are not? [Ref 277]

15. How are infectious waste liquids managed? [Refs 274, 278]

16. Describe the fiscal responsibility associated with the disposal of infectious and noninfectious waste. [Ref 280]

17. What is one criterion for determining if an item contaminated with blood is considered infectious waste? [Ref 281]

18. What items are cleaned/disinfected following each procedure? [Refs 284–286]

19. When does terminal cleaning occur in the operating room? [Ref 289]

20. What operating room items should be cleaned daily? [Ref 290]

21. What operating room items are cleaned only periodically? [Ref 292]

22. How does the cleaning procedure following a patient known to be infected with the hepatitis or HIV virus differ from cleaning after other procedures? [Ref 294]

23. What makes *C. difficile* a significant challenge for environmental cleaning? [Ref 297]

24. What is the protocol for hand hygiene following caring for a patient with *C. difficile*? [Ref 298]

25. What is a prion and how do we manage procedures for patients with known or suspected prion disease? [Refs 300, 302]

References

Association of the Advancement of Medical Instrumentation (AAMI). (2015). *Relative Humidity Levels in the Operating Room: Joint communication to healthcare delivery organizations*. Retrieved from: http://s3.amazonaws.com/rdcms-aami/files/production/public/FileDownloads/News/Humidity_in_OR_Joint_Communication_to_HDOs_January_2015.pdf

Association of periOperative Registered Nurses (AORN). (2015). *Guidelines for Perioperative Practice*. Denver, CO: Author.

Centers for Disease Control and Prevention (CDC) (2002). *Guideline for hand hygiene in healthcare settings: Recommendations of the healthcare infection control practices advisory committee and the HICPAC/SHEA/APIC/IDSA Hand Hygiene Task Force*. Retrieved from http://www.cdc.gov/mmwr/preview/mmwrhtml/rr5116a1.htm

Centers for Disease Control and Prevention (CDC). (2015a). *Multidrug-resistant organism & Clostridium difficile infection (MDRO/CDI) module*. Retrieved from http://www.cdc.gov/nhsn/PDFs/pscManual/12pscMDRO_CDADcurrent.pdf

Centers for Disease Control and Prevention (CDC). (2015b). *Surgical site infection (SSI) event*. Retrieved from http://www.cdc.gov/nhsn/PDFs/pscManual/9pscSSIcurrent. pdf

Centers for Disease Control and Prevention (CDC). (2015c). *Healthcare-associated infections: Clostridium difficile*. Retrieved from http://www.cdc.gov/HAI/organisms/cdiff/Cdiff_clinicians.html

Centers for Disease Control and Prevention (CDC). (2015d). *Prion diseases*. Retrieved from http://www.cdc.gov/prions/index.html

Centers for Disease Control and Prevention (CDC). (2012) *Updated CDC recommendations for the management of hepatitis B virus–infected health-care providers and students*. Retrieved from: http://www.cdc.gov/mmwr/preview/mmwrhtml/rr6103a1. htm

Centers for Medicare and Medicaid Services (CMS). (2015). *State operations manual: Appendix A—Survey protocol, regulations and interpretive guidelines for hospitals* (Rev. 78). Retrieved from https://www.cms.gov/Regulations-and-Guidance/Guidance/Manuals/downloads/som107ap_a_hospitals.pdf

Cruse, P. H.,&Foord, R. (1980). The epidemiology of wound infection. A 10-year prospective study of 62,939 wounds. *The Surgical Clinics of North America, 60*(1), 27–40.

Environmental Protection Agency (EPA) (2002). *Using microfiber mops in hospitals*. Retrieved from: http://www3.epa.gov/region9/waste/p2/projects/hospital/mops.pdf.

Facility Guidelines Institute (FGI), U.S. Department of Health andHuman Services (HHS), & American Society for Healthcare Engineering (ASHE). (2014). *Guidelines for design and construction of hospitals and outpatient facilities*. Chicago, IL; American Society for Healthcare Engineering of the American Hospital Association.

Food & Drug Administration (FDA) (2011). *FDA issues warning about powdered gloves*. Retrieved from: http://www.infectioncontroltoday.com/news/2011/02/fda-issues-warming-about-powdered-gloves.aspx

Food & Drug Administration (FDA) (1997). *Medical glove powder report*. Retrieved from: http://www.fda.gov/MedicalDevices/DeviceRegulationandGuidance/GuidanceDocuments/ucm113316.htm

Joint Commision (TJC) (2015). *National patient safety goals*. Retrieved from: http://www.jointcommission.org/topics/hai_standards_and_npsgs. aspx

Magill, S., Edwards, J. R., Bamberg, W., Beldavs, Z. G., Dumyati, G., Kainer, M.A., . . . Fridkin, S. K. (2014). Multistate point-prevalence survey of health care-associated infections. *New England Journal of Medicine, 370*(13), 1198–1208.

National Institutes of Health (NIH).(2015). *Genetics home reference (GHR): Prion disease*. Retrieved from http://ghr.nlm.nih.gov/condition/prion-disease

Occupational Safety and Health Administration (OSHA). (2015). *Bloodborne pathogens* (CFR 1910.1030). Retrieved from: https://www.osha.gov/pls/oshaweb/owadisp.show_document?p_table=standards&p_id=10051

Occupational Safety and Health Administration (OSHA). (2011). *Bloodborne pathogens*. In: Standard 1910.1030 (d) (4)(iii)(b). 56 Fed.Reg. 64004. Retrieved from https://www.osha.gov/pls/oshaweb/owadisp.show_document?p_table=STANDARDS&p_id=10051

Petersen, P. (2006). Clinical issues: Air exchanges in the OR. *AORN Journal, 84*(4), 647–648.

Rutala, W., & Weber, D. (2010). Guidelines for disinfection and sterilization of prion-contaminated medical instruments. *Infection Control and Hospital Epidemiology, 21*(2), 107–117.

Siegel, J., Rhinehart, E., Jackson, M., & Chiarello, L. (2007). *Guidelines for isolation: Preventing transmission of infectious agents in healthcare settings*. Atlanta, GA: Centers for Disease Control and Prevention. Retrieved from http://www.cdc.gov/hicpac/2007IP/2007isolationPrecautions.html

Webster, J., & Osborne, S. (2015). *Preoperative bathing or showering with skin antiseptics to prevent surgical site infection*. The Cochrane Library. Retrieved from http://onlinelibrary.wiley.com/doi/10.1002/14651858.CD004985.pub5/abstract

World Health Organization (WHO). (2009). *World Health Organization guidelines on hand hygiene in health care*. Retrieved from http://whqlibdoc.who.int/publications/2009/9789241597906_eng.pdf

Post-Test

Part 1

1. Which of the following is an activity in the operating room designed to prevent infection?
    a. Managing the exogenous sources of infection
    b. Reducing the presence of microorganisms
    c. Creating a sterile field
    d. Preventing a mode of transmission of microorganisms

2. What is the most common type of surgical site infection?
    a. Organ/space
    b. Deep incisional
    c. Superficial incisional
    d. Muscle and fascia

3. Asepsis means
    a. the absence of pathogenic organisms.
    b. creating a sterile field.
    c. scrubbing, gowning, and gloving.
    d. the prevention of infections.

4. The key to prevention of surgical site infections in the operating room is
    a. strict adherence to aseptic practices.
    b. preoperative patient showers with an antimicrobial soap.
    c. operating room attire.
    d. traffic patterns in the operating suite.

5. Which of the following is an endogenous source of infection?
    a. A break in sterile technique
    b. A large number of microorganisms found on the patient
    c. A very long surgical procedure
    d. An extremely complicated surgical procedure

6. What is the patient's primary defense against the entry of microorganisms into the body?
    a. Overall good health
    b. Intact skin
    c. Preoperative antibiotics
    d. Poor nutritional status

7. What is the best way to handle a surgical patient with an infection?
    a. Be sure that the patient has been cleared for surgery by his physician.
    b. Cover the infection site to be sure that it is isolated during the surgical procedure.
    c. Ensure that the anesthesiologist has given preoperative antibiotics.
    d. Recommend that the surgery be postponed until the infection is resolved.

8. Which of the following risk factors for increasing microorganisms would be difficult for the perioperative nurse to control?
   a. Laughing and talking unnecessarily
   b. Artificial nails
   c. Shedding from skin and hair
   d. Length of the surgical procedure

9. When is colonization of the patient with healthcare-associated microorganisms most likely?
   a. When the patient is extremely young or very old
   b. When the patient has an extensive preoperative or postoperative stay
   c. When the patient has community-acquired MRSA
   d. When there is a break in technique during a surgical procedure

10. What is one reason that artificial nails are prohibited in patient care areas?
    a. Artificial nails are especially prone to colonization with microorganisms.
    b. Artificial nails break easily and harbor microorganisms
    c. Wearers of artificial nails frequently limit hand hygiene to protect their manicure
    d. Alcohol-based hand rubs dissolve the artificial nail adhesive

11. What is the first thing the perioperative nurse does when opening a room for a surgical procedure?
    a. Wipe all horizontal surfaces with a damp cloth.
    b. Check the casecart against the surgeon's preference card.
    c. Test equipment that will be used during the procedure.
    d. Begin to open supplies for the scrub person.

12. What differentiates standard precautions from universal precautions?
    a. OSHA defined universal precautions; the CDC refined them later into standard precautions.
    b. Universal precautions relate to blood and body fluid contamination.
    c. Standard precautions are the same as transmission-based precautions.
    d. Standard precautions apply to all patients whether or not they are known to be infectious.

13. Choose the single *best* response. The purpose of standard precautions is to
    a. protect patients and personnel from exposure to pathogenic microorganisms found in blood and body fluid.
    b. protect personnel from exposure to patients with AIDS.
    c. be sure that all patients get the same standard of care.
    d. protect patients from surgical site infections.

14. Transmission-based precautions
    a. is another term for standard precautions.
    b. are designed to protect patients from exogenous sources of infection.
    c. describe the protocols used in the operating room to protect patients from infection.
    d. include specific precautions for pathogens transmitted via the airborne, droplet, and contact routes.

15. Airborne precautions would be used for which of the following diseases?
    a. Rubeola, tuberculosis, varicella
    b. Hepatitis B, HIV
    c. Mumps, influenza
    d. C. *difficile*

16. Droplet precautions require wearing a mask within
    a. 3 feet of the patient.
    b. 5 feet of the patient.
    c. 10 feet of the patient.
    d. 15 feet of the patient.

17. Which of the following is *not* one of the three components of OSHA's mandatory practice standard?
    a. Use of protective personal barrier
    b. Proper hand washing
    c. Preoperative patient prep
    d. Proper management of sharps

18. How do we determine what PPE to wear?
    a. Consult the facility policy and procedure.
    b. Determine the likelihood of exposure to blood and body fluid.
    c. Read the OSHA list of procedures and the PPE required.
    d. Wear the same PPE for all procedures.

19. What distinguishes the operating room from other clinical areas?
    a. Scrub attire
    b. Traffic patterns
    c. Invasive procedures
    d. Aseptic practices

20. Which of the following best describes the *surgical conscience*?
    a. Personal commitment to adhere strictly to aseptic practices
    b. Policy and procedure that describe aseptic practices required in the facility
    c. Speaking up when you think there has been a break in technique
    d. Doing the right thing whenever you're precepting someone

21. What is the most important reason for creating a sterile field?
    a. To organize the supplies and equipment that are needed for the surgical procedure
    b. To separate the scrubbed personnel from the unscrubbed personnel
    c. To isolate the operative site from contamination from the surrounding area
    d. To remove any potential for the patient to get a surgical site infection

22. What is the purpose of the preoperative patient skin prep?
    a. Sterilize the skin.
    b. Define the operative site.
    c. Reduce the number of microorganisms at the surgical site.
    d. Remove pathogens.

23. Which statement about preoperative hair removal is correct?
    a. Hair at the incision site should always be removed.
    b. Hair removal has been associated with increased risk of surgical site infection.
    c. Hair should be removed the night before surgery.
    d. Use clippers—never a razor—and remove hair in the operating room immediately prior to surgery.

24. Which of the following is not considered when determining the area to be included in the preoperative patient skin prep?
    a. The possibility of extending the intended incision
    b. The possibility of drains
    c. An additional incision site
    d. The type of dressing planned

25. Which of the following statements is *true* about preoperative patient skin prep?
    a. It is recommended to start at the periphery and work toward the incision site.
    b. Pooling of prep fluids can cause patient injury.
    c. Drapes can be applied immediately following the prep.
    d. There is evidence that a sterile prep kit and sterile gloves have better outcomes than a clean prep kit and clean gloves.

Part 2

26. Dressing rooms are in which area of the surgical suite?
    a. Adjacent to the unrestricted area
    b. Unrestricted area
    c. Semi-restricted area
    d. Restricted area

27. What differentiates the restricted area from the semi-restricted area?
    a. It cannot be accessed from a non-restricted area.
    b. Only sterile items are allowed in the restricted area.
    c. It is considered restricted only if sterile supplies are open.
    d. There is a red line on the floor.

28. Which statement is (are) true about scrub attire?
    a. Scrub caps should be worn in unrestricted areas.
    b. Personal clothing should be completely covered by scrub attire.
    c. Scrub tops should be worn over scrub pants, not tucked in.
    d. Scientific studies have shown that home laundering is just as effective as commercial laundering in preventing the transmission of infection.

29. Which statement is *not true* about surgical masks?
    a. Pinching the metal strip to conform to the nose will prevent venting.
    b. Masks should be on or off, never left dangling around the neck or saved in a pocket.
    c. Used masks should be removed and handled only by the ties.
    d. Masks must fit securely to prevent the escape of microorganisms.

30. Which of the following statements about hand washing and hand hygiene is true?
    a. Hand washing refers to practices outside of the operating room.
    b. Hand hygiene refers to the use of alcohol-based preparations.
    c. Hand hygiene refers to washing hands with soap and water.
    d. Hand hygiene refers to all measures related to hand condition and decontamination.

31. What is the single most important practice to prevent the transmission of microorganisms?
    a. Washing hands at the start of a shift before doing anything else
    b. Hand hygiene
    c. Performing a surgical scrub
    d. Using an alcohol-based hand product

32. Which statement about surgical hand antisepsis (surgical scrub) is true?
    a. It removes all transient microorganisms from the hands before donning sterile gown and gloves.
    b. It can be performed without removing a watch and rings.
    c. It is sometimes performed using the "timed" or "stroke" method.
    d. Brushless, alcohol-based antiseptic has replaced the old sponge/brush method.

33. Which of the following is a correct statement about alcohol-based surgical hand products?
    a. Alcohol-based products are more effective than traditional scrub products in killing microorganisms.
    b. Water-aided alcohol scrub has greater efficacy than waterless alcohol scrub.
    c. Manufacturers' IFU are the same for all alcohol-based hand scrubs.
    d. A soap and water hand wash is not necessary when using alcohol-based surgical scrubs.

34. How do indicator gloves work?
    a. The indicator glove prevents the under glove from being punctured.
    b. A dark-colored patch is visible through the outer glove when there is a puncture.
    c. Indicator gloves are a size larger than regular gloves and are worn underneath.
    d. The inner indicator glove turns color when a puncture occurs.

35. Closed gloving
    a. is the preferred method of gloving.
    b. begins with the hands pushed through the knit cuff of the gown sleeve.
    c. is the best way to glove other members of the scrubbed team.
    d. affords a bit less opportunity for contamination than open gloving.

36. When donning a gown
    a. hold the gown with the neckline up and the outside of the gown facing you.
    b. shake the gown open so it is easy to see how to get arms into gown sleeves.
    c. place hands in sleeve slots, step backward and allow the gown to unfold.
    d. pull hands through the stockinette and complete closed gloving.

37. Why is it important to let go of the glove before the person you are gloving lifts his/her hand?
    a. To keep from snapping the glove too hard on the person's wrist
    b. To avoid contaminating your hand
    c. To let the other person know that the glove is in place
    d. To ensure that the stockinette is completely enclosed in the glove

38. Incise drapes are
    a. drapes applied directly to the skin at the operative site.
    b. drapes with adhesive strips used to seal off contaminated areas.
    c. plastic drapes with pouches to collect fluid.
    d. plastic drapes for draping irregular body parts.

39. Once the sterile members of the team have been gowned and gloved, which part of the gown is considered sterile?
    a. Neckline
    b. Chest to level of the sterile field
    c. Elbow
    d. Stockinette cuff

40. When there is doubt about the sterility of an item
    a. double-check the external monitor.
    b. reexamine the package, and then open and check the internal monitor.
    c. ask someone else what they think.
    d. consider the item to be contaminated and discard.

41. Which statement about delivering solutions to the sterile field is correct?
    a. Deliver solutions into receptacles, then label them.
    b. Recap the unused portion carefully, because the outside of the cap is contaminated.
    c. Lean carefully over the back table so you can reach the receptacle without dripping water on the table.
    d. Remove the cap from the medication vial carefully with utility scissors.

42. Which statement about the sterile field is true?
    a. If the surgery is canceled, close the room door and save the field for the next case.
    b. Covering the sterile field is permitted, but for no more than 2 hours.
    c. The sterile field is set up as close to the time of use as possible.
    d. A covered field does not need to be monitored.

43. How do personnel navigate in the presence of a sterile field?
    a. Scrubbed personnel can sit on a stool until the procedure begins.
    b. Unscrubbed personnel should never walk between two sterile fields.
    c. Unscrubbed personnel must remain at least 24 inches from the sterile field.
    d. Scrubbed personnel should keep arms folded and hands tucked into axillae.

44. The minimum standard for air exchanges recommended by the CMS, FGI, HHS, and ASHE in the operating room is _____ air exchanges per hour with at least _____ exchanges of outside air.
    a. 10; 3
    b. 12; 3
    c. 15; 3
    d. 20; 4

45. Which of the following is a correct statement about positive and negative pressure in operating rooms?
    a. Doors must be kept shut to maintain the pressure.
    b. A sign outside the room indicates if the room has positive or negative pressure.
    c. Excess talking and laughing affect the room pressure.
    d. A patient with TB should be placed in a positive-pressure room.

46. Laminar airflow is used under what circumstances?
    a. For patients with communicable diseases
    b. In cities where the outside air is highly contaminated
    c. When the patient is suspected of having CJD
    d. When the risk of infection is high

47. Products used for cleaning inanimate surfaces in the operating room are approved by the
    a. FDA.
    b. EPA.
    c. CMS.
    d. CDC.

48. For a procedure where the patient is known to have HIV
    a. the room is cleaned with hypochlorite solution.
    b. the case is scheduled for the end of the day.
    c. routine cleaning is sufficient as long as it is adequate and thorough.
    d. additional PPE such as a second gown provides additional protection.

49. Which statement is true about *C. difficile*?
    a. Hands should be disinfected with an alcohol-based hand rub.
    b. *C. difficile* forms spores that cannot be removed from surfaces.
    c. Hands should be washed with soap and water.
    d. Surfaces should be cleaned only with chlorine-containing cleaning agents.

50. Which statement about prions is *not* true?
    a. Use as many disposable supplies and instruments as possible.
    b. Prions bind tightly to surfaces and are difficult to remove by cleaning.
    c. There are no cleaning formulations that effectively eliminate prions.
    d. High-risk tissue includes the brain, spinal cord, and eye.

Competency Checklist: Asepsis

Under "Observer's Initials," enter initials upon successful achievement of the competency. Enter N/A if the competency is not appropriate for the institution.

Name_____

	Observer's Initials	Date

Standard and Universal Precautions

1. Blood and body fluids of all patients are considered infectious. Standard precautions are practiced as follows:

   a. Gloves worn when direct contact with blood and body fluids is expected to occur   _____ _____

   b. Masks and protective eyewear worn when aerosolization or splattering of blood and body fluids is anticipated   _____ _____

   c. Gowns worn that provide a barrier appropriate to the procedure   _____ _____

   d. Needles not recapped   _____ _____

   e. Sharps deposited in sharps containers   _____ _____

   f. Infectious waste correctly differentiated from noninfectious waste   _____ _____

   g. Infectious waste deposited in designated container   _____ _____

   h. Contaminated laundry deposited in designated laundry bags   _____ _____

   i. Performs hand hygiene as appropriate   _____ _____

Skin Prep

2. Skin condition and sensitivities are assessed and assessment is documented.   _____ _____

3. Prep is implemented as follows:

   a. Awake patient is informed.   _____ _____

   b. Unnecessary exposure is avoided.   _____ _____

   c. Follows the manufacturer's IFU.   _____ _____

   d. Prep progresses from clean to dirty or according to manufacturer's IFU.   _____ _____

   e. Prep solutions are not permitted to pool.   _____ _____

   f. Dirtiest areas are prepped last.   _____ _____

   g. Prep is allowed to dry for the appropriate amount of time.   _____ _____

4. Prep is documented for:

   a. Skin assessment   _____ _____

   b. Solution used   _____ _____

   c. Person performing prep   _____ _____

   d. If hair removed—site, method, time, and person   _____ _____

   e. Person who performed prep   _____ _____

   f. Patient response to prep   _____ _____

Attire

5. Hat/hood is worn so that all head and facial hair are covered.   _____ _____

6. Surgical attire that becomes visibly soiled is removed and fresh attire is donned.   _____ _____

	Observer's Initials	Date

7. Mask:

   a. Covers nose and mouth and does not permit venting   _____ _____

   b. Is either ON or OFF—not left to dangle around the neck   _____ _____

   c. Changed between cases   _____ _____

   d. Worn in presence of open supplies   _____ _____

8. Appropriate attire is worn in restricted and semi-restricted areas.   _____ _____

Surgical Scrub

9. Jewelry is removed.   _____ _____

10. Scrub includes all surfaces of nails, subungual areas, hands, and arms to inches above the elbow.   _____ _____

11. Timed anatomical, stroke-count scrub, or alcohol-rub procedure adheres to institutional policy.   _____ _____

Gowning and Gloving

12. Hands are dried without contamination of towel.   _____ _____

13. Gown is donned correctly and without contamination.   _____ _____

14. Closed gloving is performed correctly and without contamination.   _____ _____

15. Open gloving is performed correctly and without contamination.   _____ _____

16. Assistance in gowning and gloving other team members is performed without contamination.   _____ _____

17. At end of procedure, gown is removed before gloves, containing contamination.   _____ _____

18. Gloves are removed in manner that prevents bare skin from touching contaminated glove.   _____ _____

19. Hand hygiene performed after gown and glove removed.   _____ _____

Draping

20. Equipment is draped without contamination: _____ _____

   a. Back table   _____ _____

   b. Mayo stand   _____ _____

   c. Ring stand   _____ _____

21. Patient is draped without contamination: _____ _____

   a. Abdomen   _____ _____

   b. Perineum (lithotomy)   _____ _____

   c. Extremity   _____ _____

   d. (Other)   _____ _____

22. Patient is draped from the operative site to the periphery.   _____ _____

23. A cuff is formed from a drape to protect gloved hand.   _____ _____

24. Drapes are applied after sufficient prep solution contact and dry time.   _____ _____

25. Drapes are not repositioned once placed.   _____ _____

	Observer's Initials	Date

Aseptic Practices

26. Gloved hands are kept in sight at or above the level of the sterile field.	_____	_____
27. (*Circulating role*) Items are checked for sterility prior to being dispensed to the sterile field (package integrity, chemical indicator, evidence of strike-through, expiration date if applicable).	_____	_____
28. (*Scrub role*) Sterility of items is checked prior to accepting for delivery to sterile field (packaging, chemical indicator, expiration date).	_____	_____
29. Items are dispensed to the sterile field without contamination.	_____	_____
30. Items of questionable sterility and unsterile items are not delivered to the sterile field.	_____	_____
31. Sterile field is monitored for contamination.	_____	_____
32. (*Circulator*) Ungloved hands and arms are not extended over the sterile field.	_____	_____
33. Fluids:		
a. Are dispensed to a receptacle placed at the edge of the sterile field	_____	_____
b. Are poured carefully to prevent splashing	_____	_____
c. Empty bottle or bottle with remaining fluid is discarded.	_____	_____
34. Sterile field:		
a. Is set up as close to the time of surgery as possible	_____	_____
b. Is not left unattended	_____	_____
c. If covered, is covered according to approved protocol	_____	_____
35. Scrubbed nurse touches only sterile items.	_____	_____
36. Scrubbed nurse remains close to the sterile field.	_____	_____
37. Movement around the sterile field is back to back and front (sterile) to front (sterile)	_____	_____
38. Circulating nurse maintains a safe distance from the sterile field.	_____	_____
39. Circulating nurse faces the sterile field when approaching.	_____	_____

Sanitation

40. Spills or splashes of blood and body fluids that occur in the immediate vicinity of the sterile field are promptly absorbed and cleaned with an EPA-registered disinfectant.	_____	_____
41. Soiled sponges are discarded into a plastic-lined bucket, placed into a transpired count bag, counted, and sealed in an impervious package.	_____	_____
42. Specimen containers are wiped as needed with EPA-registered hospital germicide.	_____	_____

Observer's Signature   Initials   Date

_____

Orientee's Signature

_____

5

Positioning the Patient for Surgery

LESSON OUTLINE

Overview

1. The primary reason for placing a patient in a specific surgical position is to give the surgeon access to the operative site.

2. Two important responsibilities associated with positioning are stabilizing the patient to prevent inadvertent movement and protecting the patient from injury.

3. Safe patient positioning is a critical component of perioperative nursing practice. Ideally, the surgeon will orchestrate positioning of the patient; however, it is often the experienced perioperative nurse who coordinates the positioning process.

4. A variety of factors impact the degree of risk for injury related to positioning: the type of anesthesia; the type and length of the surgical procedure; the position required for exposure of the operative site; the patient's age, height, weight, nutritional status, level of mobility; comorbidities; the patient's overall condition at the time of surgery; and whether the patient is positioned correctly and safely.

5. General anesthetic and regional blocks prevent the patient from responding to pain and discomfort, the body's natural warning signals when body parts are stretched, twisted, or compressed. Damage to nerves and vascular structures, as well as respiratory and circulatory compromise, can occur without the patient being aware.

Desired Patient Outcomes

6. Following a surgical procedure, the patient will be free of signs and symptoms of injury related to positioning (Association of periOperative Registered Nurses [AORN], 2011, p. 178):

   - Skin—intact; smooth; free of ecchymosis, cuts, abrasions, shear injury, rash, or blistering

   - Cardiovascular status—heart rate and blood pressure within expected ranges; peripheral pulses present and equal bilaterally; skin warm to touch, capillary fill less than 3 seconds

   - Neuromuscular status—flexes and extends extremities without assistance; denies numbness or tingling of extremities

7. To protect the patient from injury related to positioning, the perioperative nurse must have knowledge of:

   - Principles of anatomy and physiology

   - The surgical procedure to be performed

   - Anatomical and physiologic changes related to anesthesia, surgical position, prolonged immobility, and pressure

   - Selection and proper use of positioning equipment

   - Proper positioning technique

8. Proper positioning includes maintaining the patient's anatomical body alignment, ensuring optimal airway accessibility, and adequate exposure of the surgical site.

9. Preserving the patient's dignity by preventing unnecessary exposure is also a perioperative nursing responsibility.

Impact of Surgical Positioning: Overview of Injuries

10. The five basic positions used for surgery are supine, lithotomy, sitting, prone, and lateral. Improper technique can lead to injury in any of these positions.

11. Complications from improper positioning include postoperative musculoskeletal pain, joint dislocation, nerve damage, injury to the skin and underlying tissues, and cardiovascular and respiratory compromise.

12. Positioning injuries can be severe, sometimes resulting in permanent damage to the patient.

Respiratory and Circulatory System Compromise

13. Extreme or unnatural positions such as the Trendelenburg position, where the head and upper body are lower than the feet and lower body, affect circulation and oxygen–carbon dioxide exchange. Gravity impacts pulmonary capillary blood volume and the amount of blood available for oxygenation.

14. Unnatural positions or positioning equipment may decrease compliance or excursion of the lung and the ability of the thoracic cage to expand. Reduced lung capacity diminishes the amount of oxygen available for gas exchange. With compromised respiratory mechanics, muscles become fatigued as the patient attempts to compensate, and hypoventilation may occur. Hypoxia and hypercarbia can occur even where respiratory function is supported through mechanical assistance.

15. In the Trendelenburg position, gravity causes abdominal contents to push against the diaphragm, making chest excursion more difficult.

16. The prone position may compress the ribs or sternum, decreasing lung expansion.

17. General and regional anesthetics may disrupt normal vasodilation and constriction. Dilation of peripheral blood vessels can result in a drop in blood pressure. Dilated vessels allow venous blood to pool in dependent areas, reducing the amount of blood returned to the heart and lungs for oxygenation and redistribution.

18. In procedures where body parts are placed in a dependent position for an extended period of time, a significant amount of pooling may occur.

19. Both positioning and anesthetic agents may interfere with the heart's ability to contract, resulting in relaxation of the skeletal muscles that normally support vein walls and help to propel blood, causing in a decrease in cardiac output.

20. Any restriction of flow of blood in the legs has the potential to result in the formation of a blood clot, limiting blood flow, particularly in the deep veins (deep vein thrombosis or DVT). DVT occurs primarily in the lower extremities and is a risk factor for developing a pulmonary embolism (PE).

21. Patients should be assessed for the risk of DVT.

22. Virchow's triad (venous stasis, vessel wall injury, hypercoagulability) can cause formation of a DVT. Other factors contributing to DVT include acute medical illness, acute infectious process, inflammatory conditions, and smoking (AORN, 2015, p. 471).

23. The following conditions place patients at high risk for DVT formation:
    - History of previous DVT
    - Prolonged hospitalization
    - Malignancy or immobility

- Heart failure
- Varicose veins
- Leg ulcers
- Stroke
- Age older than 40 years
- Lengthy procedure
- Total hip procedure or revision of total hip procedure

24. Sequential compression devices (SCDs) can venous stasis in the immobile patient (**Figure 5-1**). An SCD consists of a sleeve that encompasses the leg and is sequentially inflated and deflated

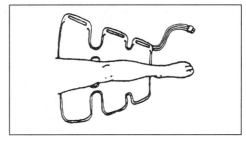

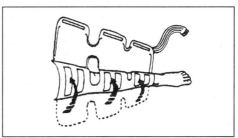

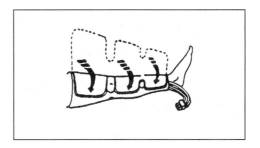

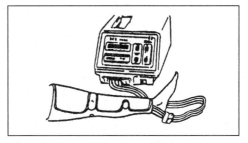

Figure 5-1 Application of sequential compression device.
Courtesy of Kendall Healthcare Prodcuts, Mansfield, MA.

automatically along the extremity. This device promotes blood flow and discourages pooling of blood.

25. Many facilities have implemented policies requiring that SCDs be utilized for all adult patients unless specifically contraindicated.

26. Sequential compression devices should be applied and activated before the induction of general anesthesia.

Section Questions

1. What is the primary objective for positioning the patient for a surgical procedure? [Ref 1]

2. What are the two responsibilities associated with positioning the surgical patient? [Ref 2]

3. Identify factors that impact the patient's degree of risk for injury related to positioning. [Ref 4]

4. Why is the anesthetized patient at greater risk for positioning injury? [Ref 5]

5. What types of injuries are associated with positioning? [Ref 5]

6. What three body systems are assessed for injuries related to positioning? [Ref 6]

7. Identify three components of proper positioning. [Ref 8]

8. What are the five basic surgical positions? [Ref 10]

9. What types of complications are associated with improper positioning? [Ref 11]

10. How does gravity affect respiration and circulation in the Trendelenburg position? [Refs 13–15]

11. How can general anesthesia disrupt normal circulation? [Refs 17, 19]

12. What is the significance of Virchow's triad? [Ref 22]

13. What are the three components of Virchow's triad? [Ref 22]

14. Identify patients at risk for the development of DVT. [Ref 23]

15. How does a sequential compression device help to prevent a DVT? [Ref 24]

Neuromuscular Injury

27. When the patient is awake, pain and pressure receptors warn against unnatural stretching and twisting of tendons, ligaments, and muscles. Opposing muscle groups prevent strain on muscle fibers. The anesthetized patient is unable to respond to an exaggerated range of motion.

28. Anesthetic agents and muscle relaxants exacerbate the potential for injury by reducing muscle tone and interfering with the patient's normal defense mechanisms.

29. Prolonged stretching or compression of nerves may result in postoperative numbness, tingling, or pain. Severe injury can result in permanent loss of sensation and paralysis.

30. Proper alignment, adequate stabilization, and support of the extremities with sufficient padding minimize musculoskeletal injury. Extremities should be secured and not allowed to hang unsupported over the edge of an armboard or the operating table.

31. Lower extremities should be positioned slowly and simultaneously to prevent sacroiliac joint dislocation. Should resistance be met in positioning, do not force the movement.

32. Fingers, toes, ears, and nose can be crushed or compressed between two surfaces when the operating table, instrument table, or Mayo stands are adjusted. Team members must maintain a mental image of the location of body parts when the patient's body is hidden by drapes. Neither furniture nor personnel should lean on the patient during the procedure.

Facial Nerves

33. Injury to the facial nerve (buccal branch), causing motor injury to the mouth, can occur when the nerve is compressed by an improperly fitting or poorly positioned facemask.

34. Pressure from endotracheal tube connectors can injure the suborbital nerve, causing numbness of the forehead.

Upper Extremity Nerves

35. The brachial plexus is vulnerable to injury because of its superficial position and close proximity to bony structures.

36. The supine position, with one or both arms extended on armboards, is the most common surgical position. Brachial plexus injury can occur when the arm is extended at an angle greater than 90°. Place the armboard at an angle less than 90° The patient's palm should be facing up with the fingers extended (AORN, 2015, p. 570).

37. Even when the arm is positioned carefully prior to surgery, unintentional hyperextension of the arm during the procedure might not be noticed when the armboard is hidden by surgical drapes.

38. Shoulder braces, sometimes used to keep patients in the Trendelenburg position from slipping from the table, may cause compression of the brachial plexus. Shoulder braces should be very well padded and should not be located too far medially or laterally.

39. Brachial plexus injury might be evidenced postoperatively by motor and sensory deficits in the arm and shoulder.

40. Ulnar neuropathy, caused by external compression or excessive flexion of the elbow, accounts for approximately one-third of postpositioning nerve injuries. It is more common in men than in women.

41. Pronation of the hand and forearm exerts more pressure on the ulnar nerve (**Figure 5-2**), while supination decreases pressure (Gerken, 2013).

42. Padding the elbow can relieve pressure on the olecranon process.

43. The radial or ulnar nerve may be injured if the elbow slips off the mattress and the nerve is compressed between the table and the medial epicondyle by personnel leaning against the table.

44. Tucking the patient's arm with a draw sheet can minimize the possibility of the arm slipping from the table. The draw sheet is secured under the patient, never under the mattress.

45. Symptoms of ulnar nerve injury include tingling, pain, and numbness in the fourth and

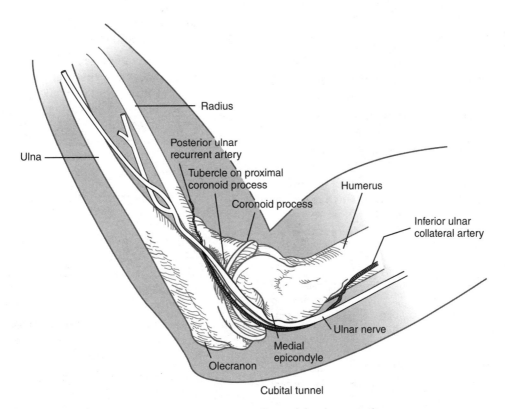

Figure 5-2 Ulnar nerve—most common postoperative peripheral neuropathy.

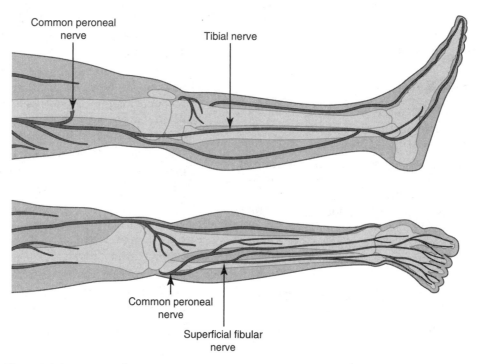

Figure 5-3 Lower extremity nerves.

fifth fingers. Severe injury can result in a weak grip or contractures, leading to a "claw hand."

46. Radial nerve damage may be evidenced by wrist drop.

Lower Extremity Nerves

47. The peroneal, posterior tibial, femoral obturator, and sciatic nerves (**Figure 5-3**) are at risk for injury in the lithotomy position.

48. Legs improperly placed in stirrups or improperly moved can cause extension, flexion, compression, or stretching injuries to lower extremity nerves.

49. Improper positioning in stirrups can compress the peroneal nerve between the fibula and the stirrup, resulting in foot drop. Stirrups today are designed to prevent this injury if they are used properly.

50. Injury to the femoral obturator nerve, resulting in paralysis and numbness of the calf muscles, can occur if the nerve is compressed between a metal popliteal knee support stirrup and the medial tibial condyle. Adequate padding can prevent this injury.

51. Foot drop from injury to the sciatic nerve can occur if the nerve is compressed or stretched by fully extending the legs in the high lithotomy position and flexing the thighs more than 90° on the trunk.

Integumentary System Injury

52. Goal #14 of The Joint Commission's (TJC) 2015 patient safety goals is to *prevent healthcare-associated pressure ulcers*. TJC estimates the cost for treatment of a pressure ulcer is $14,000 to $40,000 per ulcer.

53. Every facility must have a plan for prediction, prevention, and early treatment of pressure ulcers that includes identifying patients at risk, maintaining and improving tissue tolerance, protecting against adverse effects of external mechanical forces, and staff education (TJC, 2014), all of which are relevant to the perioperative nurse.

54. In 2008, the Centers for Medicare and Medicaid Services (CMS) implemented the Present on Admission (POA) indicator (CMS, 2015). Under this CMS policy, a hospital will not receive additional funds to care for a patient who has acquired a pressure ulcer during hospitalization. This groundbreaking policy provides a significant financial impetus for ulcer prevention.

55. Soft tissues are at risk for injury as a result of the combination of *immobility*, *pressure*, and *time*; the risk for tissue damage increases with:

- The length of time the patient has been immobile

- Increased pressure on bony prominences

- The length of the procedure

56. The anesthetized patient is immobile and subjected to uninterrupted pressure during a surgical procedure. External pressure restricting blood flow can cause tissue ischemia that exacerbates the potential for tissue injury. If the patient has been immobile for any length of time prior to the surgery, the risk for tissue damage is higher.

57. Friction and shearing can also cause tissue injury. Friction injuries occur when coarse surfaces such as bed linens or blankets rub against the skin, causing abrasions or blisters. These wounds, though usually superficial, can contribute to the more serious injury of a pressure ulcer.

58. Shearing injuries occur when gravity holds the skin stationary against a surface while the tissues beneath it move. This can occur when the patient is pulled rather than lifted, or when linen or blankets are pulled from beneath the patient.

59. An anesthetized patient who is repositioned incorrectly, or slides up or down on the table, can experience a shear injury. Shearing stretches and tears the subcutaneous capillaries, leading to tissue ischemia and cell death.

60. Deep tissue injury (DTI), or tissue necrosis occurring in the tissues under intact skin, is not uncommon in surgical patients (**Figure 5-4**). The damage occurs when capillaries are compressed against bony prominences, causing tissue ischemia, cell death, and necrosis (NPUAP, 2012). Prolonged, unrelieved pressure during surgery can occlude blood flow, causing ischemia in even the healthiest of patients.

61. DTI differs from a Stage IV pressure ulcer in that the damage begins deep in the tissue and migrates toward the surface. Muscle closest to the bone is affected first, while the skin remains intact. Over time, as the damage progresses to include subcutaneous tissue and eventually skin, the DTI appears as a bruise and rapidly progresses to an ulcer.

62. A DTI that begins in surgery can go unnoticed for days; hence, the connection between the injury and surgery is often missed. DTIs that appear within 72 hours postoperatively most likely can be attributed to the surgical procedure (Primiano et al., 2011, p. 556).

63. An area on the patient's skin that appears reddened after surgery may be an indication of the beginning of a superficial pressure ulcer, which can progress to involve deeper tissues. A reddened area may also be an indication of a self-healing transient reaction to pressure. In either case, the area should not be massaged. Massage may, in fact, compromise circulation to the affected area.

64. Areas most at risk for pressure ulcer formation are heels, elbows, scapula, sacrum, coccyx, occiput, iliac crest, ear, medial knee, malleolus, and toes, where there is little padding between skin and bone.

65. Intrinsic patient risk factors for pressure injury include age (older patients have less elastic, smaller blood vessels that hinder blood flow); weight (obesity causes additional pressure on bony prominences); nutritional status (malnourished patients); and presence of

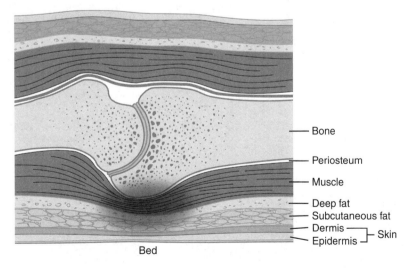

Figure 5-4 Deep tissue injury (DTI) from compression at the bone-tissue interface.
Reprinted with permisison from T. Goodman (2012 p. 15). Positioning: A Patient Safety Initiative: Study Guide for Nurses. Dallas, TX: Terri Goodman and Associates.

diabetes, vascular disease, or hypertension (the latter two conditions are associated with diminished circulation).

66. Other intrinsic factors affecting the risk for pressure injury include immobility, infection, incontinence, and impaired sensory perceptions.

67. Extrinsic factors that increase the risk of tissue damage include temperature, friction, shear, and moisture.

68. Extrinsic factors related to the surgical procedure that place patients at risk for injury include sedation, anesthetic agents, retractors, warming devices, and pooled prep solutions.

69. Adequate padding with effective pressure-relieving products is essential to protect bony prominences and prevent pressure ulcer formation. (**Figures 5-5, 5-6,** and **5-7**).

70. An individual can withstand a large amount of pressure for a short period of time more successfully than a small amount of pressure over a longer period of time.

71. In one meta-analysis of studies involving surgical patients over a 5-year period, the average incidence of pressure ulcers was estimated at 11% (Chen, Chen, & Wu, 2012), an increase from 8.5% in an earlier study (Aronovich, 2007). Reported incidences in the studies analyzed varied from 11% to 22%, demonstrating that risk factors such as the type of surgery, the quality of positioning equipment, and endogenous patient characteristics have a significant impact on outcomes.

72. It is well documented that the incidence of pressure ulcers in all patient populations rises markedly in procedures lasting for more than 2 to 2.5 hours (Goodman, 2012).

73. Commercial operating room table pads and positioning devices are designed to reduce pressure and help prevent tissue injuries in the surgical patient. In 2014, the Rehabilitation

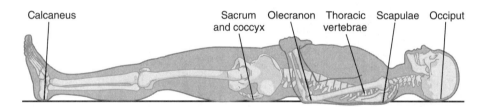

Figure 5-5 Potential pressure points in the supine position.

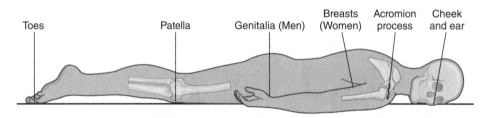

Figure 5-6 Potential pressure points in the prone position.

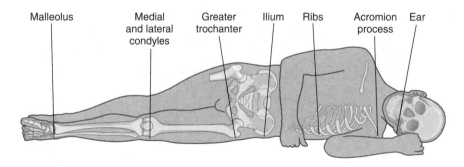

Figure 5-7 Potential pressure points in the lateral position.

Engineering and Assistive Technology Society of North America (RESNA) published the first *American National Standard for Support* *Surfaces*, which provide an objective means for evaluating and comparing support surface characteristics (Hermans, Weyl, & Reger, 2014).

Section Questions

1. How do anesthetic agents and muscle relaxants increase the likelihood of positioning injury during surgery? [Refs 27–28]

2. What steps can be taken to minimize the potential for injury? [Ref 30]

3. How should lower extremities be handled? [Ref 31]

4. What damage can be done to a patient hidden under drapes? [Ref 32]

5. Describe approaches to preventing injury to the brachial plexus. [Refs 36–38]

6. What positioning techniques can prevent ulnar neuropathy? [Refs 41–42]

7. Contrast the symptoms of ulnar nerve injury with injury to the radial nerve. [Refs 45–46]

8. What types of nerve injuries can occur in the lower extremities? [Ref 48]

9. Contrast symptoms of injury to the peroneal nerve with obturator nerve injury. [Refs 49–50]

10. How can positioning injure the sciatic nerve? [Ref 51]

11. What three factors combine to place surgical patients at risk for tissue injury? [Ref 55]

12. Describe friction and shear injuries and how they can be avoided. [Refs 57–59]

13. Explain how deep tissue injury (DTI) differs from a Stage IV pressure ulcer. [Refs 60–61]

14. Describe both intrinsic and extrinsic factors that predispose patients to tissue injury. [Refs 65–68]

15. Surgical procedures of what duration increase the likelihood of tissue damage, even in healthy patients? [Ref 72]

Responsibilities of the Perioperative Nurse Patient Advocate

74. The patient undergoing surgery is vulnerable to positioning injury, particularly when the procedure is performed under general anesthesia and lasts longer than a few hours. Neuromuscular, musculoskeletal, integumentary, and physiologic systems can be severely compromised at a time when the patient is unable to identify and address the problem.

75. Although the surgeon, surgical assistants, anesthesia personnel, and other members of the nursing team may participate in patient positioning, it is most frequently the perioperative nurse who positions the patient.

76. The perioperative nurse is a crucial patient advocate, and at no time should the responsibility to ensure proper positioning be assumed to belong to another team member. The unconscious surgical patient is unable to respond to pain or discomfort, and responsibility for patient safety becomes a perioperative nursing responsibility.

Nursing Considerations
Patient Assessment

77. Planning for positioning begins with a nursing assessment of the patient, including the following considerations:

- Age
- Height, weight, and body mass index (BMI)
- Skin condition
- Presence of jewelry
- Nutritional status
- Allergies (including latex allergy, because tape is sometimes used as a positioning aid)
- Preexisting conditions (e.g., vascular, respiratory, circulatory, neurologic, immune system suppression)

- Physical or mobility limitations
- Prosthetic, corrective, or implanted devices
- Activity level (immobility places the patient at higher risk for pressure damage)
- Peripheral pulses
- Level of consciousness
- Perception of pain
- Psychosocial or cultural issues (AORN, 2015, pp. 565–566)

78. Several risk assessment scales for pressure ulcer development are available (e.g., Braden, Gosnell, Abruzzese); however, no scale specific for the intraoperative patient population has been accepted. Efforts have been made to modify the Braden scale for the perioperative environment with some success. For example, Galvin and Curley (2012) had success with the Braden Q + P in the pediatric population (**Exhibit 5-1**).

79. In a number of studies, increasing age, a diagnosis of either diabetes or vascular disease, and vascular procedures were found to be the most frequent predictors of perioperative pressure ulcers (Goodman, 2012, pp. 23–26). Reduction in blood perfusion may be responsible for increased incidence of pressure ulcers in patients undergoing vascular procedures lasting more than 2.5 hours.

80. Extrinsic risk factors include type and length of procedure, position, anesthetic agents, retractors, warming devices, and pooled prep solutions. The quality of the operating room bed mattress and positioning devices play a significant role in preventing pressure damage (Goodman, 2012, pp. 40–48). In a number of studies, the most significant extrinsic risk factor was time on the operating room mattress.

81. The surgical procedure will determine the desired patient position. Lengthy procedures under anesthesia require extended periods of immobility and increase the risk for injury. Surgeries performed on areas where access is difficult may result in unnatural positions that increase the risk for injury.

82. Elderly patients have decreased muscle tone, poor skin turgor, and less subcutaneous fat and muscle to cushion bony prominences. These factors place elderly patients at increased risk for impaired skin integrity.

83. Height and weight are useful to determine appropriate positioning aids. Activity level and muscle tone provide information about how well the patient moves and the degree to which the patient may participate in transfer to and from the operating room bed.

84. Drugs and anesthetic agents can alter the patient's ability to move. Baseline data provide information that is useful for evaluating the impact of drugs and anesthesia on movement and muscle tone.

85. Patients with poor nutritional status are at increased risk for tissue injury. Malnourished patients lack the protein reserves necessary to maintain healthy skin cells and are at increased risk for skin impairment.

86. Obese patients may trap moisture and fluids from skin-prep solutions in tissue folds, which may lead to skin breakdown. Adipose tissue is not well vascularized, and the pressure resulting from positioning can cause a decrease in circulation to peripheral body areas. Excess body weight increases the strain on joints and ligaments. Respiratory function is compromised in obese patients because of increased weight on the chest. Obesity also places an increased workload on the heart and circulatory system.

87. Anesthetic agents and positioning for surgery place additional strain on respiratory function.

88. Positioning that increases venous blood return to the heart can further compromise circulation.

89. Underweight patients experience greater than normal pressure on bony prominences and, therefore, are at greater risk for impaired skin integrity.

90. Patients with existing integumentary damage are at increased risk for further skin impairment. Diminished body fat provides little protection for peripheral nerves, and the underweight patient is at high risk for nerve damage.

91. Certain preexisting injuries or conditions and certain surgical procedures may require additional planning to prevent injury. Preexisting conditions requiring additional considerations include the following:

- Demineralized bone conditions such as osteoporosis and malignant metastasis—increased risk of fracture
- Diabetes, anemia, and paralysis—increased risk for skin breakdown
- Arthritis and joint prosthesis—limited joint movement

Exhibit 5-1 Braden Scale for Predicting Risk for Pressure Damage

BRADEN SCALE FOR PREDICTING PRESSURE SORE RISK

Patient's Name _____ Evaluator's Name _____ Date of Assessment _____

SENSORY PERCEPTION ability to respond meaningfully to pressure-related discomfort	**1. Completely Limited** Unresponsive (does not moan, flinch, or gasp) to painful stimuli, due to diminished level of consciousness or sedation. OR limited ability to feel pain over most of body.	**2. Very Limited** Responds only to painful stimuli. Cannot communicate discomfort except by moaning or restlessness OR has a sensory impairment which limits the ability to feel pain or discomfort over ½ of body.	**3. Slightly Limited** Responds to verbal commands, but cannot always communicate discomfort or the need to be turned. OR has some sensory impairment which limits ability to feel pain or discomfort in 1 or 2 extremities.	**4. No Impairment** Responds to verbal commands. Has no sensory deficit which would limit ability to feel or voice pain or discomfort.		
MOISTURE degree to which skin is exposed to moisture	**1. Constantly Moist** Skin is kept moist almost constantly by perspiration, urine, etc. Dampness is detected every time patient is moved or turned.	**2. Very Moist** Skin is often, but not always moist. Linen must be changed at least once a shift.	**3. Occasionally Moist:** Skin is occasionally moist, requiring an extra linen change approximately once a day.	**4. Rarely Moist** Skin is usually dry, linen only requires changing at routine intervals.		
ACTIVITY degree of physical activity	**1. Bedfast** Confined to bed.	**2. Chairfast** Ability to walk severely limited or nonexistent. Cannot bear own weight and/or must be assisted into chair or wheelchair.	**3. Walks Occasionally** Walks occasionally during day, but for very short distances, with or without assistance. Spends majority of each shift in bed or chair.	**4. Walks Frequently** Walks outside room at least twice a day and inside room at least once every two hours during waking hours		
MOBILITY ability to change and control body position	**1. Completely Immobile** Does not make even slight changes in body or extremity position without assistance	**2. Very Limited** Makes occasional slight changes in body or extremity position but unable to make frequent or significant changes independently.	**3. Slightly Limited** Makes frequent though slight changes in body or extremity position independently.	**4. No Limitation** Makes major and frequent changes in position without assistance.		
NUTRITION usual food intake pattern	**1. Very Poor** Never eats a complete meal. Rarely eats more than ⅓ of any food offered. Eats 2 servings or less of protein (meat or dairy products) per day. Takes fluids poorly. Does not take a liquid dietary supplement OR is NPO and/or maintained on clear liquids or IVs for more than 5 days.	**2. Probably Inadequate** Rarely eats a complete meal and generally eats only about ½ of any food offered. Protein intake includes only 3 servings of meat or dairy products per day. Occasionally will take a dietary supplement OR receives less than optimum amount of liquid diet or tube feeding	**3. Adequate** Eats over half of most meals. Eats a total of 4 servings of protein (meat, dairy products) per day. Occasionally will refuse a meal, but will usually take a supplement when offered OR is on a tube feeding or TPN regimen which probably meets most of nutritional needs	**4. Excellent** Eats most of every meal. Never refuses a meal. Usually eats a total of 4 or more servings of meat and dairy products. Occasionally eats between meals. Does not require supplementation.		
FRICTION & SHEAR	**1. Problem** Requires moderate to maximum assistance in moving. Complete lifting without sliding against sheets is impossible. Frequently slides down in bed or chair, requiring frequent repositioning with maximum assistance. Spasticity, contractures or agitation leads to almost constant friction	**2. Potential Problem** Moves feebly or requires minimum assistance. During a move skin probably slides to some extent against sheets, chair, restraints or other devices. Maintains relatively good position in chair or bed most of the time but occasionally slides down.	**3. No Apparent Problem** Moves in bed and in chair independently and has sufficient muscle strength to lift up completely during move. Maintains good position in bed or chair.			

Total Score _____

- Edema, infection, obstructive pulmonary disease, and other conditions that reduce respiratory and cardiac reserves
- Immunocompromise—increased risk of skin breakdown

92. Surgical procedures requiring additional considerations include:

- Surgeries lasting 2 hours or longer—increased risk for tissue damage
- Vascular surgery compromises blood perfusion to tissues—increased risk for skin breakdown
- Surgeries where prolonged traction or sustained pressure is required—increased risk for skin breakdown and nerve damage
- Warming devices placed under the patient may increase the potential for pressure ulcer (Seaman et al., 2012)

Planning Care

93. The perioperative nurse should communicate with surgical and anesthesia personnel to determine any specific needs related to patient positioning. This information, the procedure, assessment data, and nursing diagnoses serve as the basis for planning the care necessary to correctly position the patient. The perioperative nurse selects appropriate positioning equipment and makes decisions regarding the number of persons needed to assist with positioning and whether aspects of positioning can be assigned to ancillary personnel.

Impact of Anesthesia

94. Patients who are awake or lightly sedated are able to communicate when they experience pain or discomfort. In contrast, patients under general anesthesia are totally dependent on the surgical team to protect them from injury. Patients who receive regional anesthesia will not feel or report pain and are at risk for injury to anesthetized regions that are improperly positioned.

95. The anesthesiologist or nurse anesthetist will perform a patient assessment prior to delivering anesthesia. The assessment data coupled with the specialized body of knowledge of anesthesia will determine the limitations to positioning with regard to anesthesia.

96. Anesthesia personnel (anesthesiologist or nurse anesthetist) are concerned with airway access, respiratory and circulatory functions, and monitoring lines. Anesthesia has a profound effect on cardiac and respiratory function.

Patient Dignity

97. Patient dignity should be a significant consideration during positioning. The patient should not be exposed unnecessarily, and, once positioning is complete, a final check should be made to ensure that the patient is appropriately covered. Patients should be comfortable with the idea that, even when they are anesthetized, they will be appropriately covered. Traffic in the room should be limited, and the doors kept closed.

98. Provide privacy for the patient to speak openly to the perioperative staff while awake (AORN, 2015, p. 568).

99. For some patients, the response to entering the operating room is to relinquish control to their caregivers. Even an awake patient who feels a loss of dignity when exposed during positioning may not feel confident enough to cover an area inadvertently left exposed. The perioperative nurse, as patient advocate, must preserve the patient's dignity whether the patient is awake or asleep.

Positioning Devices

100. Even good positioning techniques can result in tissue damage when poorly designed positioning devices are used. When positioning equipment is purchased, manufacturers should provide evidence of the efficacy of products; evidence should demonstrate that a product provides proper support and reduces pressure as expected.

101. Some type of operating bed or table is used for every surgical procedure. Most procedures use a standard operating table with attachments that facilitate the positioning required for the procedure.

102. Positioning equipment should be clean, in good repair, and used only by staff who are knowledgeable of the intended use of each piece of equipment.

- As soon as the patient is transferred to the operating room table, a safety strap is placed across the thighs to remind the patient that the bed is narrow.

- A draw sheet under the patient's body can serve as a lift sheet. A draw sheet may be used to secure the patient's arms at the sides.

- Blankets and sheets are for patient warmth. They should not be folded or rolled and used as positioning devices. They may provide stability for the patient, but they do not reduce pressure on patient tissues.

- Sheets and blankets provide privacy and preserve patient dignity.

- A pillow or contoured foam or gel headrest is used to position the patient's head and to protect the ears and nerves of the head and face.

- Donuts are not recommended as headrests or to support other high-pressure areas (Goodman, 2012, p. 41).

- Sandbags are used for immobilization.

- Pillows or foam or gel pads may be used to support and elevate body parts.

  – The firmness and density of foam padding determines its support capability. Soft foam "bottoms out" under pressure, providing little protection. Only foam that is specifically engineered to reduce pressure should be use for positioning.

  – Gel pads are made from oil-based chemical compounds or polymers sealed in a sturdy membrane-like, water-repellent covering.

- Tape is sometimes used to secure the patient or an extremity in position. Avoid placing tape directly on the patient. Assessment for tape allergy should precede the use of tape as a positioning aid.

- Eye pads may be used to protect the eyes and keep them closed.

103. Pneumatic SCDs, elastic bandages, or anti-embolectomy stockings reduce venous pooling and are frequently used to prevent DVT. In some facilities, these devices are used for every patient.

104. Table attachments are available to maintain the stability of body parts. Personnel must demonstrate competence in use of operating tables and utilize attachments appropriately.

- Head rest—protects patient from tissue injury and also from unintentional dislodging of airway management devices

- Anesthesia screen—holds surgical drapes away from patient's face and helps to prevent the trapping of oxygen under drapes

- Armboard—supports patient's arms and provides the anesthesia provider access to peripheral intravenous lines and monitoring equipment

- Shoulder braces—prevent the patient from sliding in Trendelenburg position

- Kidney brace—elevates the flank in lateral position for kidney procedures

- Table strap—helps to secure the patient on the table

- Table extensions—extend the length of the table for tall patients

- Foot board—table extension placed at a 90° angle to the table to keep the patient from sliding downward in reverse Trendelenburg position

Operating Tables and Positioning Accessories

105. Unique positioning accessories and entire complex tables have been designed to achieve specific positions and to provide patient safety and support. Each special table has a variety of accompanying equipment and accessories (**Figures 5-8** and **5-9**). Equipment associated with each type of table must be readily available for a procedure. Locating missing pieces can result in costly delays, and using the wrong pieces can result in injury to the patient.

106. Stirrups are used to elevate the legs off the surface of the operating table for gynecology, urology, and orthopedic procedures (**Figure 5-10**). Legs should be lifted into

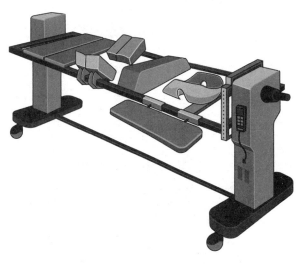

Figure 5-8 Jackson-type table with accessories.

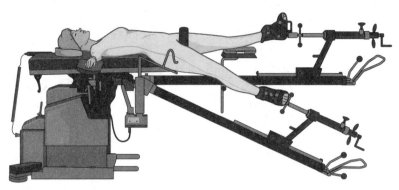

Figure 5-9 Hana fracture table.

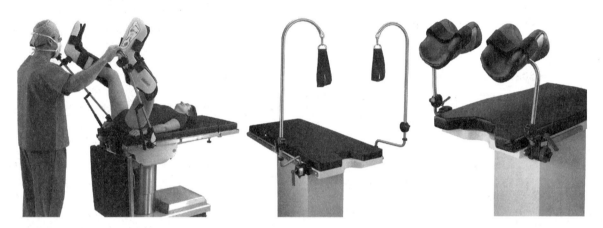

Figure 5-10 Stirrups.

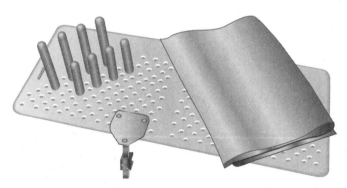

Figure 5-11 Pegboard for lateral positioning.

stirrups and lowered from stirrups simultaneously and slowly to avoid joint and nerve injury. Legs should be positioned and padded to avoid pressure on nerves or skin.

107. A pegboard is a device attached to the table for lateral positioning (**Figure 5-11**). Padding is required both the pegboard surface and the posts used to hold the patient in place.

108. A beanbag positioner is a pillow-type device filled with small particles. The patient is positioned on the device, which is molded around the patient and remains in place when the air is suctioned out. These are commonly used for lateral positioning (**Figure 5-12**)and to stabilize the patient in the steep Trendelenburg position that is common in robotic procedures.

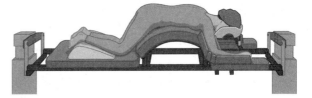

Figure 5-13 Laminectomy frame.

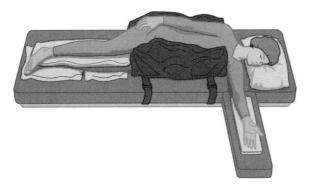

Figure 5-12 Beanbag immobilizer.

109. Newer beanbag technology has straps to hold the device securely to the bedframe, provides a softer envelope for the patient, and preserves skin integrity with a single-use cover that wicks away moisture and eliminates the pressure from wrinkled linen otherwise used to cover the device.

110. A laminectomy frame (**Figure 5-13**; or chest rolls that extend from the acromioclavicular joint to the iliac crest) supports the body in the prone position. Positioning must permit adequate excursion of the chest for effective respiration. Breast tissue must be arranged carefully to avoid unnecessary compression.

Section Questions

1. Why must the nurse assume responsibility for protecting the patient from injury during a surgical procedure? [Refs 75–76]

2. What patient factors do the nurses assess when planning for patient positioning? [Ref 77]

3. What is the most significant extrinsic risk factor for tissue injury related to surgery? [Ref 80]

4. What factors place elderly patients at higher risk? [Ref 82]

5. What about malnutrition places a patient at risk for tissue injury? [Ref 85]

6. What risk factors are specifically associated with obese patients? [Ref 86]

7. What factors affect respiration and circulation during surgery? [Refs 87–88]

8. What preexisting patient conditions require additional planning for positioning? [Ref 91]

9. What types of procedures require additional considerations for protecting patients? [Ref 92]

10. What two body systems are profoundly impacted by anesthesia? [Ref 96]

11. What is the nurse's responsibility for protecting the patient's dignity during positioning? [Refs 97–99]

12. What evidence should be available before purchasing any positioning equipment? [Ref 100]

13. Discuss the use of pillows, sheets, blankets, foam and gel padding, and tape as positioning aids. [Ref 102]

14. What can be used to prevent DVT during a surgical procedure? [Ref 103]

15. Explain the purpose for commonly used table attachments. [Ref 104]

16. Discuss responsibilities associated with specialty surgical procedure tables. [Ref 105]

17. What are some of the nursing responsibilities associated with using stirrups for positioning the patient? [Ref 106]

18. What is the purpose of the pegboard attachment for the operating table and what are some nursing considerations when it is used? [Ref 107]

19. How does the beanbag position hold the patient in the desired position? [Refs 108–109]

20. What are some nursing responsibilities associated with using beanbag positioning devices? [Ref 110]

Implementation of Patient Care

. . . .

Transportation and Transfer

111. The patient's identity should be verified, the surgical site should be marked, the procedure should be verified with the patient or a qualified patient representative, and the consent form should be signed—all before the patient is transported to the operating room.

112. The patient's condition, the presence of invasive lines, the planned procedure, and institutional policy determine whether the patient may ambulate to the operating room or whether a wheelchair or stretcher is required.

113. Stretchers used for transportation should have side rails and a locking mechanism, and the head should elevate to alter the patient's position. Pediatric transport crib rails should be high enough to prevent a standing child from falling out (AORN, 2015, p. 567).

114. During transport, stretcher side rails are kept up and the safety strap, if present, is secured. The patient is covered to maintain body temperature and to preserve dignity. The stretcher is pushed by the staff member at the head of the stretcher who is in close proximity to the patient's airway.

115. The nursing assessment will determine whether the patient's condition requires special equipment for transport, and whether additional personnel are required. (For example, patients on ventilators are transported to the operating room in a bed rather than on a stretcher, and additional personnel are required to wheel the bed and maintain the patient's respirations during transport.) Institutional policy may require the presence of nursing and/or medical personnel during transport of critically ill or ventilator-dependent patients.

116. Patient transfer from the stretcher to the operating table begins only when sufficient personnel are available. The stretcher is first brought adjacent to the operating table, and the side rail that is proximal to the table is lowered. Both the stretcher and the table are locked in place and raised or lowered to equal height. All patient intravenous lines and catheters need to be visible and free from entanglement. All team members must be ready for patient transfer.

117. During transfer to the operating table, one team member stands at the far side of the table to receive the patient. Another team member stands at the near side of the stretcher to assist the patient's move onto the operating room bed, and to ensure that the stretcher does not move away from the table should the lock fail. Operating room personnel must use good body mechanics to prevent injury to themselves.

118. If the patient is unable to move unaided, he or she is lifted from stretcher to bed; alternatively, the patient may be transferred with a roller or lateral transfer sheet/device. A patient lift may be more appropriate for obese patients. The patient is lifted—never pushed or pulled. Pushing and pulling create a shearing effect that compromises blood vessels and obstructs blood flow, creating the potential for a pressure ulcer.

119. Intravenous lines, monitoring devices, and endotracheal tubes are supported during transfer. The anesthesia provider typically supports the patient's head and indicates readiness for any move.

Initial Position Techniques

120. The safety strap is placed immediately when the patient is transferred to the operating-table. The patient is never left unattended while on the operating table.

121. Prior to being anesthetized, the patient is positioned supine with careful attention to proper body alignment. Legs are secured with the table strap, which is applied 2 inches above the knees. Venous thrombosis can result when superficial veins are occluded by pressure, straps, or other positioning devices. Safety straps should be tight enough to secure the patient but not so tight as to impair superficial venous return.

122. If necessary, the arms may be initially secured at the patient's side, with a draw sheet drawn over the arm and tucked under the patient (not under the mattress). The elbow should be padded, the palm should face the patient, and the arm should not be secured so tightly that it interferes with circulation or monitoring devices.

123. If the patient is awake, all actions should be explained. The patient should be asked if he or she is comfortable; if the patient is not comfortable, make appropriate adjustments.

124. Because the temperature in the operating room is generally cool, a warm blanket should be available to the patient. Forced-air warming blankets are available in a variety of configurations and can cover the patient to help

prevent hypothermia. Forced-air devices are never used without the appropriate blanket, because the air coming directly out of the hose is hot and can cause a burn. Maintaining normothermia can also help to prevent postoperative infection (Seamon, 2012).

125. Many patients are uncomfortable lying flat on their backs. In such a case, pillows can be placed under the patient's knees and head.

126. To reduce the potential for compression injury and/or electrical burn, no part of the patient should contact a metal surface.

127. All body parts are supported and not allowed to hang free where they may be compressed or stretched.

128. To prevent compression and trauma to blood vessels, skin, and the tibial nerve, legs must not be crossed at the ankles.

Section Questions

1. When is the surgical site marked and consent form signed? [Ref 111]

2. Describe stretchers and cribs appropriate for transporting patients to the operating room. [Refs 113–114]

3. Which situations might require special equipment or personnel for transport? [Ref 115]

4. Describe the process for transferring the patient safely to the operating room bed. [Refs 116–119]

5. What is the proper technique for placing the safety strap on the patient? [Ref 120]

6. What is the proper way to secure the patient's arm at the side? [Ref 122]

7. What is an important caution about using forced-air devices with forced-air blankets? [Ref 124]

8. Other than comfort, what is an important reason for keeping the patient warm? [Ref 124]

9. What can be done to relieve pressure on the back in the supine position? [Ref 125]

10. Why is it important to be careful not to leave the patient's legs crossed at the ankles? [Ref 128]

Basic Surgical Positions

Supine (Dorsal Recumbent)

129. The supine position is the most common surgical position (**Figure 5-14**). Procedures in this position include abdominal surgeries and those that require an anterior approach. Head, neck, and most extremity surgeries, as well as most minimally invasive procedures, are done in the supine position.

130. In the supine position, the patient is positioned flat on the back with the head and spine in a horizontal line. Hips are parallel to each other, and the legs are positioned in a straight line, uncrossed, and not touching each other.

131. The head is supported by a headrest or pillow to prevent stretching of neck muscles.

132. Arms may rest on padded armboards or at the patient's side. When the arms are extended, armboards are positioned at less than a 90° angle from the body and palms are supinated (facing upward) to prevent ulnar and radial nerve compression.

133. When the arms are positioned at the patient's sides, the palms should rest against the patient and the elbows should be padded and must not be flexed or extend beyond the mattress. The arm is secured with a draw sheet that extends above the elbows and is secured under the patient (AORN, 2011, p. 345).

134. Take extra caution to be sure the sheet securing the arm is not so tight that it will interfere with the blood pressure cuff or intravenous line. The risk for infiltration of the intravenous line or compartment syndrome exists with the arms tucked.

135. A small pillow may be placed under the lumbar curvature to prevent the back strain that occurs when paraspinal muscles are relaxed

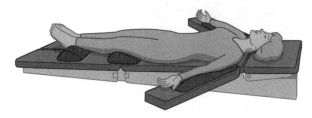

Figure 5-14 Supine position.

from anesthetic and muscle-relaxant agents. An anesthetized patient lying on the back for hours will likely experience temporary lumbar pain without a lumbar support.

136. The table strap is applied loosely at least 2 inches above the knees to prevent hyperextension of the knees. The strap should be secure, but not constricting, and should never be placed over a bony prominence.

137. Appropriate protective padding is placed at pressure points. To prevent plantar flexion and crushing injuries to the toes, the table must extend beyond the toes. A table extension may be required for tall patients.

138. Pressure points at risk for skin injury in the supine position include skin over bony prominences: occiput, spinous processes, scapulae, styloid process of the ulna and radius (elbow), olecranon process, sacrum, and calcaneus (heel). Skin breakdown from pressure is most common on the elbow, the sacrum, and the heel (Figure 5-5).

139. Nerves or nerve groups at risk include the brachial plexus, radial, ulnar, median, common peroneal, and tibial nerves.

140. Vital capacity can be reduced because of restriction of posterior chest expansion. If the patient is pregnant, a wedge may be placed under the patient's right side to prevent

hypotension caused by pressure from the uterus on the aorta and vena cava.

Trendelenburg

141. Trendelenburg (**Figure 5-15**) is a supine position in which the table is tilted head down so that the patient's head is lower than the feet. This position is used for providing additional visualization of the lower abdomen and pelvis and is also indicated for patients who develop hypovolemic shock. Patients having robot procedures are frequently placed in the Trendelenburg position.

142. The patient is positioned supine with knees over the lower break in the table. All safety measures are initiated before the table is tilted. To help maintain this position, the lower part of the table may be adjusted so that the patient's legs are parallel with the floor.

143. Take particular care when using shoulder braces because they pose a risk for brachial plexus injury unless they are positioned very carefully against the acromion and spinous process of the scapula.

144. Check the position of the patient's arm and hand to make certain that the elbow does not extend beyond the table and that the fingers are not too close to the lower break in the table where they might be crushed when the table is adjusted.

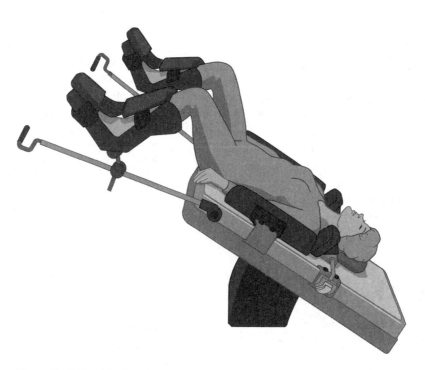

Figure 5-15 Trendelenburg.

145. Before the table is tilted into Trendelenburg position, Mayo stands, tables, and other equipment are adjusted.

146. All movements are done slowly to allow the body enough time to adjust to the change in blood volume, respiratory exchange, and displacement of abdominal contents.

147. Before the procedure begins, ensure that the Mayo stand and other equipment are not touching the patient.

148. Respiratory and circulatory changes occur as a result of redistribution of body mass. Abdominal contents press against the diaphragm, limiting expansion and decreasing the ventilation–perfusion ratio.

149. Trendelenburg position increases intrathoracic and intracranial pressure. Because of these changes, the patient should remain in Trendelenburg position for as short a time as possible.

Reverse Trendelenburg

150. In reverse Trendelenburg, the table is tilted feet down. This position is used for head and neck procedures and to provide visualization in laparoscopic procedures in the upper abdomen.

151. The patient's feet should rest firmly on a padded footboard, preventing the patient from sliding down on the table.

152. A pneumatic sequential compression device, elastic bandages, or anti-embolectomy stockings prevent pooling of blood in the legs.

153. Movement in and out of reverse Trendelenburg is done slowly to allow sufficient time for the heart to adjust to change in blood volume.

Section Questions

1. Describe the proper positioning of the patient in supine position. [Refs 130–137]

2. What is important about positioning the patient's arm on an armboard? [Ref 132]

3. What is one danger of securing the arms tightly at the patient's side? [Ref 134]

4. What might happen if the patient's feet extend beyond the operating room table? [Ref 137]

5. Name the bony prominences at risk for pressure injury in the supine position. [Ref 138]

6. Which nerves are at risk for injury in the supine position? [Ref 139]

7. How do we relieve pressure on the vena cava when positioning a pregnant patient? [Ref 140]

8. How does the Trendelenburg position differ from the supine position? [Ref 141]

9. In which instances is the Trendelenburg position appropriate? [Ref 141]

10. What is the danger in using shoulder braces to keep the patient from sliding in Trendelenburg position? [Ref 143]

11. Why are changes in position done slowly? [Ref 146]

12. How are the patient's anatomy and physiology affected in Trendelenburg position? [Refs 148–149]

13. For which types of procedures is the reverse Trendelenburg position used? [Ref 150]

14. What can we use to keep the patient from sliding in the reverse Trendelenburg position? [Ref 151]

15. Why is the patient moved in and out of reverse Trendelenburg slowly? [Ref 153]

Lithotomy

154. In lithotomy position, the patient is supine with the legs elevated, abducted, and supported in stirrups (**Figure 5-16**). The buttocks are even with the lower break in the table.

155. This position is used primarily for procedures involving the perineum region, pelvic organs, and genitalia.

156. Arms are secured on padded armboards to prevent crushing fingers and hands when the bottom section of the table is lowered or raised. Armboards should be positioned at an angle less than 90° to the body.

157. Stirrups are attached securely to the table, positioned according to the manufacturer's instructions, and adjusted to the length of the

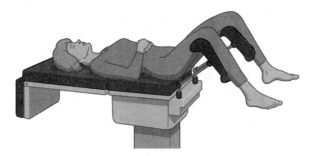

Figure 5-16 Lithotomy position.

patient's legs to prevent pressure at the knee and lumbar region of the spine.

158. Various types of stirrups are available, and their selection should be made carefully based on patient size and the type and length of the surgical procedure (Figure 5-10).

159. At-risk pressure points vary according to the type of stirrups used. Pay particular attention to the femoral epicondyle, tibial condyles, and lateral and medial malleoli.

160. Padding protects the legs from pressure from the stirrup itself, and from external compression of nerves. To prevent injury to the femoral and obturator nerves, the inner thigh should be free of pressure from the stirrup.

161. Although rare, compartment syndrome—characterized by pain, muscle weakness, and loss of sensation—has been reported as a complication of the lithotomy position (AORN, 2015, p. 572).

162. To prevent hip dislocation or muscle strain from an exaggerated range of motion, the legs are raised and lowered slowly and simultaneously by two members of the surgical team. During leg elevation, the foot is held in one hand and the lower part of the leg in the other hand. The legs are flexed slowly, and the padded foot is secured in the stirrup.

163. Padding may be placed under the sacrum to prevent lumbosacral strain.

164. After the legs are safely secured, the bottom section of the table is lowered or removed.

165. Following the procedure, the lower section of the table is raised or replaced to align with the rest of the table. The patient's legs are removed from the stirrups simultaneously, extended fully to prevent abduction of the hips, and lowered slowly onto the table. The table strap is then applied.

166. When the legs are lowered, 500 to 800 mL of blood is diverted from the visceral area to the extremities, which can cause hypotension. Lowering the legs slowly will prevent severe sudden hypotension.

167. Lithotomy position can reduce respiratory efficiency if pressure from the thighs on the abdomen and pressure from the abdominal viscera on the diaphragm restrict thoracic expansion. Lung tissue becomes engorged with blood, and vital capacity and tidal volume are decreased.

168. If nursing assessment suggests a limited range of hip motion because of contractures, arthritis, prosthesis, or another condition, the patient may be placed in lithotomy position while awake so the patient can participate and ensure that the position is comfortable.

Sitting, Beach Chair

169. The sitting position (**Figure 5-17**) is primarily used for shoulder surgery, often with the beach-chair table attachment that allows half of the backrest on the affected side to be removed for improved access to the surgical site.

170. During breast reconstruction, the patient is sometimes raised into the sitting position to assess breast symmetry, and occasionally the patient remains in the sitting position for the remainder of the surgery.

171. The sitting position has been used for certain craniotomies and cervical laminectomy, but this is rarely done, because the negative venous pressure in the head and neck places these patients at risk for air embolism that can be fatal. When done, a central venous catheter with a Doppler ultrasound flowmeter monitors the

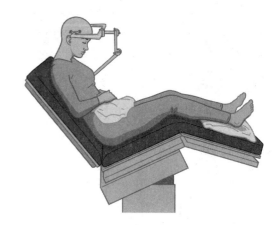

Figure 5-17 Sitting position.

sitting patient. The Doppler device is used to detect an air embolism, and the central venous pressure line is used to extract the air.

172. The patient is initially positioned supine. The head is supported in a secure headrest. The feet are usually supported on a padded footrest. The foot of the table is slowly lowered, flexing the knees and pelvis. The upper portion of the table is raised to become the backrest, and the torso reaches an upright position.

173. The arms may be flexed at the elbows and rest on a pillow on the patient's lap or on an adjustable padded platform in front of the patient. The arms should not fall into a dependent position.

174. Pressure points are similar to the supine position; however, the operating table should have a well-constructed, pressure-reducing pad because most of the patient's body weight rests on the ischial tuberosities and the sacral nerve.

175. Additional padding will protect other pressure points at increased risk for injury including the scapulae, olecranon process, back of the knees, sacrum, ischial tuberosities, and calcaneus.

176. Antiembolism stockings or a sequential compression device prevent postural hypotension and pooling of blood in lower extremities.

Semi-Sitting, Semi-Fowler's, Lawn-Chair Position

177. The Semi-Fowler's position is essentially a supine position with the table adjusted to emulate a lawnchair. The patient's body is flexed at the pelvis and knees. While the patient is in a reclining position, the back of the table can be adjusted from nearlyflat to nearly sitting, depending upon the procedure.

178. With the back raised to different levels, this position is used for nasopharyngeal, facial, neck, and breast surgery.

179. A roll may be placed under the patient's neck to hyperextend the neck and provide better access to the surgical site.

Section Questions

1. Describe the lithotomy position. [Ref 154]

2. Why should the patient's arms be positioned on armboards? [Ref 156]

3. Which pressure points are at risk for injury when the patient's legs are in stirrups? [Ref 159]

4. Describe compartment syndrome. [Ref 161]

5. Why are the patient's legs raised and lowered slowly and simultaneously? [Ref 162]

6. What is the procedure for removing legs from stirrups at the conclusion of the procedure? [Ref 165]

7. How can lowering the legs cause hypotension, and what can be done to prevent this? [Ref 166]

8. How can the lithotomy position reduce respiratory efficiency? [Ref 167]

9. What patient conditions represent a challenge to placing a patient in the lithotomy position? [Ref 168]

10. For what procedures can the sitting position be used? [Refs 169–171]

11. Describe the danger of air embolism in the sitting position, and explain how this risk is managed. [Ref 171]

12. How are the arms managed with the patient in the sitting position? [Ref 173]

13. What bony prominence bears the majority of the patient's weight in the sitting position? [Ref 174]

14. Identify other pressure points are at risk for injury in the sitting position. [Ref 174]

15. Describe the semi-Fowler's position. [Ref 177]

Prone

180. In the prone position, the patient lies face down (**Figure 5-18**). This exposure of the posterior body is used for procedures of the spine, back, rectum, and the posterior aspects of extremities.

181. The patient will either lie on a special table engineered for prone positioning, or on a regular table with a laminectomy frame (Wilson Frame) or chest rolls. All of the necessary positioning equipment must be collected and

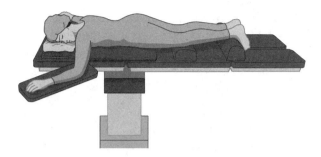

Figure 5-18 Prone position.

available prior to intubation and transfer of the patient.

182. The anesthesia provider induces the patient on the stretcher.

183. The stretcher height is raised slightly higher than the operating table to facilitate moving the patient from stretcher to table. The side rail closest to the operating table is lowered, and the stretcher is positioned adjacent to the operating table and locked.

184. Following intubation, the anesthesia provider secures the endotracheal tube to prevent dislocation and applies ointment to the eyes and tapes them shut to prevent corneal abrasion. The other side rail is lowered. The anesthesia provider will indicate when the patient is ready to be moved onto the operating room table.

185. A minimum of four persons is necessary to safely turn the adult patient from a supine position on the stretcher to a prone position on the operating table. The anesthesia provider supports and manages the head, one person supports and rotates the torso while the person on the other side of the bed positions the patient on the frame or chest rolls. The fourth person supports and moves the lower body.

186. All movement of the patient is done slowly and gently to allow the body time to adjust to the change in position. During turning, the patient's arms and hands are placed at the sides. The body is maintained in anatomical alignment, and all team members work in concert to turn the patient in a single motion.

187. The patient is placed either on the pads on the special table specifically designed for chest, hips, and thighs or onto chest rolls or a laminectomy frame (e.g., Wilson frame), positioned lengthwise on the operating table from the acromioclavicular joint to the iliac crest. This positioning lifts the patient's chest off the operating table and facilitates respiratory expansion.

Female breasts and male genitalia must be arranged to avoid unnecessary compression.

188. Chest rolls that are too small or that are improperly positioned can result in restricted lung expansion. Female breasts and male genitalia must be free and not compressed.

189. After the patient is supine, the arms are brought down and forward in a normal range of motion and placed on armboards positioned next to the head. The arms are flexed at the elbows with the hands pronated (palms down) and elbows padded.

190. The anesthesiologist either turns the patient's head to one side or places it in a headrest designed to protect the airway, and then checks that the patient's eyes are closed to prevent corneal abrasion and are free from pressure that can cause permanent eye injury. The ears must be not folded unnaturally. Neck and spine must be in good alignment.

191. A pillow under the ankles lifts the toes off the mattress and prevents stretching of the anterior tibial nerve to prevent plantar flexion and foot drop.

192. The table strap helps to hold the patient in position on the table. It is placed across the mid-thighs, which are first covered with a sheet, pad, and/or a blanket to protect the skin. The strap should be at least 2 inches above the knees to promote superficial venous return.

193. A small pillow or foam padding under the knees prevents pressure on the patellae.

194. If the patient has a stoma, take precautions to prevent ischemic compression of the stoma against the frame or chest rolls that can lead to tissue necrosis and sloughing.

195. Pedal pulses are assessed to assure circulation to the lower extremities.

Mayfield Headrest (with Pins)

196. If a Mayfield headrest (**Figure 5-19**) is used, the surgeon will attach the head brace with pins to the patient after induction while the patient is still supine on the stretcher.

197. After the patient has been placed in the prone position, the surgeon will hold the patient's head in the brace while the nurse removes the head attachment from the operating table and replaces it with the Mayfield table attachment.

198. The nurse will adjust the table attachment until it is aligned perfectly with the patient's head, which the surgeon is holding in the

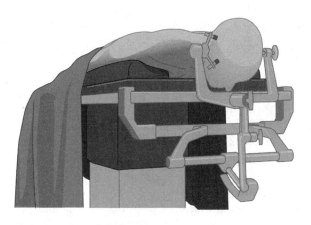

Figure 5-19 Mayfield headrest.

desired position for surgery. The nurse will then secure the headpiece in place.

199. The patient must never be repositioned on the table while the head brace is secured to the table attachment.

Kraske (Jackknife) Position

200. The jackknife position is used for rectal procedures (**Figure 5-20**).

201. The patient is first placed in the prone position on chest rolls with the hips over the center table joint. Chest rolls are not necessary if the patient is awake. The table is flexed to a 90° angle, causing the hips to be raised and the head and legs to be lowered.

202. All precautions appropriate for the prone position are applicable to the jackknife position.

203. Venous pooling in the chest and feet can cause a decrease in mean arterial blood pressure. Restriction of diaphragm movement combined with increased blood volume in the lungs can cause a decrease in ventilation and cardiac output. Because of its adverse effect on the respiratory and circulatory systems,

the jackknife position is considered one of the most precarious surgical positions.

Lateral

204. In the lateral (or lateral decubitus) position (**Figure 5-21**), the patient lies on one side. In the right lateral position, the patient lies on the right side for surgery on the left side of the body. The reverse is true for the left lateral position.

205. The lateral position is used to access the thorax, kidney, retroperitoneal space, and hip.

206. Lateral position is often supported with a pegboard (Figure 5-11) or beanbag vacuum-positioning device (Figure 5-12).

207. The patient is induced in the supine position. A team of four persons then lifts and turns the patient onto the nonoperative side. The patient is lifted in the supine position toward the edge of the operative side of the table then turned onto the side toward the center of the table.

208. The anesthesia provider supports the head and neck and guards the airway. The person standing on the operative side lifts and supports the chest and shoulders. The person on the patient's other side lifts and supports the hips, while the fourth person supports and rotates the legs.

209. The patient's head is supported with a pillow or headrest, and the body is checked for proper alignment with the head in cervical alignment with the spine.

210. The lower leg is flexed. The lateral aspect of the lower knee is well padded to prevent peroneal nerve damage that might result in foot drop caused by pressure from the fibula on the nerve. A pillow is placed between the legs, and the upper leg is extended. Feet and ankles are padded and supported to prevent foot drop and pressure injuries of the malleolus. The patient is secured with the table strap or with wide tape applied across the upper hip and fastened to the table.

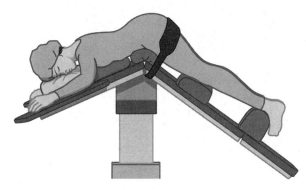

Figure 5-20 A jackknife position.

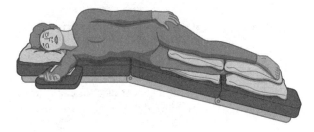

Figure 5-21 Lateral.

211. A small roll or padding is placed under the patient's lower axilla to relieve pressure on the chest and axilla, to allow sufficient chest expansion, and to prevent compression of the brachial plexus by the humeral head. The lower arm is slightly flexed and placed on a padded armboard. The upper arm may rest on a padded elevated armboard or other padded support. Take care not to abduct the arm more than 90°, because an angle greater than 90° can cause injury to the brachial plexus.

212. For kidney procedures, it is important that the patient's flank be positioned over the kidney elevator (kidney rest) with the iliac crest just below the table break. The table may be flexed at the center break. The kidney rest is raised to provide greater exposure of the area from the 12th rib to the iliac crest. Kidney braces that fit over the kidney elevator may be used to support and maintain the patient in this position. These devices must always be well padded.

213. Respiratory efficiency is affected by pressure from the weight of the body on the lower chest. The lower lung receives more blood from the right side of the heart in the lateral position, so it has increased perfusion but less residual air because of mediastinal compression and weight from abdominal contents.

214. Circulation is compromised by pressure on abdominal vessels and pooling of blood in the lower extremities. In the right lateral position, compression on the vena cava impairs venous return. If the kidney elevator is raised, additional pressure on abdominal vessels can further compromise circulation.

215. Injury of the eye or ear is a special concern with the patient in the lateral position. The ear must lie flat and the eyelid must be closed.

Section Questions

1. What procedures are commonly done in the prone position? [Ref 180]

2. What positioning equipment options are available for the prone position? [Ref 181]

3. Describe the process of moving the supine patient into the prone position. [Refs 182–186]

4. What specific responsibilities are associated with positioning the patient on a laminectomy frame or chest rolls? [Ref 187]

5. Describe the proper method for positioning the arms in prone position. [Ref 189]

6. How does the anesthesia provider protect the head and maintain the patient's airway? [Ref 190]

7. Describe positioning of the legs and feet. [Refs 191, 193]

8. Why is it important to assess pedal pulses with a patient in the prone position? [Ref 195]

9. What are special considerations associated with the Mayfield headrest with pins? [Refs 196–199]

10. Why is the jackknife position considered precarious? [Ref 203]

11. The patient will be placed in the right lateral position for surgery on which kidney? [Ref 204]

12. What positioning devices are available for lateral positioning? [Ref 206]

13. Describe the transition from the supine position to the lateral position. [Refs 207–211]

14. What is the purpose of the kidney rest? [Ref 212]

15. Describe the impact on respiratory efficiency and circulation in the lateral position. [Refs 213–214]

Positioning the Morbidly Obese Patient

216. The morbidly obese patient is an individual with a BMI of greater than 40.

217. The operating room bed must be capable of supporting the patient's weight and must be wide enough to contain the patient. Side extensions may be necessary. The manufacturer's instructions for use must be followed for weight restrictions.

218. Obesity places an increased workload on the heart and circulatory system, and respiratory

function is compromised in obese patients because of increased weight on the chest.

219. The supine position may cause the patient to have difficulty breathing due to pressure of the viscera on the diaphragm. A wedge should be placed under the right flank to relieve pressure on the vena cava.

220. The lithotomy and Trendelenburg positions should be avoided, because they may also cause respiratory and circulatory compromise.

221. The prone position may cause pressure on the diaphragm.

222. Skin breakdown is a challenge with obese patients, because moisture and fluids from skin-prep solutions may become trapped in tissue folds. Adipose tissue is not well vascularized, and the pressure resulting from positioning can cause a decrease in circulation to peripheral body areas.

223. The safety strap must be long enough and wide enough to secure the patient. Two safety straps may be necessary—one for the upper portion of the legs and one for the lower portion.

224. Lifting devices should be used to transfer the patient.

Evaluating the Positioned Patient

225. The anesthetized patient cannot report discomfort or pain related to positioning, and the effects of improper positioning will usually not be identified until the patient recovers from anesthesia and is able to report pain and injury. The patient relies on the surgical team to ensure that positioning injuries do not occur.

226. Once the patient is in position for the surgery, and before prepping and draping the patient, the perioperative nurse should do a thorough, once-over check to ensure that the patient's body is in alignment, extremities are not extended beyond their natural range of motion, bony prominences are appropriately padded, nerves where injury can occur are protected, respiratory and circulatory efforts are restricted as little as possible, and positioning devices are appropriately positioned and padded and holding the patient's body securely without excessive restriction on body structures.

227. Intermittent reevaluation of the patient's position throughout the procedure is important. If the patient is repositioned during the procedure, a thorough reevaluation is critical, with adjustments made as necessary.

Postoperative Transfer

228. When surgery is completed and the anesthesia provider indicates that the patient is stable and can be moved, the postoperative bed or stretcher is brought adjacent to the operating table. It is raised or lowered to the level of the operating table and locked into place.

229. Ideally, four people should be available to transfer the anesthetized adult patient slowly and smoothly to the bed or stretcher with a roller or lateral transfer sheet/device, maintaining the airway and proper body alignment. Lines and catheters must be protected and kept free from entanglement.

230. The patient is lifted or rolled onto the bed or stretcher, avoiding pushing and pulling. Side rails are raised and locked for safe patient transfer.

Documentation of Nursing Actions

231. Nursing documentation related to positioning should include the following information:

- Assessment and considerations for positioning—desired outcomes
- Overall skin condition on arrival and discharge from the perioperative suite
- Position
- Placement of extremities
- Type and placement of positioning equipment and devices, such as stirrups, rolls, padding, and restraints
- Precautions to protect eyes
- Presence and placement of safety strap or equivalent
- Who positioned the patient
- Any changes made in positioning during the procedure
- Patient condition following surgery—whether desired outcomes were met
- Signature

Section Questions

1. How can you tell if a bed is designed to support the weight of your patient? [Ref 217]

2. What are some of the challenges the obese patient faces with positioning? [Refs 218–219]

3. How might pressure on the vena cava be relieved to promote improved circulation? [Ref 219]

4. What challenges for the obese patient are associated with prone, lithotomy, and Trendelenburg positions? [Refs 220–221]

5. Why are obese patients at high risk for skin breakdown? [Ref 222]

6. What is the purpose of a "once-over check" following positioning of the patient? [Ref 226]

7. Which member of the surgical team determines when the patient can be moved following surgery? [Ref 227]

8. How many people should participate in transferring the patient from the operating table to bed or stretcher? [Ref 229]

9. What safety considerations are associated with moving the patient onto the stretcher or bed? [Ref 229]

10. Which elements should be included in the nurse's documentation of positioning? [Ref 231]

References

Aronovich, S. (2007). Intraoperatively acquired pressure ulcers: Are there common risk factors? *Ostomy/Wound Management, 53*(2), 57–69.

Association of periOperative Registered Nurses (AORN). (2011). *Perioperative nursing data set* (3rd ed.). Denver, CO: AORN.

Association of periOperative Registered Nurses (AORN). (2015). *Guidelines for perioperative practice.* Denver, CO: AORN.

Centers for Medicare and Medicaid (CMS). (2015) *Hospital-acquired conditions (present on admission indicator).* Retrieved: https://www.cms.gov/Medicare/Medicare-Fee-for-Service-Payment/HospitalAcqCond/index.html

Chen, H., Chen, X.,& Wu, J. (2012). Incidence of pressure ulcers in surgical patients in the last 5 years: A systematic review.*Wounds, 24*(9), 234–241.

Galvin, P.,& Curley, M. (2012).The Braden Q+P: A Pediatric perioperative pressure ulcer risk assessment and intervention tool. *AORN Journal,96*(3), 261–270.

Gerkin, S. (2013). Preventing positioning injuries: An anesthesiologist's perspectives. *AAOS Now.* Retrieved from http://www.aaos.org/news/aaosnow/jan13/managing7.asp

Goodman, T. (2012). *Positioning: A patient safety initiative: Study guide for nurses.* Dallas, TX: Terri Goodman & Associates.

Hermans, M., Weyl, C., & Reger, S.(2014). Performanceparameters of support surfaces: Setting measuring and presentation standards.*Wounds, 26*(1)28–36. Retrieved from http://www.woundsresearch.com/article/performance-parameters-support-surfaces-setting-measuring-and-presentation-standards

The Joint Commission. (2012). *National patient safety goals* (Goal 14). Retrieved http://www.lovell.fhcc.va.gov/about/2012PatientSafetyGoals.pdf

National Pressure Ulcer Advisory Panel (NPUAP) (2012). Deep Tissue Injury. Retrieved: http://www.npuap.org/wp-content/uploads/2012/01/DTI-White-Paper.pdf

Primiano, M., Friend, M., McClure, C., Nardi, S., Fix, L., Schafer, M., . . .McNett, M.(2011). Pressure ulcer prevalence and risk factors during prolonged surgical procedures.*AORN Journal, 94*(6), 555–566.

Rehabilitation Engineering and Assistive Technology Society of North America (RESNA)(2014). *American national standard for support surfaces.Volume 1: Requirements and test methods for full body support surfaces.* Arlington, VA: Author.

Seaman, M., Wobb, J., Gaughan, J., Kulp, H., Kamel, I., & Dempsey, D. (2012, April). The effects of intraoperative hypothermia on surgical site infection. *Annals of Surgery, 224* (4): pp 789–795.

Post-Test

Read each question carefully. Each question may have more than one correct answer.

1. What is the primary reason for selecting a specific surgical position?
   a. Preventing tissue damage
   b. Providing exposure to the operative site
   c. Keeping the patient comfortable
   d. Following facility policy

2. What are the two primary nursing responsibilities associated with positioning the patient?
   a. Stabilizing the patient to prevent inadvertent movement
   b. Preserving the patient's dignity
   c. Protecting the patient from injury
   d. Assisting anesthesia with maintaining the patient's airway

3. Ideally, which member of the surgical team orchestrates the positioning process?
   a. Surgeon
   b. Anesthesiologist
   c. Scrub nurse
   d. Circulating nurse

4. Which factors influence the potential for injury related to surgical positioning?
   a. Type of procedure
   b. Age of the patient
   c. Position required for the procedure
   d. Comorbidities

5. Which of the following positions is most likely to affect circulation and oxygen–carbon dioxide exchange?
   a. Supine
   b. Sitting
   c. Trendelenburg
   d. Reverse Trendelenburg

6. What physiologic outcomes are associated with compromised respiratory mechanics?
   a. Hypoventilation
   b. Hyperkalemia
   c. Hypercarbia
   d. Hypoxia

7. What are the three components of Virchow's triad that contribute to the formation of DVT?
   a. Venous stasis
   b. Hypercoagulability
   c. Small-diameter vessels
   d. Vessel wall injury

8. Which of the following procedures places patients at high risk for DVT formation?
   a. Coronary artery bypass
   b. Laparoscopic cholecystectomy
   c. Craniotomy
   d. Total hip replacement

9. Which of the following is likely to cause injury to the brachial plexus?
   a. Tucking the arms too tightly at the patient's sides
   b. Hyperextension of the arm on an armboard
   c. An automatic blood pressure cuff cycling too often
   d. Pressure on the acromion process of the elbow

10. Injury to which nerve accounts for one-third of nerve injuries related to positioning?
    a. Brachial plexus
    b. Radial nerve
    c. Peroneal nerve
    d. Ulnar nerve

11. Which of the following are symptoms of an ulnar nerve injury?
    a. Pain, tingling, or numbness in the ring finger and little finger
    b. Weakness of grip leading to a "claw hand"
    c. Pain, tingling, or numbness in the first and middle fingers
    d. Wrist drop

12. What three primary factors impact the risk for sustaining tissue damage?
    a. Surgical procedure
    b. Immobility
    c. Pressure
    d. Time

13. Which of the following injuries occurs when the skin remains stationary when the patient is moved?
    a. Shear
    b. Friction
    c. Pressure
    d. DVT

14. What is a deep tissue injury?
    a. A red area over a bony prominence that progresses from skin to deep tissues
    b. Stage IV ulcer
    c. Damage to the large muscles
    d. Necrosis at the bone–tissue interface that does not become evident until days after surgery

15. Extrinsic factors that contribute to pressure injuries include
    a. sedation.
    b. warming devices.
    c. length of surgery.
    d. obesity.

16. Which of the following place(s) the elderly at great risk for tissue damage?
    a. Decreased muscle tone
    b. Less subcutaneous tissue to protect bony prominences
    c. Heightened sensitivity to heat
    d. Poor skin turgor

17. What is the most critical component when preparing to transfer the patient from the stretcher to the operatingtable?
    a. Suction on and available
    b. A sufficient number of personnel
    c. Raising the stretcher to equal the height of the operating table
    d. Lifting device

18. How can blankets and sheets be used in positioning the patient?
    a. Draw sheet to reposition patient
    b. Provide warmth
    c. Provide privacy
    d. Rolled up to provide support

19. The table strap should be placed
    a. as soon as the patient has been transferred to the operating table.
    b. snugly across the patient's knees.
    c. 2 inches above the patient's knees.
    d. across the patient's hips.

20. Which of the following represents correct positioning of the patient's hands?
    a. Palms up on padded armboard
    b. Palms up when arms are at the patient's side
    c. Palms down on padded armboard
    d. Palms facing patient when arms are at the patient's side

21. Pressure points associated with the supine position include which of the following?
    a. Occiput
    b. Acromion process of the shoulder
    c. Sacrum
    d. Heel

22. The Trendelenburg (head down) position is used
    a. to provide good visualization of the lower abdomen and pelvis.
    b. to manage hypovolemic shock.
    c. for obese patients, to keep them from sliding off the table.
    d. for robotic surgery.

23. Why is movement out of the Trendelenburg position done slowly?
    a. To keep the patient from getting dizzy
    b. To prevent nausea and vomiting
    c. To prevent headache and increased intracranial pressure
    d. To allow the patient to adjust to the changes in blood volume and respiratory exchange

24. Some challenges in the Trendelenburg position include
    a. decreased intrathoracic pressure.
    b. decreased ventilation–perfusion ratio.
    c. increased intracranial pressure.
    d. Mayo stand placing pressure on the patient's legs and feet.

25. For what circumstances is the reverse Trendelenburg position appropriate?
    a. Head and neck procedures
    b. Obese patients
    c. Laparoscopic procedures of the upper abdomen
    d. Craniotomy

26. What steps are taken to prevent hip dislocation and muscle strain in the lithotomy position?
    a. Legs are raised quickly, one at a time.
    b. Legs are raised slowly, one at a time.
    c. Legs are raised and lowered slowly and simultaneously.
    d. Legs are raised and lowered quickly and simultaneously.

27. What is a serious potential complication associated with the sitting position?
    a. Postural hypotension
    b. Air embolism
    c. Iliac crest compression
    d. Increased intracranial pressure

28. How is cardiorespiratory expansion preserved in the prone position?
    a. Pillows are placed under the patient's chest.
    b. Shoulder braces hold the patient in place.
    c. Chest rolls or a laminectomy frame lift the patient's chest from the table.
    d. The patient's weight rests on knees and shoulders.

29. How are the patient's arms managed in the prone position?
    a. Arms are at the sides when the patient is turned onto the bed.
    b. Arms are extended on padded armboards at an angle less than 90°.
    c. Arms are tucked at the sides with palms facing the patient.
    d. Arms are rotated down and forward onto armboards next to the patient's head.

30. What is one very important principle related to positioning in a Mayfield headrest with pins?
    a. The surgeon will attach the head brace before the induction of anesthesia.
    b. The patient must never be repositioned while the head is secured to the table attachment.
    c. Final positioning of the patient on the table will be completed after the head brace has been secured in the table attachment.
    d. The surgeon aligns the patient's head in the head brace with the table attachment that the nurse is holding.

31. Which of the following are challenges related to the jackknife position?
    a. Restriction of diaphragm movement
    b. Increased blood volume in the lungs
    c. Increase in ventilation and cardiac output
    d. Venous pooling in the chest and feet

32. Which areas are at risk for injury in the lateral position?
    a. Eye
    b. Ear
    c. Peroneal nerve
    d. Brachial plexus

33. Which of the following are challenges that an obese surgical patient faces?
    a. Respiratory restriction from visceral contents pushing against the diaphragm
    b. Circulatory compromise due to the increased workload obesity places on the heart
    c. Skin break because adipose tissue is poorly vascularized and pressure can cause a further decrease in circulation
    d. Moisture trapped in skin folds, which can accelerate tissue breakdown

34. Describe the reason for the "once-over" check of the patient following positioning.
    a. Once the drapes are in place and the surgery has begun, it is too late to spot and correct positioning errors.
    b. The circulating nurse is ultimately responsible for any adverse outcomes of positioning.
    c. Any improvements in patient positioning can be made prior to prepping and draping of the patient.
    d. A thorough reevaluation of the patient's position is important if the patient is repositioned during the surgical procedure.

35. Nursing documentation related to positioning should include:
    a. the patient's skin condition before positioning.
    b. the patient's position and positioning equipment used.
    c. the presence and placement of a safety strap.
    d. who positioned the patient.

Competency Checklist:
Positioning the Patient for Surgery

Under "Observer's Initials," enter initials upon successful achievement of competency. Enter N/A if competency is not appropriate for institution.

Name _____

	Observer's Initials	Date
1. Table operation		
a. Armboards—attach, remove, adjust	_____	_____
b. Rotation—right, left, Trendelenburg, reverse Trendelenburg, flex	_____	_____
c. Lower leg portion of table and remove section (lithotomy position)	_____	_____
d. Attach/remove side rail stirrup holders	_____	_____
e. Other	_____	_____
2. Patient transfer		
a. Side rails up and secure during transport	_____	_____
b. Patient covered	_____	_____
c. Stretcher adjacent to table with proximal side rail lowered	_____	_____
d. Stretcher and table locked	_____	_____
e. Stretcher and table are equal height	_____	_____
f. Two team members present during transfer	_____	_____
g. Patient lifted or rolled, not pulled; lift/transfer device as appropriate	_____	_____
3. Supine		
a. Patient is flat on back with head and spine in a straight, horizontal line.	_____	_____
b. Hips are parallel and legs are in a straight line and uncrossed.	_____	_____
c. Safety strap is placed at least 2 inches above the knees (secure but nonconstricting).	_____	_____
d. Small pillow is placed beneath the patient's head.	_____	_____
e. Arms extended on armboards are at less than a 90° angle from the body and supinated.	_____	_____
f. Arms at patient's side are not flexed and do not extend beyond the mattress; arms are secured with a draw sheet, not too tightly.	_____	_____
g. Protective padding is placed at pressure points.	_____	_____
4. Trendelenburg		
a. Patient is positioned supine.	_____	_____
b. Knees are over lower break of the table.	_____	_____
c. Table is tilted head down.	_____	_____
d. Following table tilt, patient's toes are checked.	_____	_____
5. Reverse Trendelenburg		
a. Patient is positioned supine.	_____	_____
b. Table is tilted feet down.	_____	_____
6. Lithotomy		
a. Equipment assembled	_____	_____
• Appropriate stirrups	_____	_____
• Operating table stirrup holders	_____	_____
• Padding	_____	_____

    b. Patient is initially positioned supine. _____ _____

    c. Buttocks are positioned directly above the break in the table. _____ _____

    d. Both legs are simultaneously and slowly raised and positioned in stirrups by two people. _____ _____

    e. Both stirrups are at even height. _____ _____

    f. Fibular head is free of pressure from stirrups. _____ _____

    g. Stirrups are not exerting pressure against the upper inner aspect of the calf. _____ _____

    h. Padded stirrups do not compress vascular structures in the popliteal space. _____ _____

    i. Padding is placed beneath the sacrum. _____ _____

    j. Both legs are slowly and simultaneously lowered to the bed by two people. _____ _____

7. Sitting

    a. Patient is initially positioned supine. _____ _____

    b. Foot of table is slowly lowered. _____ _____

    c. Upper portion of table is raised. _____ _____

    d. Feet are supported on a padded footrest. _____ _____

    e. Torso and shoulders are secured with table strap. _____ _____

    f. Arms are flexed and positioned on a pillow on the patient's lap. _____ _____

    g. Pressure points are padded. _____ _____

8. Prone

    a. Equipment assembled _____ _____

       • Chest roll or laminectomy frame _____ _____

       • Donut _____ _____

       • Pillows and padding _____ _____

    b. Patient is logrolled from the stretcher to the operating table onto chest rolls or laminectomy frame by four people. _____ _____

    c. Arms are rotated through their normal range of motion and positioned on padded armboards next to the patient's head. _____ _____

    d. Arms are not abducted beyond 90°. _____ _____

    e. Elbows are padded. _____ _____

    f. Patient's head is positioned to one side and supported on a donut. _____ _____

    g. Eyes and ears are checked for pressure points. _____ _____

    h. Male genitalia are checked for pressure points. _____ _____

    i. Female breasts are checked for pressure points. _____ _____

    j. Knees and toes are protected with padding. _____ _____

9. Jackknife (Kraske's)

    a. Patient is positioned prone. _____ _____

    b. Hips are placed over the center table break. _____ _____

    c. Arms are positioned on padded armboards next to the patient's head. _____ _____

    d. Elbows are flexed; palms are pronated. _____ _____

    e. Pillow is placed beneath the ankles. _____ _____

    f. Table strap is placed across thighs. _____ _____

    g. Table is flexed to a 90° angle. _____ _____

	Observer's Initials	Date

10. Lateral

   a. Equipment is assembled (all components, attachments, pillows, etc.). _____ _____

   b. Patient begins in supine position. _____ _____

   c. Patient is turned onto the nonoperative side by four people. _____ _____

   d. Patient's head is in cervical alignment with the spine. _____ _____

   e. Bottom leg is flexed. _____ _____

   f. Lateral aspect of lower knee is padded. _____ _____

   g. Upper leg is extended. _____ _____

   h. Pillow is placed between the legs. _____ _____

   i. Patient is secured with table strap or tape across hips. _____ _____

   j. Axillary roll is placed at the lower axilla. _____ _____

   k. Lower arm is flexed on a padded armboard. _____ _____

   l. Upper arm is supported on a padded elevated armboard/pillow/padded support. _____ _____

   m. Arms are not abducted more than 90°. _____ _____

   n. Lower ear is flat and eyes are closed. _____ _____

11. Assembles appropriate positioning devices for morbidly obese patient _____ _____

12. Documentation

   a. Preoperative assessment of skin _____ _____

   b. Assessment—considerations for positioning _____ _____

   c. Position _____ _____

   d. Placement of padding _____ _____

   e. Safety strap _____ _____

   f. Who positioned patient _____ _____

   g. Intraoperative changes made to position _____ _____

   h. Outcome _____ _____

   i. Signature _____ _____

Observer's Signature   Initials   Date

_____

Orientee's Signature

_____

6

Prevention of Retained Surgical Items

LEARNER OBJECTIVES

1. Identify the desired patient outcome for counts in surgery.
2. Discuss nursing responsibilities for counts in surgery.
3. Describe the procedures for soft goods, sharps, and instrument counts.
4. List documentation requirements for counts.

LESSON OUTLINE

Overview

1. Retained surgical items (RSIs)—soft goods, sharps, instruments—occur in an estimated 1 in 5,500 surgeries. Gauze sponges account for 48% to 69% of RSIs. Steelman and Cullen (2011) identify the abdomen as the cavity most often involved. In abdominal surgeries, the incidence is 1 in every 1,000 to 1,500 operations (American Hospital Association, 2011). The Association of periOperative Registered Nurses (AORN, 2015) cites the abdomen and pelvis as sites where retained items are most frequently found.

2. A retained surgical item is considered a sentinel event or "never event"—an unexpected occurrence involving death or serious injury that is reasonably preventable by following evidence-based guidelines. The Joint Commission (TJC, 2014b) identified RSIs as the most frequently reported sentinel event every year since 2010 (Table 6-1).

3. RSI is first on the Centers for Medicare and Medicaid Service's (CMS, 2014, p. 10) list of hospital-acquired, non-reimbursed conditions.

4. Items opened and delivered to the sterile field that could be retained in the surgical wound are counted to prevent patient injury. Counted items include soft goods (radiopaque sponges and towels); sharps such as blades, needles, drill bits; instruments; and miscellaneous items such as vessel loops and vein introducers.

5. The purpose of a count is to reconcile everything delivered to the sterile field before the initial incision and during the procedure with what remains at the end of surgery.

Definitions

Gossypiboma: Unintentional retention of soft goods.

Never event: Medical errors that should never occur because they are entirely preventable.

Radiopaque marker: Thread or patch sewn into a sponge or towel that can be visualized on X-ray.

Retained surgical item (RSI): A preventable occurrence of leaving soft goods, sharps, or an instrument in a patient following a surgical procedure.

RF technology: Radiofrequency chip embedded in the fabric of soft goods that can be identified by a wand, connected to a detection console, that is passed over the patient.

Sentinel event: An unexpected patient safety event that reaches a patient and results in death, permanent harm, or severe temporary harm and intervention required to sustain life.

Soft goods: Sponges and towels used on the surgical field; each must have a radiopaque marker.

Table 6-1	Sentinel Events				
Sentinel Event	**2010**	**2011**	**2012**	**2013**	**2014**
Retained foreign body	**133**	**168**	**115**	**102**	**112**
Wrong pt/site/procedure	93	152	109	109	67
Delay in treatment	95	138	107	113	73
Suicide	67	131	85	90	82
Op/postop complication	86	133	83	77	52
Falls	56	96	76	82	91

Data from The Joint Commission. (2015). Summary Data of Sentinel Events Reviewed by the Joint Commission. SE Statistics as of 1/14/2015; The Joint Commission. (2012). Summary Data of Sentinel Events Reviewed by The Joint Commission. SE Statistics as of 12/31/2012.

6. AORN (2015, p. 348) asserts that a standardized, transparent, verifiable, and reliable system that accounts for all items opened and used during a surgical procedure is a primary and proactive injury-prevention strategy. Such a system recognizes that the entire surgical team is responsible for preventing RSIs, that clear and accurate communication is essential, and that unnecessary activities, distractions, and multitasking can interfere with the proper implementation of any process and must be controlled.

7. Many healthcare facilities have established count policies that reflect the AORN's guidelines for prevention of retained surgical items; however, there are also facilities whose count policies differ from the AORN guidelines (**Exhibit 6-1**). Count policies should specify when counts are to be taken, by whom, and what is counted.

8. According to TJC (2013), the most common root causes of RSIs are the absence of policies and procedures and failure to comply with existing policies and procedures.

9. Policies specify what is counted based on the nature of the procedure, the anticipated size of the incision, the probability of a retained item, and the supplies required for the procedure. It identifies who participates in the count, what

Exhibit 6-1 Facility Count Policy

POLICY TITLE: PROCEDURAL COUNTS: SPONGES, SHARPS, MISC. ITEMS AND INSTRUMENTS
DEPARTMENT: SURGICAL SERVICES
POLICY MANUAL: PATIENT CARE
CORPORATE REFERENCE: NONE
EFFECTIVE DATE: 1.1.15   REVISED DATES:
POLICY NUMBER: PC. 701.107   REPLACES POLICY NUMBER (S):

POLICY:

Sponges, sharps, miscellaneous items and instruments (as appropriate for the case) on the operative field will be counted on every surgical and/or invasive procedure and every vaginal delivery to prevent unintended retention of a surgical item in a patient.

PURPOSE:

To establish a proactive injury prevention process that will help to avoid injury to patients when the possibility exists for objects to be unintentionally retained after a surgical and/or invasive procedure. All items need to be accounted for at the end of a procedure so that all team members can be sure that a surgical item is not left in the patient.

PROCEDURE:

All counts will be performed in a standard approach.

An initial sponge, sharp, miscellaneous item count and instrument inventory is initiated prior to the beginning of all surgical procedures to establish a baseline for reference. All like items will be counted together at one time, i.e., all sponges, all laps, all needles, etc.

The Circulating Nurse and the scrub person are responsible to perform the surgical/procedural counts. All items will be counted audibly by the Scrub person and Circulating Nurse while concurrently viewing each item and instrument as it is counted. Unnecessary activity and distraction such as radios, pagers, and conversation will be curtailed during the counting process to allow the Scrub person and the Circulating Nurse to focus on counting.

1. When counting instruments, the instrument menu count list will be used to establish an accurate baseline count.
2. The circulating nurse is responsible for counting and recording the count on the work sheet and/or white board, which is maintained throughout the procedure. The Scrub Tech is responsible to verify the integrity and completeness of all counted items during the baseline count and as items placed within the patient are removed. The Circulating Nurse is responsible for recording the results of the final counts on the operative/procedure record and informing the surgeon/proceduralist and surgical team of the count results. Both the Circulating Nurse and the Scrub person must verify the presence of a radiopaque element in all sponges. Completion of the proper counting procedure is the responsibility of the entire Operative/Procedural team.
3. Surgical procedural counts will include:
   a. Sponges: separated and counted on all procedures
   b. Sharps: counted on all procedures, suture needles will be counted
      i. according to the number marked on the outer package and verified by the
      ii. scrub person when the package is opened.
   c. Miscellaneous items: counted on all procedures
   d. Instruments: counted on all procedures in which a body cavity is entered.
      i. All parts of a broken or disassembled instrument must be accounted for in its entirety by members of the surgical team.
4. Counts will be performed in the following sequence:
   a. Wound
   b. Operative field
   c. Mayo
   d. Back table and/or any other sterile tables
   e. Any sponge, sharp, miscellaneous items or instruments off the sterile field.
5. Sponge, sharps, and miscellaneous item counts are performed at the following times:
   a. Before the procedure to establish a baseline
   b. When additional items are added to the sterile field they will be counted and the number added to the baseline count .
   c. Before closure of a cavity within a cavity
   d. Before wound closure begins
   e. At end of procedure when counted items are no longer in use and with all sponges off the field.
   f. At the time of relief of the scrub personnel and/or circulating nurse
   g. Anytime a member of the surgical team requests to count
   h. When procedures require the patient to be placed in the lithotomy position, an additional sponge count will be done after the patient is returned back to the supine position.
6. Instrument counts are performed at the following times:
   a. Before the procedure to establish a baseline
   b. When additional items are added to the sterile field the additional items will be added to the baseline count.
   c. Before wound closure begins

continues

Exhibit 6-1 Facility Count Policy (continued)

    d. When feasible, at the time of permanent relief of the scrub person and/or circulating nurse (although direct visualization of all items may not be possible, the scrub person should return instruments to their designated set and maintain as accurate accounting of the location of various items in the wound and on the sterile field and verbalize to the relief).

7. When the count from the package of sponges, laps, or miscellaneous items is incorrect prior to placement of the patient in the room the Circulating Nurse will:
    a. Discard the entire package.
    b. Remove the package from the room.

8. When the count is incorrect after the patient is in the room the Circulating Nurse will:
    a. Not use any of the items.
    b. Remove that entire package of items from the sterile field.
    c. Place sponges and/or items in a plastic bag and mark the bag appropriately.
    d. Tie/secure the opening in the plastic bag and keep the plastic bag in the room.
    e. Document the information on the worksheet and/or white board.

9. Types and sizes of sponges in the sterile environment are kept to a minimum. Additional supplies will be opened on an "as needed" basis only.

10. A hanging sponge counter bag will be used anytime laps and/or raytec sponges leave the sterile filed.

11. All items are to be counted in the same numbers as presented in their original configuration. (Raytec by 10s, Laps by 5, etc.)
    a. Sponges and laps, etc. must be left in their original configuration and the bands or paper tape not cut or broken until they are counted.
    b. The string and/or x-ray tape must be visible. Lap sponges will be stretched out to their full length to avoid the inadvertent hiding of a smaller item.
    c. Non-x-ray detectable sponges will not to be brought into the sterile field until final counts are completed and the incision is closed.
    d. Used Lap sponges will be placed in the designated pockets of the hanging sponge counter bags.
    e. Only X-Ray detectable towels will be used for large cavity cases.
    f. Used Raytec sponges are placed in designated pockets of the hanging sponge counter bags in multiples of ten (10) per hanging bag if/whenever Raytec sponges leave the sterile field.
    g. Sponges must be separated and pulled apart so that the x-ray blue line is visible when/if they are being placed in the appropriate pockets of the hanging sponge counter bags.
    h. Suture needles are counted during the initial count according to the number marked on the outer package. This number is verified by the scrub person and circulating nurse when the package is opened.
    i. Scrub personnel are responsible for maintaining a current inventory of all needles and their location on the sterile field and through the final count.
    j. Miscellaneous items are counted as needed. These items are to remain on the sterile field in a sterile basin, in a designated area.
    k. When miscellaneous items, sponges, towels, lap pads used in the surgical procedure are cut into pieces, each piece will be counted when cut and accounted for in the final count.
    l. Items placed in an endocavity (throat, vagina) will be recorded on the white board when the item is placed in the cavity and recorded when it si removed.

12. Sponges, sharps, miscellaneous items, and instruments should remain in the room until all counts are correct. Linen and/or trash containers will not be removed from the room until all counts are correct and the dressing applied.

13. Needles, sharps, or instruments broken during a procedure are accounted for in their entirety. Broken items may be handed off the sterile field and maintained by the circulating nurse.

14. Sharps are contained in a puncture-resistant impervious container.

15. Once the final count has begun do not discard any item from the sterile field until the count is completed.

16. The Circulating Nurse is responsible to document in the operative record the name of both individuals completing each count and the type of items counted (sponges and misc. items, or instruments, or none).

17. Medical devices, stents, catheters that will be used in the procedure will be inspected before use for damage during shipment or storage or out of box defects.

A. **Responsibility of Surgeon and First Assistant**
The Surgeon and First Assistant should maintain awareness of all soft goods, instruments, and sharps used in the surgical wound during the course of the procedure. The Surgeon does not perform the count but should facilitate the process by:
    1. Using only radiopaque surgical items in the wound;
    2. Communicating placement of surgical items in the wound to the perioperative team;
    3. Acknowledging awareness of the start of the count process;
    4. Moving unneeded soft goods and instrumentation from the surgical field at the initiation of the count process to the back table to facilitate counting;
    5. Performing a methodical wound exploration when closing counts are initiated;
    6. Accounting for and communicating about surgical items in the surgical field.

B. **Responsibility of Anesthesia Care Providers**
Anesthesia care providers should maintain situational awareness and engage in safe practices that support the prevention of retained surgical items.
    1. Anesthesia care providers must not use counted items;
    2. Anesthesia care providers should verify that throat packs, bite blocks, and other similar devices are removed for the oropharynx and communicate to the perioperative team when these items are inserted and removed.

continues

Exhibit 6-1 Facility Count Policy (continued)

C.   **COUNT DISCREPENCY**

When a discrepancy in any of the counted items occurs, the entire count of that item is in discrepancy and must be repeated for verification. The Circulating Nurse will announce to the surgical team that the count is incorrect, request a temporary stop and document the time the team is notified.

1.   The operative site is searched by the surgeon/proceduralist.
2.   The sterile field is searched by the Scrub person.
3.   The Non-sterile area, including all linen and waste receptacles and all appropriate areas within the room are searched by the Circulating Nurse.
4.   All sponges in the counter bags are opened and recounted.
5.   Linen is emptied and searched.
6.   Waste receptacles are emptied and searched.
7.   If the item is not found and the final count is unresolved, a two opposing view X-ray of the entire operative site will be taken before continuing with closure. If closure is complete two opposing view x-rays will be taken before the patient leaves the room. The Radiologist and/or surgeon/proceduralist will review the x-ray immediately and report the results to the surgical team. An X-ray for count discrepancy does not require a physician order and the reason for the x-ray , the description of the missing surgical item and the name of the surgical procedure will be noted by the Circulating Nurse when ordering the x-ray and documented in the intra-operative record (13mm or smaller needles may not be detectable on x-ray). If the Radiologist is unfamiliar with the missing surgical item an x-ray will be taken of the missing item for comparison identification.
8.   If the count remains incorrect after all the steps to locate the missing item(s) have been exhausted, the Circulating Nurse will document on the Intraoperative Record "unresolved", what actions were taken and the time the actions were taken.
9.   The Circulating Nurse will complete an occurrence report.

D.   **Intra-Operative Count X-Rays**

In cases of extreme patient emergency that necessitate omission of a pre-procedural/procedural count a post-operative two opposing view x-ray will be obtained of the operative site before the patient leaves the OR/procedure room. If the Surgeon determines any delay in transferring the patient to the next level of care will compromise the patient's critical condition the x-ray may be obtained at the next level of care (ICU, PACU). The Circulating Nurse will document the reason for the count omission (emergency or trauma procedures), the reason for the x-ray and the results of x-ray. Once the x-rays are obtained the Surgeon and/or Radiologist will immediately review and validate the films.

E.   **Methods to help prevent occurrences of retained device fragments:**

1.   Use medical devices in accordance with its labeled indications and the manufacturer's instructions for use, especially during insertion and removal;
2.   Inspect the medical device before use for damage during shipment or storage, and any out-of-box defects that could increase the likelihood of fragmentation during a procedure;
3.   Retain any damaged medical device to assist with analysis of the event, including original packaging.

F.   **INTENTIONALLY RETAINED PACKING**

When the surgeon/proceduralist intentionally places surgical packing:

1.   Sponges counted and used in the procedure will not be used for postoperative packing. Non-radiopaque towels will not be used for surgical packing.
2.   When the surgeon/proceduralist intentionally places surgical packing the Circulating Nurse will open and count with the scrub person a separate pack of sponges documenting the number and the type of sponges and/or laps and/or gauze used for intentionally retained packing in the operative record.
3.   Handoff communication between the Circulating Nurse and the receiving nurse will include verbal verification and a completed Intentionally Retained Packing form documenting the intentionally retained packing including the location, type, and number left in place.
4.   The nurse caring for the patient is responsible to assess at the beginning of each shift that the intentionally retained packing remains in place documenting this information in the nurse's notes.
5.   If at any time the intentionally retained packing is removed by the physician outside of the OR the nurse caring for the patient at that time is responsible to document the removal of the packing including the number and type of sponges and/or laps and/or gauze removed on the Intentionally Retained Packing form. The nurse will reconcile the number and type of sponges and/or laps and/or gauze removed with the number and type of sponges and/or laps and/or gauze used for the packing and document in the nurses notes the confirmation that the packing removed matches what the surgeon placed in the OR. Two opposing view x-rays of the entire operative site(s) will be taken.
6.   If the patient is discharged home with the intentionally retained packing in place the discharge nurse will document the status of the packing in the nurse's notes, on the Intentionally Retained Packing form and on the patients discharge instructions and inform the patient that the packing has been left in place.
7.   If the patient returns to surgery for the removal of intentionally retained packing the number and type of sponges and/or laps and/or gauze removed are reconciled with the number and type of sponges and/or laps and/or gauze documented on the intra-operative record placed during the initial procedure. The removed sponges/gauze/laps will be isolated from the sponges/gauze/laps counted and used for the procedure. Prior to closing a body cavity or skin and prior to transporting the patient from the OR to the next level of care two opposing view x-rays of the entire operative site will be taken, unless patient requires immediate transport to a higher level of care.

documentation is required, and how to manage a situation when the count policy must be suspended.

10. The perioperative nurse should be familiar with the intended surgical procedure and the risk associated with it to be able to assess the risk of a retained item. Facility policies provide clear direction even when the nurse does not have extensive experience.

11. Compliance with facility policy and an understanding of the principles of and the techniques for surgical counts can provide a foundation for patient safety.

12. In an extreme emergency situation, such as major trauma, there may be no time to perform a count before the procedure. Facility policy should provide guidance for such situations. This policy should be followed, and documentation should reflect omission of the count and the rationale.

13. Surgical counts are not a guarantee that items will not be retained in a patient. When an RSI occurs, it is not unusual for the count to have been documented as correct. The false "correct count" usually represents a process failure or failure in communication related to distractions or multitasking.

14. The sensitivity of intraoperative radiographs is only 67%; therefore, a negative X-ray is not a completely reliable indication that the patient is free from a retained surgical item (Cima, et al., 2008).

15. In addition to causing harm to the patient, RSIs can result in malpractice litigation. Because a retained surgical item in a patient is almost always indefensible based on the doctrine of *res ipsa loquitur* ("the thing speaks for itself"), such cases usually do not come before a jury. Any or all members of the surgical team may be held liable.

Nursing Diagnosis: Desired Patient Outcome

16. Patients undergoing surgery are at risk for injury related to an unintentionally retained surgical item (AORN, 2011, pp. 146–149; 2015, p. 347).

17. One desired outcome following a surgical procedure is that the patient is free from signs and symptoms of injury caused by RSIs (AORN, 2011, p. 146).

18. A retained surgical item can cause unnecessary pain and suffering, extended stay or readmission to the hospital, additional surgery, delayed healing, and a significant increase in healthcare costs. According to TJC (2013), the average total cost of care related to an RSI is about $166,000.

19. Reactions to gossypiboma can be either acute or delayed. Acute presentations generally follow a septic course, with abscess or granuloma formation. Often these symptoms do not occur until after the patient has returned home. Delayed presentation may occur months or years after surgery with adhesion formation and encapsulation (AORN, 2015, p. 349).

20. In addition to the abdomen and pelvis, there have been reports of items retained in the vagina, thorax, spinal canal, face, brain, and extremities (AORN, 2015, p. 347).

21. As patient advocates, perioperative nurses have a responsibility to ensure that count protocols are carried out according to facility policy. Protocols should include minimizing distractions of any kind while a count is in progress.

Challenges

22. Steelman and Cullen (2011, p. 135) discovered four general themes that represented challenges to correct counts: distraction, multitasking, not following procedure, and time pressure.

23. Unkempt, messy, or cluttered sterile field and disorganized documentation can also be challenges to the count process.

24. One example of disorganized documentation is failure to document an item that is delivered to the field by someone other than the circulating nurse.

25. Common challenges can be difficult to address. The best approach to prevention of a retained surgical item is meticulous attention to the processes intended to prevent its occurrence:

   • Distractions such as interruptions, conversations, loud music, telephones, and pagers interfere with concentration. Managing distractions requires a concerted effort by the entire surgical team.

   • Sponges saturated with blood are not easily visualized in the wound.

- Sponges placed in cavities for packing can be forgotten or overlooked.

- Each change in personnel during a procedure requires a count; with multiple changes in personnel, it is not always possible to perform a complete relief count each time.

- Emergency surgery does not always allow for the time to follow usual procedures. An RSI is 9 times more likely when an operation is performed as an emergency (TJC 2013).

- An unplanned change in the procedure can interrupt protocol and make an RSI 4 times more likely (TJC, 2013).

- Patients with high body mass index represent an additional significant challenge (TJC, 2013).

26. If counted sponges are used to pack the wound and will remain in the wound until the patient returns for a subsequent procedure, the number and type of sponges must be documented on the intraoperative record and the sponge count is noted as "incorrect." When the sponges are subsequently removed, the count will be revised to "correct."

Assistive Technologies

27. Technologies available to supplement manual counting include radiofrequency (RF) detectable sponge systems and bar coded sponge systems. An assessment of RF device technology by Steelman and Alasagheirin (2012), found the "sensitivity and specificity much higher than those of surgical sponge counts or published findings on the use of intraoperative radiographs to identify retained surgical sponges."

28. Some facilities use adjunct technology (RF; bar code) in addition to the surgical count. These technologies must be used according to the manufacturer's instructions for use.

29. When using bar code technology, soft goods should be scanned after they are removed from the sterile field and no longer in use.

30. When using RF technology, if the sponge count is incorrect and scanning indicates that the sponge is not in the patient, in most cases the sponge will be found by proceeding with a scan around the operating room table and trash and linen hampers.

Section Questions

1. Define a "sentinel event." [Ref *Definitions*]

2. Define "soft goods." [Ref *Definitions*]

3. Which items have been identified as having potential for being retained in a surgical wound? [Ref 1]

4. What is a "never event"? [Ref 2]

5. What is the purpose of the surgical counts? [Refs 4–5]

6. What are some components of a facility policy for prevention of retained surgical items? [Refs 6–7]

7. What does TJC consider the primary root causes of RSIs? [Ref 8]

8. On what does a facility policy base its decision on what is counted? [Ref 9]

9. Explain how a correct count and a negative X-ray do not guarantee that the patient is free from an RSI. [Refs 13–14]

10. What are some of the consequences to the patient of a retained surgical item? [Refs 18–19]

11. What are the most common sites for an RSI? [Ref 20]

12. What are the four major categories of challenges to correct counts identified by Steelman and Cullen (2011)? [Ref 22]

13. Discuss some of the specific situations that can lead to an RSI. [Refs 23–25]

14. How are sponges used to pack the wound managed in the count process? [Ref 26]

15. Describe some of the assistive technologies available to augment the counting process. [Refs 27–30]

Soft Goods

31. Soft goods are materials incorporating a radiopaque marker that are designed to absorb blood and fluids. Soft goods include:

    - Laparotomy pads (also referred to as lap sponges, tapes, and lap pads)—square or rectangular gauze pads with an X-ray-detectable tape sewn to the corner of the sponge. These sponges are used where moderate to large amounts of blood or fluid are encountered.

    - Gauze sponges (also referred to as Raytec, X-rays, and 4×4's)—commercially folded into approximately 4¾-inch squares and used where a small amount of blood or fluid is anticipated. They may also be folded and clamped to ring forceps (sponge stick) to be used for swabbing or deep dissection.

    - Kitner dissectors (Peanuts)—a small ball of cotton tape about the size of a pea that is held in the jaws of a forceps and used for dissection or absorption.

    - Cherry dissectors—slightly larger and softer than Kitner dissectors; used for dissection and absorption.

    - Tonsil sponges—cotton-filled gauze in the shape of a ball with a long tape attached, used in tonsil surgery. They are inserted into the mouth to absorb blood and stop bleeding from the tonsil bed. The tape extends outside the mouth and is used for retrieval.

    - Cottonoid patties (also referred to as neuro sponges)—strips of compressed cotton in a variety of sizes that incorporate a radiopaque thread down the center of the sponge and may or may not have a radiopaque string attached. They are used for surgeries on delicate structures such as the brain and spinal cord. When patties become saturated with blood, they are difficult to see; the string facilitates their location.

32. All soft goods admitted into the sterile field should incorporate a radiopaque marker (**Figure 6-1**). If the count remains unresolved, an intraoperative X-ray might be ordered to see if the radiopaque marker on a sponge can be located in the wound.

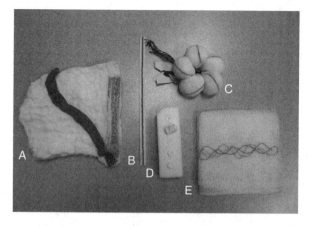

Figure 6-1 Sponges with radiopaque markers: (A) Laparotomy sponge (B) ¼" Cottonoid (C) Tonsil sponges (D) Kittner sponges (Peanuts) (E) Raytec (4 × 4; X-Ray sponge)
Courtesy of Medical City Dallas, Dallas, TX.

33. Softgoods should never be altered:

    - The radiopaque strip should never be removed (e.g., never pull the radiopaque thread from gauze sponges or cut the tails from lap sponges).

    - Sponges must never be cut into more than one piece.

34. Sponges are generally supplied from the manufacturer in packs of five or 10 and are held together with a paper strip. Never assume that the amount indicated on the package label is accurate. The paper strip must be removed, and the sponges must be separated and counted individually.

Counts

35. Counted items should never be removed from the operating room before final counts have been completed.

36. If a commercially prepared package of sponges is found to have more or fewer sponges than indicated, it should be removed from the field, bagged, labeled as defective, and isolated from the rest of the sponges. These sponges may be removed from the room before the patient enters. If the patient was already in the room when the package was opened, the sponges must remain in the room, but are not included in the count (AORN, 2015, p. 350).

37. All counts must be performed carefully by the scrub person and the circulating nurse together; they must share the responsibility equally.

38. The scrub person and circulating nurse count items together and aloud. Both must be able to see each item being counted. It is not acceptable for the scrub person to count and tell the circulating nurse how many items are present.

39. Counts should be performed:
    - Before the procedure to establish a baseline and identify manufacturing and packaging errors (initial count)
    - When new items are added to the field
    - Before closure of a cavity within a cavity (e.g., the uterus)
    - When wound closure begins
    - At skin closure at the end of the procedure or at the end of the procedure when counted items are no longer in use (i.e., the final count)
    - At the time of permanent relief of either the scrub person or the circulating nurse, although direct visualization of all items may not be possible (AORN, 2015, p. 350)

40. Other team members should support and facilitate the count process by acknowledging the importance of the count procedure and not distracting the attention of the individuals who are counting. The entire surgical team is responsible for protecting the patient from injury.

41. Additional sponges delivered to the sterile field during the procedure must be separated and counted aloud by both the scrub person and circulator, then added to the count for the procedure.

42. Counts should be verified when either the scrub person or the circulating nurse is relieved by a new team member. A circulating nurse should never sign for a count that he or she did not perform.

43. During surgery, the scrub person discards used sponges according to facility policy. There may be a plastic-lined kick bucket or specially prepared surface for collecting used sponges. Avoid throwing used sponges on the floor.

44. Individual healthcare facility policy and the U.S. Department of Labor, Occupational Safety and Health Administration (OSHA, 2012) Bloodborne Pathogen Standards 1910-1030 should be consulted for guidelines related to personal protective equipment and disposal of infectious waste. Some state regulations for definition and disposal of regulated waste may be more stringent than the federal regulations. As a result, policies for managing soiled sponges will vary among facilities.

45. Some facilities use a wallboard where counts are recorded during the procedure. Only the final count results are documented in the permanent record.

46. Soiled sponges are never handled with bare hands.

47. The circulator should display used sponges in a pocketed sponge bag or a similar system (AORN, 2015, p. 351). When five lap sponges or 10 Raytec sponges accumulate, the circulating nurse counts them aloud with the scrub person and places the counted bag aside where it can be visualized for the final count (**Figure 6-2**).

48. As wound closure begins, the scrub person and the circulating nurse count aloud and together all sponges on the sterile field and any

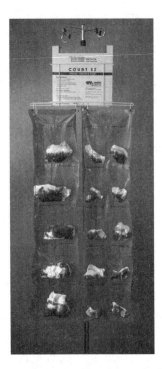

Figure 6-2 Sponge collection bag: (A) Break divider between two pockets to make one large pocket for a laparotomy sponge (B) Place one Raytec sponge in each of the ten pockets.
Courtesy of Xodus Medical, Inc.

that have been discarded from the field. The number of sponges still in use plus the number of previously counted sponges should equal the total number supplied for the surgery.

49. The procedure for counting sponges should be consistent, following the same sequence each time. Typically, the count starts at the surgical site, continues to the Mayo stand, moves to the back table, and finally goes to the discarded sponges. The count begins with the smallest type of sponge and progresses to the largest. Consistent practice promotes efficiency and continuity.

50. All sponges that were opened for the procedure should remain in the room until the procedure is completed and the patient has left the room. Trash and linen containers should also remain in the room. This practice will assist in locating a missing sponge in the event that the count cannot be immediately reconciled.

51. The circulator is responsible for documenting count information and for notifying the surgeon of the count results.

52. After the final count, the bags containing sponges are discarded in a manner that reduces the risk of bloodborne pathogen disease transmission.

53. The surgical team is informed of the results of the initial closing count. If the count is accurate, closure will continue. As skin closure begins, a final count of sponges is conducted using the same procedure. The results are reported to the surgical team and are documented.

54. If the count is incorrect at the time of wound closure, the surgical team is notified and a thorough search is initiated, beginning within the wound and including the sterile field, the room, and the trash. If the sponge cannot be located, facility policy will determine if an intraoperative X-ray is required.

55. When a surgical count cannot be resolved, facility policy will provide specific instructions for documentation and follow-up. It is the responsibility of the nurse to inform the surgeon and for all team members to assist in locating the missing item before the wound is closed.

56. A retained surgical item is one that is not found until after the last stitch or staple has been placed. When the surgeon is informed of an incorrect count, wound closure should not be completed until the item is found or all efforts to find it have been exhausted.

57. According to TJC (2014a; and many states), a retained surgical item is a sentinel event and is reportable if discovered after wound closure.

58. The search for a missing item should begin at the incision site and progress to the entire sterile field, then to the environment, including sponge-collection system, floor around and under the table, linen hamper, and the trash.

59. The following steps will minimize the possibility of an incorrect sponge count:

    • Keeping the amount, size, and types of sponges opened for a procedure to a minimum

    • Counting and bagging discarded sponges frequently

    • Containing all sponges in the room

    • Not removing any linen, trash, or supplies from the operating room until after the patient leaves the room

60. If the surgeon chooses to pack the surgical wound with counted sponges, this must be documented with rationale and the number and type of sponges, and communicated in the hand-off report. The count is documented as "incorrect". When the patient returns to surgery and the sponges are removed, the count from the original surgery should be reconciled.

61. X-ray-detectable sponges should not be used for wound dressing. Should the patient require a postoperative X-ray, the radiopaque marker on the sponge might be mistaken for a retained item.

62. Do not deliver dressing sponges to the sterile field until the surgery and the counts are complete. Dressing sponges do not contain a radiopaque marker and are not counted. Keeping these sponges separate from sponges used during the procedure prevents them from accidentally being counted and contributing to an incorrect count.

63. At the end of a procedure, all counted items should be removed from the room. Any counted item left behind might interfere with the count in a subsequent procedure in that room.

Section Questions

1. Describe the various sponges recognized as "soft goods." [Ref 31]

2. Explain the purpose of the radiopaque marker in soft goods. [Ref 32]

3. Describe behaviors related to soft goods that one should avoid. [Ref 33]

4. At what point can counted items be removed from the operating room? [Ref 35]

5. How are commercial packages of soft goods that contain an incorrect number of items handled? [Ref 36]

6. Who is responsible for actually counting soft goods? [Refs 37–38]

7. When are counts performed? [Ref 39]

8. What responsibility for the surgical count do members of the surgical team other than the scrub person and circulator have? [Ref 40]

9. How are sponges discarded from the field managed? [Refs 43–47]

10. What is the preferred sequence for counting soft goods? [Ref 49]

11. When is the final count done? [Ref 53]

12. When does an unaccounted-for sponge become a retained surgical item? [Refs 56–57]

13. Discuss some interventions that minimize the possibility of an incorrect sponge count. [Ref 59]

14. How is the sponge count documented when counted sponges are left in the wounds as packing? [Ref 60]

15. What is the best approach to managing dressing sponges? [Refs 61–62]

Sharps and Miscellaneous Items

64. Sharps include scalpel blades, suture needles, hypodermic needles, cautery blades, needles, and safety pins, among other items. Miscellaneous items include vessel loops, vein introducers, vessel clip bars, trocar sealing caps, electrosurgery tip scratch pads, and marking pens. Any item that could be inadvertently left inside the patient should be accounted for.

65. The procedure for counting sharps is the same as that for counting soft goods. Items must be visualized and counted aloud by the scrub person and circulating nurse. The circulating nurse documents the sharps count.

66. Sharps pose a risk of inflicting injury and transmitting infectious disease to patients and personnel. The scrub person should account for and confine all sharps on the sterile field until the final count is reconciled. Used sharps should be kept in a puncture-resistant container (AORN, 2015, p. 352).

67. To prevent an excess of loose needles on the field, it is good practice to keep suture packets unopened until the suture is needed.

68. When delivering suture packages containing multiple sutures to the field, it is acceptable practice to count needles according to the number indicated on the packet label; however, once the scrub person opens a suture multipack, both the scrub person and the circulating nurse must verify the number of needles inside.

69. Occasionally, a needle or blade will break during a surgical procedure. When this occurs, the sharp(s) in question must be accounted for in their entirety.

70. On occasion, the risk of injury to a patient may be greater if a needle or piece of a needle is retrieved than if it is left to encapsulate in tissue. The decision not to retrieve a needle rests with the surgeon. Individual institutional policy dictates documentation of such an occurrence.

71. A 2004 Emergency Care Research Institute (ECRI) and Institute for Safe Medical Practices (ISMP) study concluded that searching for needles smaller than 13 mm (6-0 suture size) would expose patients to unnecessary radiation for a very small chance of locating retained needles.

72. If a sharp is removed from the sterile field for any reason during a procedure, the circulating

nurse should isolate it and keep it in a designated place in the operating room until the final count is performed and the procedure is complete. Like the sponge count, the procedure for counting sharps should be consistent.

73. When a surgical procedure requires a large number of suture needles, frequent needle counts can help reduce the risk of an incorrect count.

74. Actual needles—not suture packets—should be used to verify counts. Empty suture packets should not be used to rectify a discrepancy in a closing needle count (AORN, 2015, p. 352). The actual number of needles may not be the same as the number of suture packets.

75. Following the procedure, sharps must be disposed of in containers that are leak proof, puncture resistant, and color coded, or labeled as biohazardous waste (OSHA, 2012).

Instrument Counts

76. Instrument counts are a proactive injury-prevention strategy. In procedures where risk of a retained instrument is either nonexistent or minimal, facility policy will determine whether an instrument count can be omitted.

77. Instruments can also be counted for inventory and cost-containment purposes. It is not uncommon for instruments, such as towel clips and Allis clamps used for utility purposes, to be inadvertently discarded. Instruments are less likely to be lost if they must be accounted for.

78. Instrument counts should be completed before skin closure. Facility policy will provide direction for managing situations in which an instrument count is not possible.

79. The procedure for counting instruments is essentially the same as that for counting soft goods and sharps.

80. Instruments should be accounted for in their entirety. The individual pieces of multipart instruments must all be identified and present. For instance, the Balfour retractor has a removable bladder blade and wing nut and may also have pairs of removable deep blades. The Balfour is only present if all of the parts are present.

81. As with all counts, instruments must be visualized by the scrub person and circulating nurse concurrently and counted aloud. The circulating nurse documents the instrument count results.

82. Instruments removed from the sterile field should remain in the operating room until the final count is complete and the patient leaves the room. Removal of an instrument from the room during the procedure increases the potential for an incorrect count.

83. It is helpful when instrument sets are standardized and when the number of instruments in sets is kept to a minimum. Standardization promotes consistent behaviors and reduces the likelihood of error.

Documentation

84. Count sheets may be generic, specialty specific, or set specific (**Exhibit 6-2**).

85. When instrument sets are standardized, count sheets can be preprinted; the list of instruments on the count sheet is identical to the contents of the set. The count sheet may be delivered to the operating room along with the set or retrieved from a computerized database within the operating room.

86. Computerization of instrument set lists facilitates periodic review and modification of count sheets as appropriate. Preprinted count sheets that list instruments and the number of each included in the set *cannot* substitute for performing a count.

87. Preprinted count sheets are also helpful for those healthcare personnel responsible for set assembly.

88. Documentation of counts is included in the electronic health record.

89. The intraoperative record should document the outcome of the count. Regardless of where the documentation is maintained, it must be retrievable, be traceable to the patient, and include the following information:

- Types of counts: soft goods, sharps, instruments, miscellaneous items
- Number of counts
- Names and credentials of personnel involved in the count
- Results of the counts
- Surgeon who was notified of the count results
- Any adjunct technology used and associated records
- Explanation for any waived counts
- Number and location of any instruments intentionally remaining with the patient

Exhibit 6-2 Count Sheet

Gyn Minor Set

6/24/2015 9:15 am

Prepared By: Bperry   Set ID: GynMinor-000   Set Cat: Gyn   Bar Code: 10397-000   Date Prepared: 06/24/2015

Date Set Used: _____   Tech/RN: _____   Set Was ___ Satisfactory ___ Not Satisfactory   Ster Meth: Steam

If Set was not satisfactory, please explain: _____

List Instruments needing repair/replacement: _____

Pre Cnt	Cls Cnt	Add Cnt	Qt Is	Qt Mi	SP Cnt	Description:	Man	Product#	Inst ID	Comment
—	—	—	2		—	Retractor, Senn, Rake			10236	
—	—	—	2		—	Towel Clip, Small			10658	
—	—	—	2		—	Retractor, Army Navy			10123	
—	—	—	2		—	Retractor, S			14967	
—	—	—	1		—	Forceps, DeBakey, Short			11027	
—	—	—	1		—	Forceps, Tissue, 6'', w/Teeth			11057	
—	—	—	1		—	Forceps, Adson, w/Teeth			10016	
—	—	—	1		—	Handle, Knife, #3			10341	
—	—	—	1		—	Scissors, Mayo, Curved			10318	
—	—	—	2		—	Needleholder, Crile Wood, 6''			10706	
—	—	—	2		—	Clamp, Pean			10972	
—	—	—	4		—	Clamp, Allis			10310	
—	—	—	2		—	Clamp, Ochsner, Straight			10311	
—	—	—	4		—	Forceps, Kelly, 5 1/2''	Aesc		21697	
—	—	—	1		—	Scissors, Metzenbaum, Curved, Regular		BH135R	11478	

Wrap Tray

Total Insts: 28   Creation Date: 10/13/05   Date of Last Modification: 08/29/11   Num of Changes: 1

Instruments Added by OR

Instrument	1st	2nd	Laps	Atr. Needles	Free Needles
			Raytec	Peanuts	Other

187

Courtesy of Medical City Dallas, Dallas, TX.

or radiopaque soft goods intentionally retained as therapeutic packing

- Unretrieved device fragments left in the wound

- Actions taken when count discrepancies occur

- Rationale for counts not performed or completed according to policy

- Outcome of action taken (AORN, 2015, p. 357)

Section Questions

1. What items are included in the term "sharps"? [Ref 64]

2. How are used sharps managed? [Ref 66]

3. How are multipacks of suture needles counted? [Ref 68]

4. How are broken needles and blades managed? [Refs 69–71]

5. Why are the needles themselves, not the suture packets, used for the sharps count? [Ref 74]

6. In addition to preventing an RSI, what is another reason for counting instruments? [Ref 77]

7. How are multipart instruments counted? [Ref 80]

8. Explain the value of standardizing instrument sets. [Refs 83, 85]

9. Of what value is the computerization of instrument set lists? [Ref 86]

10. What should be included in the documentation of counts? [Ref 89]

References

American Hospital Assocation (AHA). (2011). *Retained surgical items: Incidence and how to avoid*. Retrieved from: https://aharesourcecenter.wordpress.com/2011/03/29/retained-surgical-items-incidence-and-how-to-avoid/

Association of periOperative Registered Nurses (AORN). (2011). *Perioperative nursing data set* (3rd ed.). Denver, CO: AORN.

Association of periOperative Registered Nurses (AORN). (2015). Guideline for the prevention of retained surgical items. In: *Guidelines for perioperative practice* (pp. 347–363). Denver, CO: AORN.

Centers for Medicare and Medicaid Services (CMS). (2014). *Evidence-based guidelines for selected and previously considered hospital-acquired conditions*. Retrieved from http://www.cms.gov/Medicare/Medicare-Fee-for-Service-Payment/HospitalAcqCond/Downloads/Evidence-Based-Guidelines.pdf

Cima, R. R., Kollengode, A., Garnatz, J., Storsveen, A., Weisbrod, C., & Deschamps, C. (2008). Incidence and characteristics of potential and actual retained foreign object events in surgical patients. *Journal of the American College of Surgrons, 207*(1), 80.

Emergency Care Research Institute, & Institute for Safe Medical Practices. (2004). *Patient safety advisory: Use of X-rays for incorrect needle counts*. Retrieved from http://patientsafetyauthority.org/ADVISORIES/ AdvisoryLibrary/2004/jun1%282%29/Documents/05.pdf

The Joint Commission (TJC). (2013). *Sentinel event alert: Preventing unintended retained foreign objects*. Retrieved from http://www.jointcommission.org/assets/1/6/SEA_51_URFOs_10_17_13_FINAL.pdf

The Joint Commission (TCC). (2014a) *Sentinel event policy and procedures*. Retrieved from http://www.jointcommission.org/Sentinel_Event_Policy_and_Procedures/default.aspx

The Joint Commission (TJC). (2014b). *Summary data of sentinel events reviewed by The Joint Commission*. Retrieved from http://www.jointcommission.org/assets/1/18/2004_to_2014_2Q_SE_Stats_-_Summary.pdf

Occupational Safety and Health Administration (OSHA). (2012). *Toxic and hazardous substances: Bloodborne pathogens*. Retrieved from http://www.osha.gov/pls/oshaweb/owadisp.show_document?p_table=standards&p_id=10051

Steelman, V., & Alasagheirin, M. (2012). Assessment of radiofrequency device sensitivity for the detection of retained surgical sponges in patients with morbid obesity. *Archives of Surgery, 147*(10), 955–960.

Steelman, V., & Cullen, J. (2011). Designing a safer process to prevent retained surgical sponges: A healthcare failure mode and effect analysis. *AORN Journal, 94*(2), 132–141.

Post-Test

Read each question carefully. A question may have more than one correct answer.

1. The radiopaque marker in each sponge
   a. distinguishes one type of sponge from another.
   b. cannot be seen on film when the sponge is completely saturated with blood.
   c. permits X-ray visualization of a sponge that has been inadvertently left in a patient.
   d. causes a wand attached to a detection console to emit a signal.

2. The most common retained surgical item is a
   a. sponge.
   b. instrument.
   c. blade.
   d. suture needle.

3. The most frequent site(s) of a retained surgical item is/are the
   a. pelvis.
   b. cranium.
   c. abdomen.
   d. hip.

4. The primary purpose of a surgical count is to
   a. reconcile items delivered to the sterile field throughout a procedure with what remains at the end of surgery.
   b. identify the instruments used for a specific procedure.
   c. insure that instruments are not inadvertently discarded.
   d. comply with The Joint Commission standards.

5. A facility count policy specifies
   a. what items are counted.
   b. who participates in the count.
   c. what to do when a count cannot be performed.
   d. what count information is documented in the medical record.

6. According to The Joint Commission, the most common root causes of an RSI are
   a. the absence of adjunct technology to improve the count process.
   b. absence of policies and procedures.
   c. that all members of the surgical team are not committed to the process.
   d. failure to comply with facility policy.

7. Facility policies indicating what is counted are based on
   a. national and state regulations.
   b. the nature of the procedure.
   c. anticipated size of the incision.
   d. the probability of a retained item.

8. According to Cima and colleagues (2008), what is the sensitivity of an intraoperative radiograph?
   a. 58%
   b. 67%
   c. 74%
   d. 83%

9. The doctrine of *res ipsa loquitur* means
   a. no single individual is responsible.
   b. everyone is responsible.
   c. the situation must go to trial.
   d. the situation speaks for itself.

10. Which of the following will have the greatest impact on achieving a correct count?
    a. Keeping a neat sterile field
    b. Turning off the music in the room
    c. Paying meticulous attention to the process of counting
    d. Asking everyone to stop talking

11. The recommended sequence for the final count begins with what?
    a. Sealed bags of sponges that have already been counted
    b. Sponges arranged in pouches ready to be counted
    c. Sponges on the back table
    d. Sponges in use on the sterile field

12. How do OSHA requirements impact the management of infectious waste?
    a. OSHA inspects facilities periodically to be sure that counts are being done.
    b. OSHA establishes the required personal protective equipment.
    c. OSHA Bloodborne pathogen standard provides guidelines.
    d. OSHA determines what type of bags are used to collect used sponges.

13. A lost sponge that is found is considered an RSI if
    a. an X-ray is required to locate it.
    b. the last stitch has been placed to close the surgical wound.
    c. the nurse has already documented the count as "incorrect."
    d. dressings have already been delivered to the field.

14. If the surgeon leaves counted sponges in the wound as packing at the end of the procedure,
    a. identify the number of sponges left and mark the count "correct."
    b. take an X-ray before the patient leaves the room to document the number of sponges left inside.
    c. identify the number of sponges left and mark the count "incorrect."
    d. the count is left unresolved until the subsequent procedure when the packing sponges are removed.

15. How can you determine which "miscellaneous" items to count?
    a. Miscellaneous items are listed in the facility's count policy.
    b. The list of items to be counted is determined by OSHA and The Joint Commission.
    c. The surgical team decides what items will be counted at the beginning of the procedure.
    d. Any item that can inadvertently be left in a patient should be counted.

16. What is a good way to prevent an excess of loose needles on the surgical field?
    a. Don't open suture packages until the suture is needed.
    b. Count needles frequently, seal them in a puncture-proof container, and pass them off the field.
    c. Collect used needles in a medicine cup and arrange them carefully on a needle mat for the final count.
    d. Put used needles back into the packages they came from.

17. What organization determined that using X-ray to search for needles smaller than 13 mm (6-0) exposed the patient to unnecessary radiation because the chance of locating the needle was small?

    a. ECRI & ISMP

    b. OSHA

    c. TJC

    d. FDA

18. How should instruments be counted?

    a. Base the initial count on the number of instruments listed on the count sheet.

    b. The scrub person counts the instruments as he or she sets up the field and reports the number to the circulator.

    c. Count only the instruments removed from the set and used on the procedure.

    d. The scrub person and circulator together count all instruments one by one.

19. Which of the following statement(s) is/are true about instrument counts?

    a. Instruments do not need to be counted on very short cases.

    b. Instruments that are not taken out of the set do not need to be counted.

    c. Facility policy will indicate when an instrument count is not necessary.

    d. An instrument with five pieces is counted as five instruments.

20. Which of the following pieces of information should be included in the patient record?

    a. Number of counts done during the procedure

    b. Name and credentials of the individuals participating in the count

    c. Explanation for any waived count

    d. Results of the count(s)

Competency Checklist:
Preparing the Patient for Surgery

Under "Observer's Initials," enter initials upon successful achievement of competency. Enter N/A if competency is not appropriate for institution.

Name _____

	Observer's Initials	Date
1. A "no interruption" period is implemented while counting.	_____	_____
a. Ask anesthesia, surgeon, and other providers if there is anything they need prior to beginning the count.	_____	_____
b. Announce the beginning of the count as a reminder to others that interruptions will not be recognized.	_____	_____
2. Counts are performed and documented:		
a. Prior to procedure	_____	_____
b. During the procedure when items are added	_____	_____
c. Before closure of a body cavity	_____	_____
d. When closure begins	_____	_____
e. At the time of relief	_____	_____
3. Counts are performed concurrently and aloud by the scrub person and the circulating nurse.	_____	_____
4. Items being counted are separated and are visible to both the scrub person and circulating nurse.	_____	_____
5. Sharps are maintained on a needle mat (or other device designed for this purpose).	_____	_____
6. Counts are verified when personnel are relieved.		
7. Contents of multipack sutures are verified when each package is opened.	_____	_____
8. Sponges that are discarded are counted in units of five or 10 and bagged.	_____	_____
9. All sponges, sharps, or instruments opened for the procedure are retained in the room until the procedure is completed.	_____	_____
10. The count begins at the surgical site and progresses to the Mayo tray and the back table, ending with the sponges outside of the sterile field.	_____	_____
11. Sponges are handled according to OSHA guidelines.	_____	_____
12. The surgeon is notified of the count results (correct or incorrect).	_____	_____
13. Names of all persons who performed counts during the procedure are documented.	_____	_____
14. Documentation is complete.	_____	_____
15. Count results are included in the debriefing.	_____	_____

Observer's Signature   Initials   Date

_____

Orientee's Signature

_____

7

Prevention of Injury: Hemostasis, Tourniquets, and Electrosurgical Equipment

LEARNER OBJECTIVES

1. Describe the natural process of hemostasis.
2. Explore approaches to artificial hemostasis.
3. Discuss mechanical hemostasis.
4. Identify three potential patient injuries associated with tourniquets.
5. List two criteria for evaluating desired patient outcomes related to tourniquets.
6. Describe nursing interventions to prevent patient injury when a tourniquet is used.
7. Describe appropriate documentation related to the use of a tourniquet.
8. Identify three potential patient injuries related to electrosurgical equipment.
9. Define terminology associated with electrosurgery.
10. Describe potential injury related to capacitive coupling.
11. Identify the desired patient outcome relative to electrosurgery.
12. List four criteria for evaluating the desired patient outcomes related to electrosurgery.
13. Describe nursing interventions to prevent patient injury when electrosurgical equipment is used.
14. Describe appropriate documentation related to the use of electrosurgical equipment.
15. Discuss use of an ultrasonic energy device (scalpel) and an argon beam coagulator.

LESSON OUTLINE

I. Overview

II. Natural Hemostasis

III. Chemical Hemostasis

IV. Mechanical Hemostasis
   A. Instruments, Ties, Suture Ligatures, and Ligating Clips
   B. Bone Wax
   C. Pressure

D. Tourniquets

E. Nursing Diagnoses and Desired Patient Outcomes

F. Nursing Interventions
   i. Application of the Tourniquet

V. Electrical Hemostasis: Electrosurgery
   A. Electrosurgical Components
      i. Generator
      ii. Active Electrodes
      iii. Dispersive Electrodes

Overview

1. Hemostasis is the arrest or control of bleeding.

2. Historically, attempts to achieve hemostasis have included applications of egg yolk, dust, cobwebs, hot oil, cautery with hot irons, and use of crude sutures made from materials such as cotton or harp strings derived from sheep intestines. Until the advent of modern hemostatic methods, blood loss made surgery difficult and was a serious surgical complication.

3. Hemostasis may be achieved by natural or artificial methods.

4. Modern hemostatic methods, including chemical hemostasis, electrosurgery, and tourniquet application, have greatly enhanced the surgeon's ability to perform slow, deliberate surgery where control of bleeding permits excellent visualization of anatomical structures.

Natural Hemostasis

5. Injury to a blood vessel creates a roughened surface to which platelets adhere. When several layers of platelets have accumulated, a platelet plug is formed. A platelet plug is often sufficient to seal small injuries.

6. Platelet plug formation is not the same as coagulation. As the platelets break down, they release thromboplastin which is necessary for coagulation to occur. In coagulation, a fibrin clot is formed.

7. Coagulation is a complex mechanism involving multiple clotting factors and a series of reactions:

    • First, prothrombin, present in blood, reacts with thromboplastin released with the breakdown of platelets. Prothrombin, thromboplastin, and calcium ions in the blood form thrombin.

    • Thrombin then unites with fibrinogen, a glycoprotein in blood plasma, to form fibrin. Fibrin is the basic structure of the clot and reinforces the platelet plug.

    • Initially the fibrin is white. As platelets, white cells, and red cells become entangled in the fibrin, the clot becomes red, taking on the appearance we recognize as a blood clot.

8. The process of coagulation is self-regulated; coagulation ceases when the blood loss is under control.

9. In spite of the complexity of the coagulation process, it is rapid and sufficient to prevent blood loss from most small wounds.

10. Natural hemostasis is not sufficient, however, to control the gross bleeding and oozing that occur during surgery. Artificial hemostatic methods—chemical, mechanical, or thermal—may be used to control bleeding and oozing during surgery.

11. Chemical hemostasis relies on thrombin, absorbable gelatin, oxidized cellulose, microfibrillar collagen, collagen pads, and styptics. Mechanical hemostasis includes the application of direct pressure, the use of instruments, ties, suture ligatures, ligating clips, staples, bonewax, and tourniquets. Electrosurgery relies on electrical energy to control bleeding.

Chemical Hemostasis

Thrombin

12. Thrombin is an enzyme that combines with fibrinogen and accelerates the coagulation process. It is useful in controlling capillary bleeding.

13. Thrombin is supplied as a dry white powder that occasionally is sprinkled on an oozing site, but is more frequently mixed with sterile water or saline to form a solution that is used to saturate a gelatin sponge. This thrombin–gelatin combination is particularly useful in neurosurgery and in vascular surgery for controlling capillary bleeding at the site of a vascular graft.

14. Thrombin will lose its potency within 3 hours of reconstitution and should be mixed just prior to use.

15. Thrombin is for topical use only; it must never be injected.

16. Thrombin has traditionally been made from dried cow's blood. On rare occasions, bovine thrombin preparations have been associated with abnormalities in hemostasis, ranging from asymptomatic alterations in laboratory tests, such as prothrombin time (PT) and partial thromboplastin time (PTT), to severe bleeding or thrombosis. These abnormalities have rarely been fatal. Repeated clinical applications of topical bovine thrombin can increase the likelihood that antibodies against thrombin and/or factor V may be formed.

17. Thrombin derived from human plasma is now available. It is less immunogenic and will likely become more popular.

Absorbable Gelatin

18. Absorbable gelatin is made from a purified gelatin solution and is available as a powder, a compressed pad (Gelfoam), and beads. In the compressed form, it resembles Styrofoam.

19. When placed on an area of capillary bleeding, fibrin is deposited in the interstices of the pad; the pad swells, and clot formation progresses. Gelfoam pads are available in a variety of sizes and may be cut to the desired size.

20. Gelfoam may be used alone, but is frequently cut into manageable pieces and soaked in a thrombin solution. Gelfoam may also be soaked in epinephrine. In the powder form, gelatin is mixed with sterile saline to form a paste.

21. Gelfoam absorbs 45 times its weight in blood. It is not soluble. If left in the body, it will be absorbed in 20 to 40 days. Once hemostasis has been achieved, it is common practice to remove gelatin during the procedure to prevent compression of adjacent anatomic structures.

Oxidized Cellulose

22. Oxidized regenerated cellulose (Oxycel, Surgicel, Surgicel Nu-Knit) is a specially treated knitted gauze or cotton product applied directly to an oozing surface to control bleeding.

23. When oxidized cellulose contacts whole blood, it absorbs seven to eight times its own weight, forms a gel, and promotes clot formation.

24. Oxidized cellulose promotes clotting within minutes, swelling to create a pseudo-clot that puts pressure on the wound, helping to speed up the normal clotting process and preventing further blood loss. The pseudo-clot can be left in situ where it is fully absorbed after 1 to 2 weeks.

25. Oxidized cellulose must be removed when used around the optic nerve or spinal cord, because swelling of the cellulose can exert harmful pressure on these structures.

Microfibrillar Collagen

26. Microfibrillar collagen (Avitene, Instat) is a fluffy, white, absorbable material made from purified bovine dermis. It is applied as a dry product that is placed directly over the source of bleeding, usually on friable tissue, in crevices, and on areas of irregular contour. Platelets and fibrin adhere to the collagen and provide hemostasis as clot formation progresses.

27. Although it is absorbable, excess material is removed once hemostasis has been achieved.

28. Collagen is also manufactured into pads, sponges, and felt that are applied directly to a bleeding surface.

Styptic

29. Styptics are agents that cause blood vessel constriction. Epinephrine is a frequently used styptic; it is often added to a local anesthetic such as lidocaine to constrict blood vessels and decrease bleeding.

30. Silver nitrate, in the form of a stick or pencil with a silver nitrate crystal head, is another form of styptic applied topically to small vessels.

Mechanical Hemostasis
Instruments, Ties, Suture Ligatures, and Ligating Clips

31. A hemostatic clamp may be used to occlude the end of a bleeding vessel. As long as the clamp remains in place, bleeding is controlled. However, clamping is a temporary means of hemostasis and is followed by the application of a tie, a suture ligature, a ligating clip, electrosurgery, or electrocautery for permanent hemostasis.

32. A tie is a strand of suture material tied around the vessel to occlude the lumen. A suture ligature is a tie with an attached needle that is used to anchor the tie through the vessel. A ligating

clip (Hemoclip, Ligaclip, Surgiclip) is a stainless steel, tantalum, or titanium clip used to permanently seal a vessel. Except for clips made from synthetic absorbable suture, ligating clips remain permanently within the patient.

Bone Wax

33. Bone wax is made from beeswax and is used to stop bleeding from bone. Bone wax is rolled into a ball and rubbed over a cut bone surface to seal the holes and control bleeding. Bone wax is used most often in neurosurgery and orthopedic surgery.

Pressure

34. Manual pressure applied directly to small vessels may delay bleeding long enough for clot formation to begin. Pressure is applied with sponges to blot areas of bleeding. When the sponge is removed, it is possible to identify the area of continued bleeding and to use additional methods of hemostasis, if necessary.

Section Questions

1. What is hemostasis? [Ref 1]
2. Identify two general approaches to achieving hemostasis. [Ref 3]
3. Differentiate coagulation from natural hemostasis. [Ref 6]
4. Describe the process of natural hemostasis involving platelets and thromboplastin. [Refs 7–9]
5. Identify artificial methods used to achieve hemostasis in surgery. [Ref 10]
6. How does thrombin help to control capillary bleeding? [Ref 12]
7. Why must thrombin be mixed just prior to use? [Ref 14]
8. Compare bovine thrombin to recombinant human thrombin. [Refs 16–17]
9. How does absorbable gelatin promote hemostasis? [Refs 19–20]
10. How is oxidized cellulose used? [Ref 22]
11. What happens when oxidized cellulose comes in contact with whole blood? [Ref 23]
12. What special precautions are taken with oxidized cellulose when this material is used around the optic nerve or spinal cord? [Ref 25]
13. Where is microfibrillar collagen most helpful in achieving hemostasis? [Ref 26]
14. How does a styptic work to achieve hemostasis? [Ref 29]
15. Identify several products that are styptic agents. [Refs 29–30]
16. Describe mechanical hemostasis. [Refs 31–32]
17. Which items are used to produce mechanical hemostasis? [Refs 31–32]
18. How is bonewax used to achieve hemostasis? [Ref 33]
19. How does manual pressure promote hemostasis? [Ref 34]
20. What is the purpose of blotting an area of bleeding with a sponge? [Ref 34]

Tourniquets

35. A pneumatic tourniquet placed on an extremity occludes arterial and venous circulation to the extremity and, therefore, creates a bloodless surgical field, enhancing the surgeon's ability to visualize anatomical structures and preventing blood loss.

36. Once the tourniquet is released, the severed vessels will bleed, and measures to achieve hemostasis will be necessary.

37. The simplest tourniquet is a length of rubber tubing, such as a Penrose drain, that is placed around an extremity in preparation for a venipuncture. Surgical tourniquets are most

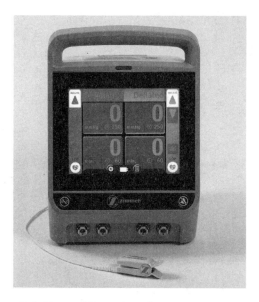

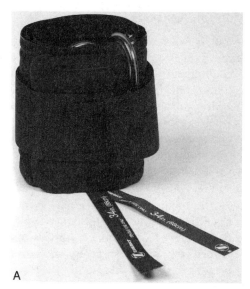

A

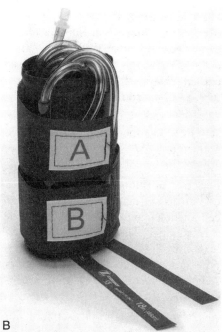

B

Figure 7-1 Zimmer ATS4000 Tourniquet.
Courtesy of Zimmer, Inc.

frequently used for orthopedic, podiatric, and plastic surgery procedures.

38. Pneumatic tourniquets contain an internal bladder housed in a pressure cuff that is attached to a system that inflates the cuff with either ambient air or compressed gas (**Figure 7-1**). Most automated systems:

- Contain a microprocessor that performs a self-test and self-calibration upon activation

- Recommend a limb occlusion pressure based on a reading from a sensor that is placed on the patient's toe or finger prior to surgery

- Include an audible indicator that reports cuff status, changes in pressure, and passage of a specified amount of time

- Contain a battery backup

39. Tourniquet cuffs are available in a variety of sizes and shapes corresponding to the wide variety in patient size (**Figure 7-2A**). The cuffs may be single use or reusable.

40. A cuff with a double bladder is used when the extremity will be anesthetized with a regional anesthetic block (Bier block) (Figure 7-2B).

Nursing Diagnosis and Desired Patient Outcomes

41. Nursing diagnosis: high risk for injury related to use of tourniquet. The Association of periOperative Registered Nurses (AORN, 2011) outcome standard states, "The patient is free from signs and symptoms of injury caused

Figure 7-2 (A) Cylindrical single tourniquet cuff and (B) Cylindrical double tourniquet cuff.
Courtesy of Zimmer, Inc.

by extraneous objects" (p. 165). The patient should not experience an injury as a result of tourniquet use.

42. Injuries from a tourniquet can include skin injury, such as a chemical burn from prep solutions soaked in the padding under the tourniquet; abrasion, bruise or blister formation; and swelling, pain, or nerve injury, including paralysis. Release of the tourniquet can have an impact on fluid shift. Tourniquet deflation must be managed carefully.

Nursing Interventions

43. Nursing interventions to prevent injury from tourniquet application require knowledge of equipment use and appropriate safety precautions. AORN guidelines (2015a, pp. 153–186) address proper care of the surgical patient when a tourniquet is used. The perioperative nurse must be able to select an appropriate tourniquet in good working order and must demonstrate competence in tourniquet application, management, and removal.

44. Facility policy and practice may dictate who has responsibility for tourniquet application. Regardless of who actually applies the tourniquet, the nurse, surgeon, and anesthesia personnel all share responsibility for patient safety with regard to tourniquet use.

45. Possible contraindications to use of a tourniquet include diabetes mellitus, vascular graft, compromised circulation, vascular disease, deep vein thrombosis (DVT), increased intracranial pressure, severe crush injury, open fracture, and infection (AORN, 2015a, p. 156).

46. Prior to tourniquet application, the nurse should assess the patient's skin for integrity and turgor, and select a tourniquet appropriate for the size of the patient's extremity.

47. Because tourniquet use can lead to circulatory stasis and acidosis, hypoxemia and sickle cell anemia can be contraindications to using a tourniquet. The anesthesiologist will take into consideration the patient's hemoglobin type and level and determine if a patient with sickle cell anemia can tolerate a tourniquet (McEwen, 2015a).

48. Medications such as prophylactic antibiotics that must be infused prior to incision should be completely infused before a tourniquet is applied.

49. All tourniquet systems are not alike. Never substitute tubing or gas for inflation. Check for compatibility of the cuff, tubing, and regulator.

50. The pneumatic tourniquet should be tested and inspected for integrity, cleanliness, and function according to the manufacturer's instructions for use and facility policy.

    • The cuff and tubing should be clean and free of cracks or holes. A cuff may have been punctured if a towel clip was used to hold it in place. Holes and cracks can result in unintentional pressure loss.

    • Tourniquet cuffs and bladders should be cleaned with an Environmental Protection Agency (EPA)–registered tuberculocidal germicide, then thoroughly rinsed to prevent skin irritation. Cuff and bladder should be thoroughly dried; moisture can promote microbial growth. Microorganisms can proliferate and debris can collect on Velcro fasteners. The gauges and pressure source should also be inspected for cleanliness and cleaned as needed.

    • Connections should be secure, and electrical cords should be intact.

    • Audible alarms and indicators should be set to a level that can be heard above other sounds in the operating room.

    • An inspection label should verify that the last inspection of the device by biomedical engineering personnel occurred within the last 12 months.

    • When nitrogen gas is used to inflate the cuff, check the level of gas in the tank to ensure that the tank contains an adequate supply for the duration of the surgery.

51. The selection of a tourniquet cuff should take into consideration the surgical site and the size of the patient's extremity (AORN, 2015, p. 159):

    • The length of the cuff should provide sufficient overlap (3 to 6 inches) and full engagement of the hook and loop fasteners.

    • Contour cuffs are appropriate in situations where there is a significant tapering of the extremity between the upper and lower edges of the cuff (**Figure 7-3**). This is frequently the case with obese patients.

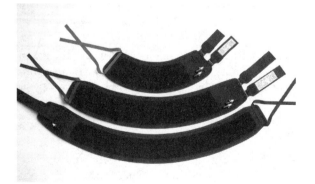

Figure 7-3 Contour tourniquet cuffs.
Courtesy of Zimmer, Inc.

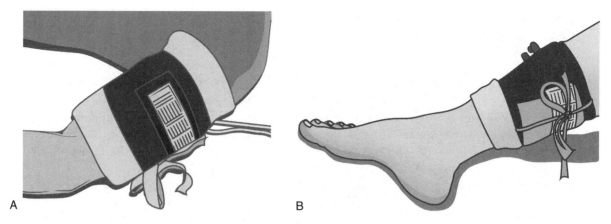

Figure 7-4 Tourniquet in place: (A) upper extremity (B) lower extremity.

- Wider cuffs minimize the potential for injury to underlying vessels, muscles, and nerves by dispersing pressure over a wider surface area.

52. The tourniquet should fit snugly. In general, a snug fit allows two fingers under the cuff. If only one finger fits under the cuff, the cuff is too tight; if three fingers fit, it is too loose (McEwen, 2015b).

Application of the Tourniquet

53. The operative limb should be verified by the surgical team.

54. The position of a tourniquet cuff should not be revised once it has been placed. If a cuff position change should be necessary, the cuff should be removed and reapplied. Moving a cuff after placement may cause shearing of underlying tissue (AORN, 2015a, p. 161).

55. Tourniquets placed on the upper arm or thigh should be placed on the limb at the point most proximal to the surgery and at the point of maximum circumference, according to the manufacturer's written instructions (**Figure 7-4A**). Calf tourniquets should be placed with the proximal edge of the cuff at the area of largest circumference (AORN, 2015a, p. 180) (Figure 7-4B). When a tourniquet is applied to the calf, take care not to compromise the head of the fibula, because this problem can result in damage to superficial nerves in the area.

56. The tourniquet should not be applied to unprotected skin. Stockinette material or Webril should be wrapped around the extremity where the tourniquet will be applied, taking care to prevent bunching or wrinkling of the material, which can cause uneven pressure against the skin with the potential for impairing skin integrity.

57. When a patient is extremely obese, an assistant should apply traction to the excess skin until the tourniquet is applied to prevent overlapping of skin and possible pressure or shearing injury.

58. Protect the area of tourniquet application from any potential or actual pooling or collection of fluids that can irritate the skin. Prepping agents, if allowed to pool and soak into the padding under the cuff, can cause a chemical burn to the skin. Protect the area from pooling of fluids during surgery by applying a protective fluid barrier—one might be included as part of the extremity drape and will be applied during the draping procedure.

59. Before application of a tourniquet, raise the extremity to permit gravity to drain blood from the extremity. A long piece of rolled latex (Esmarch bandage) can be wrapped tightly around an extremity from the distal end toward the proximal end to compress superficial blood vessels and further exsanguinate the extremity. The cuff is then inflated, and the Esmarch bandage is removed.

60. Following exsanguination, there is an increase in blood volume to vital organs. Healthy patients may experience only minor hemodynamic changes; however, elderly patients and those with cardiac conditions may experience intraoperative hypertension or other complications.

61. Although standard settings have been identified (350–350 mmHg for lower extremities and 200–250 mmHg for upper limbs), tourniquet

pressure should be based on the patient's systolic pressure and limb circumference and set at the minimum inflation pressure needed to create a bloodless field. A lower pressure is used for children and for patients whose blood supply to the extremity is diminished.

62. Insufficient pressure and subsequent prolonged venous congestion can also result in nerve injury. Excessive inflation pressure can damage underlying tissue, whereas too low a pressure can cause passive congestion of the limb, shock, and hemorrhagic infiltration of a nerve (AORN, 2015a, p. 162).

63. Inflation times should be kept to a minimum. Excessive inflation times can damage underlying tissue and cause injury as severe as permanent paralysis. For an adult, 1 hour for an upper extremity and 1.5 to 2 hours for a lower extremity are the usual maximum inflation times.

64. The surgeon and nurse should agree on the intervals intraoperatively for which the nurse reports the length of time that the tourniquet has been inflated. Most tourniquet systems automatically display pressure readings and inflation time and will sound an alarm when a predetermined time is reached. Anesthesia personnel also monitor inflation times. All team members work in concert to ensure adequate and appropriate communication regarding the tourniquet.

65. Throughout the surgery, the nurse should monitor the tourniquet gauge to recognize fluctuations in pressure that might indicate a tourniquet failure. In the case of inadvertent loss of pressure, the tourniquet should be totally deflated, and the extremity allowed to reperfuse.

66. When the surgeon instructs, the tourniquet should be deflated slowly to maintain hemodynamic stability and prevent too rapid a

decrease in blood pressure as blood is shunted back into the extremity. When bilateral tourniquets are used (e.g., bilateral arthroscopies), the nurse should confirm the sequence and timing of the deflation of each cuff.

67. Deflation of a dual bladder cuff (Bier Block) should be guided by the anesthesia provider, because the anesthetic agent released into the bloodstream may have systemic effects (AORN, 2015a, p. 166).

68. Core body temperature gradually increases following tourniquet inflation due to the decreased heat loss from the affected limb. It is important not to overheat the patient while the tourniquet cuff is inflated. Deflation leads to a transient decline in core temperature due to the redistribution of body heat. Hypothermic blood from the ischemic limb exacerbates this drop in core temperature.

69. Documentation related to use of a pneumatic tourniquet should include the following (AORN, 2015, pp. 169–170):
    - Tourniquet system and identification (serial) number
    - Limb occlusion pressure
    - Cuff pressure settings and duration of cuff inflation
    - Skin protection measures
    - Location of the tourniquet cuff
    - The assessment of skin and tissue integrity under the cuff before and after tourniquet use
    - Time of inflation and deflation
    - Identification of the person who applied the cuff
    - Assessment and evaluation of the entire extremity

Section Questions

1. What is the reason for using a tourniquet for surgery on extremities? [Ref 35]

2. What types of patient injury can occur with the use of a tourniquet? [Ref 42]

3. What are some contraindications for using a tourniquet? [Refs 45, 47]

4. How is the administration of prophylactic antibiotics coordinated with the use of a tourniquet? [Ref 48]

5. What is involved in testing a tourniquet? [Ref 50]

6. What are some considerations for selecting a tourniquet cuff? [Ref 51]

(continues)

Section Questions (continued)

7. What are some criteria for assessing the fit of a tourniquet cuff? [Ref 52]

8. When it is necessary, how should a cuff be repositioned? [Ref 54]

9. Where on the operative extremity should the tourniquet be placed? [Ref 55]

10. How is padding used in conjunction with a tourniquet? [Ref 56]

11. What is one method for avoiding skin damage when placing a tourniquet cuff on an obese patient? [Ref 57]

12. What can happen to the patient if the tourniquet padding is not protected from fluids? [Ref 58]

13. What purpose does the Esmarch bandage serve in preparing for the use of a tourniquet? [Ref 59]

14. What are the customary pressure settings and inflation times for the upper and lower extremities? [Ref 61]

15. What patient factors affect the adjustment of tourniquet inflation pressure? [Ref 61]

16. What dangers are associated with setting the tourniquet pressure too high or too low? [Refs 62–63]

17. Why should bilateral cuffs not be deflated at the same time? [Ref 66]

18. Why is it important to deflate a double cuff used for a Bier Block very slowly? [Ref 67]

19. How does using a tourniquet contribute to an increase in the patient's core temperature? [Ref 68]

20. What information should the perioperative nurse document related to tourniquet use? [Ref 69]

Electrical Hemostasis: Electrosurgery

70. Electrosurgery is used routinely in most surgical procedures as a more rapid alternative to other methods of cutting tissue and coagulating vessels.

71. The unit that supplies the current is referred to as an electrosurgical unit (ESU) or generator (**Figure 7-5**).

Electrosurgical Components
Generator

72. In the 1920s, Dr. William Bovie was instrumental in the development of the first spark-gap

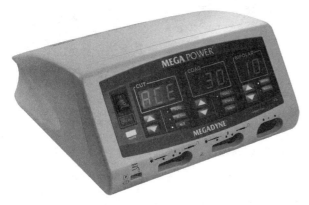

Figure 7-5 Electrosurgical generator.
Courtesy of Megadyne Medical Products, Draper, UT.

vacuum-tube generator that produced cutting with hemostasis. Bovie's design remained the basis for electrosurgical units until the 1970s, when solid-state electrosurgical units were introduced. Solid-state units with small printed circuit boards and transistors replaced the much larger vacuum-tube machines. Nevertheless, the term "Bovie" continues to be synonymous with "electrosurgical unit" regardless of the brand or style of the unit.

73. Electrosurgical units are designed to deliver a current that will coagulate vessels, cut tissue, or cut and coagulate at the same time (blend setting).

74. A single power setting is not appropriate for all surgeries. Differences in generator performance, surgical technique, active electrode size, patient size, and location of the patient return electrode all affect power settings. Generally, low power is used in neurosurgery, dermatology procedures, and oral and plastic surgery.

75. The "cut" setting is a continuous high-frequency waveform that delivers current to vaporize and sever tissue producing little heat and little coagulation (**Figure 7-6A**).

76. The "coagulation" setting is an intermittent waveform that produces higher peak voltages, meets with more tissue resistance, produces more heat, and drives current deeper into

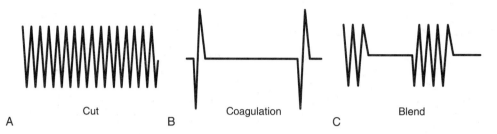

A   Cut   B   Coagulation   C   Blend

Figure 7-6 Waveform settings for electrosurgery.
Modified from Megadyne Medical Products, Draper, UT.

tissue. There is "down time" between peaks to allow the tissue to cool and form a coagulum (Figure 7-6B).

77. The "blend" setting is a modified cut waveform that adds occasional "down time" to allow tissue to cool and form a coagulum (Figure 7-6C). The "blend" is a function of cutting energy; there is no blend associated with the "coag" setting.

78. Coagulating tissue produces an eschar that must be absorbed during the healing process. If an excessive amount of coagulated tissue is present in the wound, sloughing may occur, inhibiting the healing process.

79. Desiccation and fulguration are two types of coagulation:

- Desiccation—the technique used in most surgeries—refers to coagulation produced when the active electrode contacts tissue. Desiccation results in hemostasis, slowly driving the water content out of the cells. Most surgeons will use a coagulation current low enough that it does not result in necrosis.

- Fulguration relies on sparking to coagulate bleeders and to char tissue. The active electrode is held a short distance above the tissue. Sparks cross the gap and create superficial coagulation. As the sparking continues, superficial coagulation is followed by necrosis. General surgeons use fulguration during laparoscopic cholecystectomy to control bleeding on the liver bed when removing the gall bladder; cardiothoracic surgeons may use a ball electrode to fulgurate the sternum.

80. The type of current and the amount of power are regulated by controls on the electrosurgical unit and the accessories. Selection of the type of current should be based on the procedure, the patient's size, and the surgeon's preference, using the lowest power setting that will achieve the desired electrosurgical effect.

81. There are two basic types of electrosurgery—monopolar and bipolar:

- Monopolar: The current flows through the patient from the active electrode to the dispersive electrode, which returns the current to the ESU.

- Bipolar: The current flows from one tine of the bipolar forcep through the tissue to the second tine, which returns the current to the ESU; no dispersive electrode is required.

Active Electrodes

82. Active electrodes connect by a cord to the ESU and are activated either by a control on the handpiece or a foot pedal.

83. Active electrodes may be:

- Disposable or reusable

- Monopolar or bipolar

- Designed for open or endoscopic procedures

84. Single-use, monopolar electrodes are often called "Bovie pencils" (**Figure 7-7**). They have one active tip that delivers a concentrated

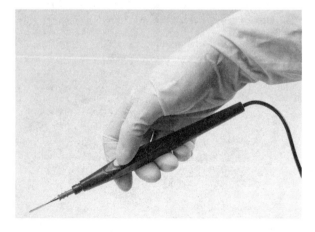

Figure 7-7 Active electrode: monopolar—hand control pencil for open procedures.
© starman963/iStockphoto.

current to the target tissue, which then travels through the body to the dispersive electrode and back to the ESU.

85. A variety of interchangeable tips (e.g., blade, ball, loop, hook, or needle) fit into the monopolar electrode for different surgical applications (**Figure** 7-8A). Similarly shaped monopolar electrodes are crafted for endoscopic procedures (Figure 7-8B).

86. Open and endoscopic bipolar forceps are shown in **Figure** 7-9. One tip acts as the active electrode, and the other tip acts as the return or dispersive

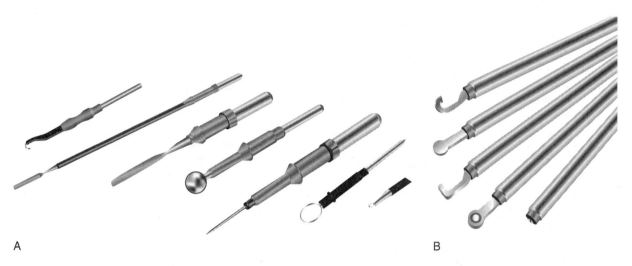

A   B

Figure 7-8 Monopolar active electrode tips: (A) Interchangeable tips for open procedures (B) Endoscopic monopolar electrodes.

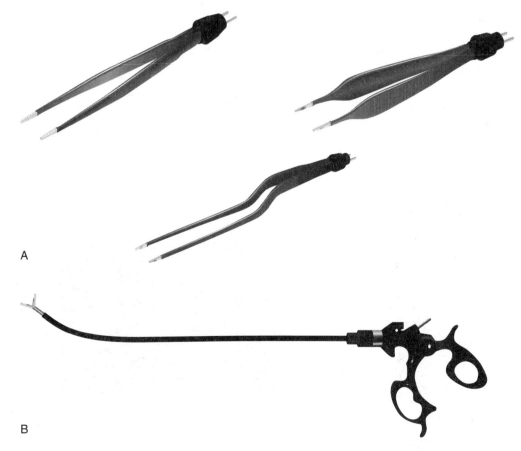

A

B

Figure 7-9 Bipolar forceps: (A) Bipolar forceps for open procedures (B) Laparoscopic Bipolar forceps.

electrode. Current flows only between the tips of the forceps and is not dispersed throughout the body. Lower voltages are required, and there is no need for a dispersive electrode.

87. Bipolar electrodes are used for delicate procedures, primarily in neurosurgery and plastic; ear, nose, and throat (ENT); and ophthalmic procedures.

88. Active electrodes may also be combined with suction, often called a "suction Bovie" or "suction cautery." (Note: These are legacy terms. "Cautery" is heat-based technology and is not synonymous with electrosurgery.) The active electrode is insulated to prevent current transfer to the suction cannula. The insulation must be examined carefully; a defect in the insulation can result in an inadvertent burn injury to the patient.

Dispersive Electrodes

89. Monopolar electrosurgery requires a dispersive electrode that returns electrical current to the generator, completing the electrical circuit.

90. The dispersive electrode either adheres to the patient (adhesive-backed electrodes often called "Bovie pads" or "grounding pads") (**Figure 7-10A**) or is in close proximity to the patient (capacitive electrode that lies on the operating room bed under the patient; (Figure 7-10B)).

91. The dispersive electrode is much larger than the active electrode to ensure that current density is low, minimizing the potential for burns.

92. The return electrode monitoring feature of the adhesive-backed dispersive electrode protects the patient from a pad-site burn in case the pad becomes detached from the patient during the procedure. When there is good contact with the patient, impedance from the two sides of the pad is virtually equal. An interrogation current from the generator measures impedance between the two foil sides and responds to impedance changes greater than 30–40% of baseline (indicating that the pad is not uniformly adhering to the patient) by triggering an alarm and deactivating the ESU.

93. Capacitive pads do not adhere to the patient. They are placed on the operating room table, usually under the sheet, promoting maximum contact with the patient's body.

94. Capacitive pads also use a patient return electrode monitoring system to prevent pad-site burns and provide a greater measure of safety because the patient contact area with the pad is many times greater than with an adhesive dispersive electrode.

95. The capacitive pad also plugs into to the generator. One pad style can be used on all patients weighing greater than 0.8 pounds (0.35 kg). Another style provides the added feature of pressure reduction and can be used on patients weighing greater than 25 pounds (11.5 kg). The manufacturer's instructions for use will describe any patient weight minimums or requirements for placement.

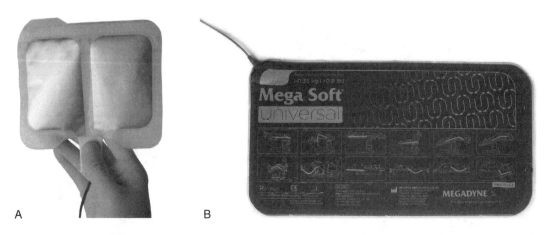

A   B

Figure 7-10 Dispersive electrodes: (A) Adhesive-backed dispersive electrode (B) Capacitive dispersive pad.
Courtesy of Megadyne Medical Products, Draper, UT.

Section Questions

1. What is the significance of the term "Bovie," which is used synonymously with "electrosurgical unit"? [Ref 72]
2. What factors affect the choice of power setting for electrosurgery? [Ref 74]
3. How do the cut and coagulation settings differ in their effect upon tissue? [Refs 75–76]
4. What is the function of the blend setting? [Ref 77]
5. How do the waveforms for cut, coagulation, and blend differ from one another? [Refs 75–77, Figure 7-6]
6. What impact does the eschar created by coagulating vessels have on wound healing? [Ref 78]
7. Differentiate between desiccation and fulguration. [Ref 79]
8. What factors affect the selection of the current and power settings? [Ref 80]
9. How do the current pathways related to the two types of electrosurgery differ from one another? [Ref 81]
10. Which component used with monopolar electrosurgery is unnecessary when bipolar electrosurgery is used? [Ref 81]
11. Why is inspecting the insulation essential before using a "suction Bovie"? [Ref 88]
12. What is the purpose of a dispersive electrode? [Ref 89]
13. Why is the dispersive electrode much larger than the active electrode? [Ref 91]
14. How does the return electrode monitoring system minimize the potential for a pad-site burn? [Ref 92]
15. Contrast the adhesive-backed dispersive electrode with the capacitive pad. [Refs 93–94]

Nursing Diagnosis

96. Nursing diagnosis for patients on whom electrosurgery is used: high risk for injury related to use of electrosurgery.

97. Electrosurgery creates high risk for fire and risk for impaired skin integrity. Not all facilities have the most modern equipment, and even the newest equipment does not eliminate the potential for injury. Dispersive electrode pads without return electrode monitoring can allow concentration of current and subsequent pad-site burns if there is poor contact between the patient and the dispersive electrode. Pads placed incorrectly can result in poor contact.

98. A patient burn or a fire can occur if the generator is accidentally activated, and the active electrode is not housed in a clean, dry, nonconductive safety holster (AORN, 2015b, p. 123).

99. There is an increased risk of burn injury during minimally invasive endoscopic surgery. In laparoscopic surgery, the active electrode is introduced into the patient through the abdominal wall through a cannula. The internal view is limited, and the shafts of the laparoscope and the cannula are not visualized. Unintended transfer of energy along the laparoscope or cannula shafts, or along the active electrode shaft, can result in an internal burn that might go unnoticed.

100. Inadvertent activation of the active electrode outside the visible field can also cause an internal burn. A burn causing perforation of the bowel can result in peritonitis—a life-threatening complication.

101. Electrosurgical complications in laparoscopic surgery can result from the following sources:
    - Insulation failure on the active electrode
    - Direct coupling between the active electrode and other metal instruments or with tissue
    - Capacitive coupling

102. When the insulation on an active electrode is cracked or damaged, current can flow to an unintended area. Even very small insulation defects can result in patient injury. Electrons can escape through holes hardly visible to the naked eye.

103. Electrical energy escaping through faulty insulation can transfer to a metal instrument that

subsequently can burn tissue, potentially causing life-threatening injury. Escaping energy can be transferred through the entire shaft of the cannula, burning the abdominal wall, skin, or structures adjacent to the cannula.

104. Direct coupling occurs when the tip of the active electrode touches another metal instrument and electrical current is transferred to the instrument that will burn tissue at the contact site. This type of injury occurs within the surgeon's field of view, should not go unnoticed, and can be repaired before the surgery is completed.

105. Capacitive coupling is the induction of electrical current from the monopolar active electrode into adjacent conductors in an effort to balance the charge of electrons oscillating at radio frequencies. When the active electrode is passed through a cannula or the working channel of a laparoscope, current can be induced onto the metal even though the insulation on the active electrode is intact. This electrifies the entire instrument and creates the potential for a burn, most likely at the abdominal wall or on external skin.

106. The risk for capacitive coupling injury increases:

   • With high-voltage settings and fulguration

   • When the surgeon activates the electrode "in open air" (without touching the tip to tissue)

   • When the mix of instrumentation does not account for the dynamics of capacitive coupling

107. The risk for capacitive coupling is diminished with:

   • Advances in endoscopic instrumentation, including laparoscopic bipolar active electrodes and shielded monopolar active electrodes with monitors designed to detect insulation failure

   • Active electrode monitoring (AEM) that detects insulation failure and capacitive coupling and will deactivate the ESU

   • Shielded monopolar monitoring systems that detect insulation failure and automatically deactivate the ESU

108. Bipolar electrodes localize current. Bipolar systems offer safety advantages and protect the patient from insulation failure and capacitively coupled electrosurgical current.

Hazards: Fire and Surgical Plume

109. Operating room fires from electrosurgical equipment that involve patient injury or death are reported every year. The active electrode provides the ignition source; drapes and sponges provide an ample source of fuel; and the oxygen-enriched surgical environment completes the first triangle. Fires in surgery can become intense in just a few minutes.

110. Plume or surgical smoke resulting from electrosurgical and laser applications can injure surgical personnel. Patients who are intubated or receive inhalation anesthetic via mask are protected from inhaling surgical plume.

111. Research studies have confirmed that surgical plume can contain toxic gases and vapors such as benzene, hydrogen cyanide, and formaldehyde; bioaerosols; dead and live cellular material (including blood fragments); and viruses (National Institute for Occupational Safety and Health [NIOSH], 1996).

112. Adverse effects of surgical smoke include eye irritation; headache; nausea; dizziness; and higher rates of respiratory symptoms, sinus infections/problems, allergies, asthma, and bronchitis (Lindsey, Hutchinson, & Mellor, 2015).

113. NIOSH (1996), the American National Standards Institute (ANSI, 2011), and AORN (2015c, pp. 130–131) recommend evacuation and filtration of surgical smoke. In the absence of a dedicated smoke evacuator, wall suction with a 0.1-micron inline (ULPA) filter can be used, but only during surgeries in which a small amount of smoke is generated and only when the flow rate of the wall suction is adequate.

114. High-filtration surgical masks (e.g., N95 masks) should not be considered a first line of protection from surgical plume, but only adjunct protection (ANSI, 2011; AORN, 2015c, p. 131).

Desired Patient Outcome/Criteria

115. Desired patient outcome: The patient will experience no injury as a result of the use of electrosurgery.

116. Criteria to evaluate successful achievement of the desired outcome include no evidence of the following complications:

   • Impaired skin integrity (burn) at the dispersive electrode site or alternate current path

   • A burn at an unintended site

- A burn at the entrance site of laparoscopic instrumentation
- Fever or abdominal pain associated with peritonitis

Nursing Interventions: Patient and Staff Safety

117. Although electrosurgery is performed by the surgeon and/or assistants, perioperative nursing interventions are critical to a safe patient outcome.

118. Prior to surgery, the patient's skin should be assessed for the placement of the dispersive electrode. The electrode should not be positioned over scar tissue, excessive adipose tissue, prosthetic implant, pacemaker, or automatic implantable cardioverter-defibrillator device (ICD).

119. The AORN (2015b) guidelines and the Perioperative Nursing Data Set (AORN, 2011, pp. 175–177) detail protective measures to prevent injury due to electrical sources. The scrub person will implement some of the measures; the circulating nurse will implement others.

120. Before the procedure:
- Use only equipment that has been inspected by biomedical engineering personnel. Inspection stickers should be visible and must not be expired.
- Prior to use, inspect the generator for frayed cords and loose connections.
- Turn the generator off between cases.
- Use only those dispersive and active electrodes that are compatible with the generator.
- Ensure the alarm system is intact and activated.
- Test the alarm; ensure that it is loud enough to be heard during surgery.
- Do not use reusable active electrodes beyond their intended life. Refer to the manufacturer's instructions for use to determine the permitted number of uses.
- In some older generators, two electrodes can be attached to a single generator. When one electrode is activated, the other is automatically activated. Avoid using this type of generator when it is anticipated that two electrodes will be required; use two separate ESUs.
- Select a dispersive electrode appropriate to the patient's size; never cut the dispersive electrode to modify its size or shape.

- Check the dispersive electrode to ensure that it is not damaged, cord connections are secure, and the expiration date has not passed.
- For adhesive dispersive pads (these steps are not necessary when using a disposable capacitive pad):
  - Place the dispersive electrode on the patient over clean, dry skin that covers a large muscle mass (well-vascularized tissue) and is as close to the operative site as possible to minimize the path of current flowing through the patient's body.
  - Avoid placing the dispersive electrode over the following areas:
    - Bony prominences and scar tissue, because they are less conductive and create resistance that can slow the passage of electrosurgical current and concentrate the current.
    - Implants, because there is usually scar tissue from the implantation surgery.
    - Excessive hair and areas where fluids can accumulate and compromise firm adhesion to the skin. If necessary to ensure adherence, hair should be clipped at the dispersive electrode site.
    - Excess adipose tissue, because this poorly vascularized tissue can impede conductivity of electrical current and dissipation of heat. Muscular areas generally have adequate circulation and promote conductivity of the electrical current. Suitable areas of placement include the anterior and posterior thigh, the calf, the upper arm, the midback, and the abdomen.
    - Areas close to electrocardiograph electrodes, because current may be attracted to these electrodes and cause an alternative-site burn. Current electrode technology minimizes this risk.
    - Tattoos, many of which contain metallic dyes that can, at least theoretically, cause a burn.
    - Between the patient and a warming device. The combination of heat at the dispersive electrode site and heat from a warming device can affect how the dispersive electrode adheres to the skin (AORN, 2015b, p. 126) and can result

in patient injury. Disposable capacitive pads have negligible heat buildup.

○ Metal implants should not be in the circuit path between the active electrode and the dispersive electrode.

– Ensure that there is no point of contact between the patient and any metal surfaces, such as the operating room table.

– Ask the patient to remove any metal jewelry that is near where the active electrode will be used or that is in the circuit path of electricity.

– If two dispersive electrodes are used, the manufacturer's instructions for use must be followed for their placement and application.

• Avoid tenting of surgical drapes that can result in an accumulation of oxygen that can create an oxygen-rich environment to enrich a fire.

• Place the ESU foot pedal in a plastic bag to keep it clean and dry.

• Prior to surgery, inspect the active electrodes for insulation defects. If a defect is noted, the device must be discarded and replaced.

121. During the procedure:

• Place the generator close enough to the patient to prevent cords from being pulled taut, creating tension at the connection sites.

• Electrical cords should be free of bends and kinks.

• Verbally confirm the power settings with the surgeon. Use the lowest possible power settings to achieve the desired electrosurgical effect. If a request is made to increase power because the present setting is no longer adequate, check for loose connections, pad placement, and generator malfunction. Replace the generator if a malfunction is discovered or suspected.

• Do not place liquids on the generator; spilled liquids may cause the equipment to malfunction.

• Position the active electrode on the sterile field close to the operative site and in a protective container or holster so that accidental activation will not cause incidental burns to the patient or ignite sponges or drapes.

• Avoid coiling cords around conductive metal objects (e.g., Allis clamp, hemostat, towel clamp), because normal leakage currents can

be induced into those instruments, and possibly present an ignition source for a fire.

• Keep the active electrode clean during surgery by periodically removing charred tissue. Eschar creates impedance that may result in a request for a higher power setting. Clean the tip with a moist (not dry) sponge or a scratch pad intended for this purpose. An active electrode inadvertently activated and in contact with a dry sponge (gauze pad) can start a fire. Nonstick active electrodes minimize the buildup of eschar.

• Do not use electrosurgery in the presence of flammable agents. Prep solutions containing flammable agents must be allowed to dry before using electrosurgery. Other factors, such as pooling of solution onto drapes, towels, and into body hair, can alter the drying time of the prep solution.

• Open suture packages containing alcohol should be kept away from the area of the active electrode.

• Sponges are flammable; use moistened sponges in the area of the active electrode.

• Be diligent when using electrosurgery in oxygen-enriched environments—including around a nasal cannula, when the patient is receiving oxygen via an oxygen mask, and when the anesthesia provider is using an uncuffed endotracheal tube.

• Methane gas, which can be present in the intestinal tract, is flammable. The active electrode should not be activated in the presence of methane gas.

• Evacuate electrosurgical smoke from the field.

• During lengthy procedures, or when the patient is repositioned during surgery, verify that the dispersive electrode continues to maintain good contact with the patient.

• In the event of the failure of any of the electrosurgical components, retain the defective items for follow-up with biomedical personnel and for reporting of medical instrumentation failure as required.

Electrosurgical Use During Endoscopic Surgery: Special Precautions

122. The following additional precautions are appropriate when using electrosurgery during endoscopic surgery:

• Prior to surgery, inspect the active electrodes for insulation defects. Some laparoscopic instruments have a double-sheathed shaft of insulation of different colors that can help to identify an insulation defect. If a defect is noted, the electrode must not be used.

- If a defect is noted during the surgery or following the procedure, inform the surgeon that the patient might have potentially sustained an inadvertent internal burn.

- Active electrode monitoring equipment should be used whenever available to detect insulation failures and capacitive coupling on active electrode instrumentation during endoscopic surgery.

- The surgeon should avoid activating the electrode before the tip is in contact with the target tissue. Without tissue contact, voltage increases, which increases the risk of current deviation or unintentionally high voltage when contact with tissue is made.

- Most trocars in use today are disposable. However, all-metal trocar systems help reduce the risk of capacitive coupling. When electrical current builds up on a metal cannula, the current will be absorbed into the abdominal wall.

Electrosurgical Use in the Presence of an Implantable Electronic Device

123. Internal cardioverter-defibrillator devices (ICDs) should be deactivated prior to surgery; the ICD should then be reactivated following the procedure. Facility procedure should detail the process for ICD deactivation and reactivation. Regardless of who is responsible for activation and deactivation, the perioperative nurse must ensure that the process is properly documented. An alternative to deactivation is bipolar electrosurgery, because it does not interfere with the ICD.

124. Electrosurgery can interfere with the operation of some pacemakers. The dispersive electrode should be placed as close as possible to the surgical site and in such a way that the pacemaker is not in the circuit path between active and dispersive electrodes. The pacemaker manufacturer's instructions for use will detail the safest practice for management during surgery. As with an ICD, a bipolar energy source is preferred.

125. Patients with a pacemaker or ICD should have continuous electrocardiogram monitoring during procedures where electrosurgery is used, and a defibrillator and a pacemaker magnet or programming unit should be readily available.

126. Bipolar electrosurgery is also recommended for other implantable devices such as cochlear implants and bone, brain, spinal cord, and vagal nerve stimulators (AORN, 2005). Device manufacturers' instructions for use provide the best guidelines for managing implanted devices during surgery.

127. Following surgery, the dispersive electrode should be removed slowly and carefully to avoid damaging the skin. The placement area should be inspected for injury.

128. Documentation of electrosurgical use should include the following information:

- Assessment of the skin preoperatively with name of individual performing assessment

- Site of dispersive electrode placement with name of individual performing assessment

- Identification of electrosurgical equipment and serial number

- Range of settings used

- Use of safety holster for the active electrode

- Postoperative assessment of skin with name of individual performing assessment

Section Questions

1. What is the purpose of the nonconductive safety holster? [Ref 98]
2. Describe the minimally invasive surgery environment that creates risk for burn injury. [Ref 99]
3. How can insulation failure result in a burn injury? [Refs 102–103]
4. What is direct coupling and how can it result in patient injury? [Ref 104]
5. Describe capacitive coupling in laparoscopic surgery and how the potential for injury can be decreased. [Refs 105–107]

(continues)

Section Questions (continued)

6. Describe the new developments in endoscopic instruments that minimize the risk of burn injuries. [Ref 107]

7. What safety advantages does bipolar electrosurgery offer? [Ref 108]

8. Explain how electrosurgery can cause a fire in the operating room. [Ref 109]

9. What interventions can protect personnel from surgical smoke or plume? [Refs 113–114]

10. What criteria are used to evaluate successful achievement of preventing harm from electrosurgery? [Ref 116]

11. Prior to the surgical procedure, describe the process of ensuring the safe use of the electrosurgery generator. [Ref 120]

12. Describe the ideal site for placement of the adhesive-backed dispersive electrode. [Refs 118, 120]

13. Explain why certain sites should be avoided when placing the adhesive-backed dispersive electrode. [Ref 120]

14. How might tenting of the drapes affect fire safety during a surgical procedure? [Ref 120]

15. What should the perioperative nurse do when the surgeon continually asks that the power setting be increased on the electrosurgical unit? [Ref 121]

16. Where should the active electrode be positioned on the sterile field? [Ref 121]

17. How can eschar on the active electrode interfere with safe electrosurgery? [Ref 121]

18. Why would you not discard a defective active electrode? [Ref 121]

19. How would you handle a situation in which you discovered faulty insulation on an active electrode following an endoscopic procedure? [Ref 122]

20. What is the best source of information for managing surgery on patients with implantable devices? [Ref 126]

Ultrasonic/Harmonic Technology

129. Ultrasonic technology cuts and coagulates simultaneously and at temperatures up to 100°C (212°F—much lower than the 150°C [302°F] or higher needed for electrosurgery) and produces less plume than electrosurgery.

130. Ultrasonic technology results in minimal char and tissue desiccation and permits precise dissection near vital structures. It can be used as an adjunct to or a substitute for electrosurgery.

131. The ultrasonic scalpel generator is a microprocessor that uses controlled high-frequency power to drive an acoustic system within a handpiece. Electrical energy is converted into mechanical energy or ultrasonic waveforms transmitted to the handpiece and a blade that vibrates at a speed of 55,500 vibrations per second. No electricity is transferred to the patient, so no dispersive electrode is required.

132. The handpiece is activated with a foot pedal. When the blade contacts tissue, it denatures the protein and creates a sticky coagulum, thereby sealing blood vessels.

133. The cutting speed and the coagulation effects are inversely related. Four factors control the effect upon tissue:

- Tissue tension: More tension produces faster cutting and less hemostasis; less tension produces slower cutting and more hemostasis.

- Blade sharpness: Shear mode cuts faster; blunt mode provides more coagulation for vascular structures.

- Power: Higher power increases cutting speed and decreases coagulation; lower power slows cutting and increases coagulation.

- Time: Shorter application of power to the tissue produces faster cutting and less hemostasis; longer application time results in slower cutting and greater hemostasis.

Argon Beam–Enhanced Electrosurgery/ Argon Plasma Coagulation

134. Argon beam–enhanced electrosurgery technology uses a beam of ionized argon to achieve rapid hemostasis by coagulation. The flow of

the argon gas clears the tissue of liquid blood and other fluid, and the energy from the ionized argon beam creates a superficial eschar directly on the tissue that helps to prevent further bleeding. Coagulation occurs from the arcing effect of electrical energy, not from the argon gas.

135. Argon beam coagulation is used for open and endoscopic procedures where coagulation and minimal tissue penetration are desired. It can control bleeding from vascular structures where large areas of coagulation are needed and to control surface bleeding of organs such as the liver.

136. The clinical benefits of argon beam coagulation include rapid, efficient coagulation; formation of a thin, flexible eschar; less charring; and less tissue damage than with traditional electrosurgical coagulation.

137. Active electrodes include blade and needle tips for open procedures and a variety of electrode tips for endoscopic surgery.

138. Argon is an inert gas and is noncombustible. It produces less plume, odor, and tissue damage than electrosurgery.

139. Because electrical current is delivered to the patient, a dispersive electrode is required.

Enhanced Monopolar Technology

140. One new electrosurgical technology that is beginning to gain footing (Megadyne® ACE Blade and Covidien® Peak Plasma Blade) involves advances in monopolar energy that produces minimal thermal damage to soft tissue. Surgeons are able to use one tool to cut, dissect, and coagulate that provides results equivalent to using a scalpel. In addition, the new technology saves a significant amount of surgical time.

Section Questions

1. How does cutting and coagulating with ultrasonic technology compare to conventional electrosurgery? [Refs 129–132]

2. What is the relationship of the cutting speed to coagulation with ultrasonic technology? [Ref 133]

3. What is the relationship of tissue tension to both cutting and coagulation with ultrasonic technology? [Ref 133]

4. Discuss the impact of alterations in blade sharpness, power, and time on cutting and coagulating with ultrasonic technology. [Ref 133]

5. How does argon beam-enhanced technology control bleeding? [Ref 134]

6. Describe the clinical benefits of argon beam-enhanced coagulation. [Ref 136]

7. How does the plume created by argon beam-enhanced coagulation compare with traditional electrosurgery? [Ref 138]

8. Explain the reason for using a dispersive electrode with argon beam-enhanced coagulation. [Ref 139]

References

American National Standards Institute (ANSI). (2011). *ANSI Z136.3: American national standard for safe use of lasers in health care facilities.* Orlando, FL: Laser Institute of America.

Association of periOperative Registered Nurses (AORN). (2005). Guidance statement: Care of the perioperative patient with an implanted electronic device. *AORN Journal, 82*(1), 74–82.

Association of periOperative Registered Nurses (AORN). (2011). *Perioperative nursing data set.* Denver, CO: Author.

Association of periOperative Registered Nurses (AORN). (2015a). Guideline for care of patients undergoing pneumatic tourniquet-assisted procedures. In: *Guidelines for perioperative practice* (pp. 153–186). Denver, CO: Author.

Association of periOperative Registered Nurses (AORN). (2015b). Guideline for electrosurgery. In: *Guidelines for perioperative practice* (pp. 121–138). Denver, CO: Author.

Association of periOperative Registered Nurses (AORN). (2015c). *Management of surgical smoke tool kit.* Retrieved from http://www.aorn.org/Secondary.aspx?id=21878&terms=smoke%20evacuation

Lindsey, C., Hutchinson, M.,& Mellor, G. (2015). The nature and hazards of diathermy plumes: A review. *AORN Journal, 101*(4), 428–442.

National Institute for Occupational Safety and Health (NIOSH). (1996). *Control of smoke from laser/electric surgical procedures* (NIOSH publication 96–128). Retrieved from http://www.cdc.gov/niosh/docs/hazardcontrol/hc11.html

Occupational Safety and Health Administration (OSHA). *eTools: Hospital – Surgical Suite.* Available online: https://www.osha.gov/SLTC/etools/hospital/surgical/surgical.html Accessed: June 2015

Occupational Safety and Health Administration (OSHA). *Safety and health topics: Laser/electrosurgery plume.* Available online: https://www.osha.gov/SLTC/laserelectrosurgeryplume/index.html Accessed: June 2015

McEwen, J. (2015a). *Contraindications to tourniquet use.* Retrieved from http://www.tourniquets.org/clinical_applications.php#contraindications

McEwen, J. (2015b). *Tourniquet use and care.* Retrieved from http://www.tourniquets.org/use_care.php#appropriate_pressure

Moss CE, Bryant C, Stewart J, et al. (1990). *NIOSH Health hazard evaluation report,* University of Utah Health Sciences Center. HETA 88-101-2008. Atlanta: NIOSH.

Raju P (2010). *Arterial tourniquets: Anaesthesia tutorial of the week 200.* Available at: http://totw.anaesthesiologists.org/wp-content/uploads/2010/10/200-Arterial-Tourniquets.pdf. Accessed September 2012.

Post-Test

Read each question carefully. Each question may have more than one correct answer.

1. Hemostasis
   a. is the arrest or control of bleeding.
   b. is accomplished both by natural and artificial means.
   c. is sometimes achieved with the formation of a platelet plug.
   d. requires that coagulation occur.

2. Which statement(s) is (are) true about coagulation?
   a. As platelets from a platelet plug break down, thromboplastin is released into the blood.
   b. Coagulation is a complex process that begins with the interaction of prothrombin and thromboplastin.
   c. Potassium ions are part of the coagulation process.
   d. Fibrin is the basic structure of a clot.

3. Which additional statement(s) is (are) true about coagulation?
   a. It is self-regulating; the process will stop on its own when bleeding stops.
   b. It is a slow process, and even small wounds need prompt attention.
   c. The clot becomes red as platelets, white blood cells, and red blood cells become entangled in the fibrin.
   d. Fibrin is red and gives the clot its characteristic color.

4. Which statement(s) is (are) true about thrombin?
   a. Thrombin is useful in controlling major artery bleeding.
   b. Thrombin is a hormone that combines with fibrin to form a clot.
   c. Thrombin is for topical use only.
   d. Thrombin made from human plasma has fewer side effects than bovine thrombin.

5. Which statement(s) is (are) true about absorbable gelatin?
   a. Absorbable gelatin is available in a compressed pad (Gelfoam), powder, or beads.
   b. Fibrin is deposited into the interstices of Gelfoam, which swells and promotes clot formation.
   c. Gelatin is sometimes used with thrombin or epinephrine.
   d. Gelfoam is soluble and is commonly left in the wound.

6. Which statement(s) is (are) true? Oxidized cellulose
   a. is placed directly on an oozing surface.
   b. swells, forms a gel, and promotes clot formation when it comes into contact with blood.
   c. forms a pseudo-clot that puts pressure on the wound to speed up the clotting process.
   d. must be removed if used near the optic nerve or spinal cord.

7. Which statement(s) is (are) true?
   a. Microfibrillar collagen is often used in crevices and sites of irregular contour.
   b. Styptics cause blood vessels to dilate.
   c. Hemostatic clamps must be replaced with a ligature or ligating clip for permanent hemostasis.
   d. Manual pressure is a form of temporary hemostasis.

8. Which statement(s) is (are) true about tourniquets?

    a. A tourniquet is used to create a bloodless field for surgery.

    b. Tourniquets create hemostasis so that when they are deflated, there is no further bleeding.

    c. An Esmarch bandage is wrapped around the extremity to force blood out and remains in place during surgery.

    d. Appropriate pressures for upper and lower extremities are determined by the tourniquet manufacturer.

9. Which of the following might be contraindications for tourniquet use?

    a. Hypertension

    b. Open fracture

    c. DVT

    d. Sickle cell anemia

10. Which of the following are appropriate nursing interventions related to tourniquets?

    a. Choosing the size of tourniquet to use

    b. Ensuring that prophylactic antibiotics are not infused until the cuff has been inflated

    c. Testing the cuff and the tourniquet

    d. Assessing the patient's skin integrity and potential for complications

11. Which statement(s) is (are) true about tourniquet cuffs?

    a. A contoured cuff is useful when the distal circumference of the extremity is very different from the proximal circumference.

    b. The cuff selected should be as narrow as possible.

    c. The cuff should overlap at least 3 to 6 inches.

    d. Padding under the cuff is necessary to prevent damage to the skin.

12. Which statement(s) is (are) true about tourniquet management?

    a. The nurse should remind the surgeon periodically how long the tourniquet has been inflated.

    b. If the tourniquet's pressure drops, it should be inflated immediately to the desired pressure setting.

    c. Bilateral tourniquets should be deflated simultaneously.

    d. Inflating the tourniquet results in an increase in core body temperature.

13. Which statement(s) is (are) true about electrosurgery?

    a. Electrosurgery can generate enough heat to vaporize tissue.

    b. Each ESU manufacturer determines the ideal power setting for each type of surgery.

    c. Both monopolar and bipolar electrosurgery require an active electrode and a dispersive electrode.

    d. Cutting tissue requires a continuous waveform; coagulating tissue requires an interrupted waveform.

14. Which statement(s) is (are) true about coagulation?

    a. A single power setting is appropriate for most surgery.

    b. Coagulated tissue produces an eschar and must be absorbed during the healing process.

    c. Fulguration and desiccation are two types of coagulation.

    d. Fulguration is more commonly used than desiccation.

15. Which statement(s) is (are) true about active electrodes?

    a. Active electrodes triggered by hand or a foot pedal deliver current from the generator to the operative site.

    b. The current from a monopolar electrode passes from the tip, through the patient, to the dispersive electrode.

c. The current from a bipolar electrode passes through the tissue between the tips of the forceps.

d. Bipolar electrosurgery requires higher voltage than monopolar electrosurgery.

16. Which statement(s) is (are) true about dispersive electrodes?

    a. The dispersive electrode is also called a grounding pad or Bovie pad.

    b. The dispersive electrode may also be a capacitive pad that lies between the patient and the operating table.

    c. The dispersive electrode is much larger than the active electrode, and current density at the dispersive electrode is low.

    d. The dispersive electrode must make good contact with the patient to work properly.

17. Which of the following statement(s) is (are) true?

    a. The use of electrosurgery creates a risk for both fire and impaired skin integrity.

    b. One important fire-prevention tactic is using a clean, dry, nonconductive safety holster to house the ESU pencil when it is not in use.

    c. There is a lower risk for patient injury related to electrosurgery in laparoscopic procedures.

    d. An ESU burn during a laparoscopic procedure will be noticed immediately, because the active electrode is in the field of view.

18. Burns to the patient can result from

    a. cracked insulation on the active electrode.

    b. inadvertent activation of a pencil in a protective holder.

    c. a dispersive electrode that is not secured to the patient.

    d. capacitive coupling.

19. Which of the following statement(s) is (are) true?

    a. Capacitive coupling occurs when the tip of an electrode touches another metal instrument.

    b. The scrub person should find insulation defects upon inspection because they are easily seen.

    c. The risk for capacitive couple increases when the surgeon activates the electrode before touching the tip to tissue.

    d. Direct coupling occurs when the active electrode transfers current to another metal instrument.

20. Which of the following statements about surgical plume is (are) true?

    a. Plume can contain toxic gases and live cellular material.

    b. Adverse effects of exposure to plume, according to Lindsey and colleagues (2015), include cancer and death.

    c. NIOSH recommends a dedicated smoke evacuator or wall suction with a 0.5-micron filter.

    d. High-filtration masks are an alternative first line of protection from surgical plume.

21. In preparation for a surgical procedure, the perioperative nurse should do which of the following?

    a. Test the alarm on the ESU to be sure that it can be heard during the procedure.

    b. Find an ESU generator that supports two active electrodes when it is anticipated that two electrodes might be necessary.

    c. Cut the dispersive electrode so that it fits the pad site on the patient perfectly.

    d. Place the dispersive electrode over clean, dry, well-vascularized muscle tissue.

22. Which of the following can fuel a surgical fire?

    a. Methane gas

    b. Alcohol from suture packages

    c. Oxygen under the drapes

    d. Vapors from prep solutions trapped under the drapes

23. Which of the following nursing interventions promote(s) electrosurgical safety?
    a. Attach two electrodes to the generator if two people will be using them simultaneously during the procedure.
    b. If the dispersive electrode is too large, trim it to fit snugly on the area you have selected.
    c. Check for frayed cords, test the alarm of the electrosurgical unit, and be sure that the alarm is loud enough to be heard during surgery.
    d. Avoid placing the dispersive electrode over scar tissue, a bony prominence, or in the vicinity of an implant.

24. Which of the following statement(s) is (are) true?
    a. The electrosurgical generator is a handy place to put saline to be delivered to the back table.
    b. Store the active electrode in a protective receptacle on the surgical field.
    c. The eschar that builds up on the active electrode tip helps to disperse the current effectively.
    d. Wall suction will remove surgical smoke from the field on most procedures.

25. Which statement(s) is (are) true about ultrasonic energy devices?
    a. An ultrasonic device has both cutting and coagulation settings.
    b. Ultrasonic devices cut and coagulate at higher temperatures than needed for electrosurgery.
    c. The effect of the ultrasonic device is affected by tissue tension, blade sharpness, generator power, and time.
    d. Ultrasonic devices and electrosurgery cannot be used at the same time.

Effective Management of Surgical Instrumentation

Nursing Diagnosis: Desired Patient Outcome

1. The patient undergoing surgery is at risk for injury and infection related to use of surgical instrumentation.

2. Potential injury includes tearing of tissue caused by an instrument that does not perform as expected and retention of a foreign body caused by a portion of an instrument that breaks or falls off inside the patient and is not retrieved.

3. Infection or a foreign-body reaction may result from an improperly processed instrument. An instrument that is inappropriately processed

may have a retained toxic residue that can harm a patient (Association for the Advancement of Medical Instrumentation [AAMI], 2011, p. 61). An improperly processed instrument or one that malfunctions can extend the length of a surgical procedure, increasing the patient's anesthesia time and interfering with the flow of the operative schedule.

4. Following surgery, the patient should be free from signs and symptoms of injury caused by extraneous objects (Association of periOperative Registered Nurses [AORN], 2011, p. 165) and should be free of signs and symptoms of infection related to improperly processed or malfunctioning instruments.

5. When a patient sustains an injury or an infection during surgery, it is sometimes difficult or impossible to identify the exact cause. For example, many factors in the surgical environment can contribute to a postoperative infection (e.g., poor aseptic technique, poor surgical technique, inadequate skin preparation, improperly cleaned and processed instrumentation, the patient's state of health, or a combination of any of these factors).

6. The effects of a toxic residue from an inadequately processed instrument might not be recognized for some time, and a cause-and-effect relationship may never be established. This inability to assign causality is an important reason to take all steps necessary to protect the patient from injury related to instrumentation.

7. Meticulous aseptic technique, coupled with proper use and care of surgical instruments, provides the best insurance against an injury or infection related to surgical instrumentation.

8. Desired patient outcomes related to surgical instruments include absence of injury or infection related to poorly processed or defective instruments and no evidence of retained instrument or instrument part.

Evolution of Surgical Instrumentation

9. There is evidence of the use of surgical instrumentation as early as the Neolithic Period (circa 10,000 BC) when stone knives and trephines were used to perform surgery. Other early surgical implements included sharpened flints used for circumcision and sharpened animal teeth used for bloodletting.

10. In medieval Europe, barbers with their sharp razors did amputations and applied leeches for bloodletting.

11. Before the 1700s, when surgery gained recognition as a scientific discipline, instruments were made by blacksmiths, cutlers, and armorers. Then, skilled craftsmen—silversmiths, wood turners, coppersmiths, and steel workers—took over the crafting of surgical instruments.

12. Instruments were made to individual specifications and often had ornate, finely carved wooden or ivory handles and were encased in velvet-lined boxes. Surgery was still barbaric—performed without anesthesia or understanding of aseptic technique.

13. The advent of anesthesia in the 1840s enabled surgeons to work slowly and deliberately and also generated the need for more precise and varied surgical instrumentation.

14. With the introduction of instrument sterilization, wooden and ivory handles were replaced by all-metal instruments that could tolerate repeated sterilization.

15. The development of stainless steel in the 1900s further enhanced manufacturers' ability to make precise surgical instruments, and instrument making evolved into a highly skilled occupation. Many craftsmen from Europe, especially Germany, came to the United States to instruct apprentices. Germany is often considered the home of high-quality surgical instruments, and many instruments used in the United States today are manufactured in Germany.

16. The majority of surgical instruments are manufactured from stainless steel, although titanium, Vitallium, and other metals are also used.

17. Recent advances, especially in minimally invasive surgery, combined with advances in technology and new materials, have led to the development of many new, precise, sophisticated, complex, delicate, and very expensive surgical instruments, scopes, and cameras.

Manufacture of Surgical Instruments

18. The majority of basic instruments is made from stainless steel, which is composed of iron ore and varying amounts of carbon and chromium. The carbon provides the necessary hardness to the steel, and chromium provides the stainless, corrosion-resistant

characteristics. Most stainless-steel instruments are made from alloys that are high in carbon and low in chromium.

19. There are more than 80 different types of stainless steel. The quality of stainless steel varies according to its composition. The American Iron and Steel Institute grades steel using a three-digit number, based on various qualities and on the amount of carbon and chromium it contains.

20. Stainless steel series 300 and 400 are commonly used for the manufacture of surgical instruments. The 300 series is used primarily for non-cutting instruments, while the 400 series is used for both cutting and non-cutting instruments.

21. Both the 300 and 400 series are high-quality stainless steel that resists rust and corrosion, has good tensile strength, and maintains a keen edge. The specific stainless steel selected for instrument manufacture is determined by the intended use and desired flexibility and malleability of the instrument.

22. The initial step in instrument manufacture is the conversion of raw steel into sheets that are milled, ground, or lathed into instrument blanks. These blanks are then forged, die-cast, molded, or machined into specific instrument pieces of various shapes and sizes. Excess metal is trimmed, and the component parts are hand-assembled, ground, and buffed.

23. Each instrument is then heat-treated, or tempered, to achieve the desired spring, temper, and balance. Balance and temper provide the flexibility that is necessary to withstand the stress of repeated use.

24. Following inspection for defects that may include X-ray or fluoroscopy, the instrument is immersed in a nitric acid bath that removes carbon steel particles and promotes the formation of a chromium oxide surface coating. This process, called passivation, minimizes the potential for corrosion.

25. In the final step, tiny pits left behind when the carbon particles are removed are polished away, leaving a smooth surface on which a continuous layer of chromium oxide forms.

26. Passivation and polishing essentially close the instrument pores and retard corrosion. The chromium oxide layer continues to form when the instrument is exposed to the atmosphere and when it is subjected to the oxidizing agents contained in cleaning agents.

27. Instruments comprised of two halves may have one of three types of joints:
    - Box lock: One half fits into a slot on the other half creating a permanent articulation; the two halves cannot be separated. This is the most common articulation (**Figure 8-1A**).
    - Semi-box: The two halves of the instrument can be separated by rotating the halves so that the lock disengages and the instrument separates into two pieces.
    - Screw joint: A screw secures the two halves of an instrument; older instruments had a thumbscrew that could be removed to separate the instrument halves (Figure 8-1B).

Instrument Finishes

28. Surgical instruments have one of three types of finish:
    - Bright, highly polished
    - Satin or dull
    - Ebony

29. The highly polished finish resists surface corrosion. It is shiny and reflects light, which, on occasion, may distract the surgeon or obscure visibility. The majority of instruments have this finish. The scrubbed person can minimize this distraction with careful placement of the overhead lights.

30. The satin finish eliminates glare but is slightly more susceptible to corrosion.

31. Ebony, the least common finish, is black and eliminates glare. It is used most often in laser surgery to prevent reflection of the laser beam.

32. Stainless steel is not completely stainless. The chemical composition and the manufacturing

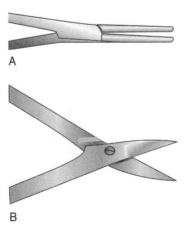

Figure 8-1 Instrument joints: (A) Box lock (B) Screw joint.

process determine the degree to which an instrument resists staining. With repeated use, some spotting or staining may occur. The degree of spotting, staining, or corrosion of stainless steel instruments also depends on the quality of water and chemicals used for processing.

33. Titanium instruments have a bluish finish. Titanium is stronger and lighter than stainless steel and is more corrosion resistant. It is also significantly more expensive. Titanium is used primarily for delicate, precise instruments used in microsurgical and neurosurgical procedures.

Instrument Nomenclature

34. Instrument names are not consistent. Different manufacturers, facilities, and individuals may identify the same instrument by different names.

35. There are some recognizable patterns in the nomenclature of surgical instruments. An instrument can be named:

    • By function: clamp, needle holder, pickups

    • By visual description: scissors, rake, hook, ribbon (retractors); knife

    • For the inventor: DeBakey forceps, Bookwalter retractor, Bishop forceps, Balfour retractor, Weitlaner retractor, Gelpi retractor, Satinsky clamp, Adson forceps, Cooley retractor, Stephens tenotomy scissors

    • Scientifically by its function in Latin, French, or other language: osteotome (Latin: bone knife), rongeur (French: gnawer), tracheotome (Latin: tracheal knife), scalpel (Latin: scraper/scratcher), speculum (Latin: mirror)

Nursing Responsibilities Related to Surgical Instrumentation

36. A large portion of the operating room budget is devoted to the purchase and repair of surgical instruments.

37. Proper instrument care and handling can preserve inventory and reduce expenditures for repair. Instruments that do not function properly, are out for repair, or are processed incorrectly can cause delays in surgery—a source of frustration for both the surgical team and the patient.

38. Proper care and handling of surgical instruments require that nurses be able to determine whether an instrument has been adequately prepared for use in surgery and have demonstrated competence in instrument care.

39. Operating room and sterile processing department (SPD) personnel share the responsibility for the care and handling of instruments. Instrument processing begins at the point of use. Personnel in the operating room are responsible for preparing instruments for processing by removing as much visible contamination as possible and sorting instruments into sets. The condition of the instruments that arrive in SPD to be processed has a significant impact on the time it takes to clean them and the degree to which they can be cleaned.

40. Dried blood, one of the biggest culprits in instrument corrosion, can be managed with meticulous care of instruments at the point of use. Instruments left covered with blood at the end of a procedure, especially those that are not transported quickly to the SPD, will corrode quickly and will have to be replaced. This represents an unnecessary and avoidable waste of resources.

41. In addition to the inspection of instruments in the SPD prior to packaging and sterilization, the scrub person setting up for a procedure must inspect instruments to determine that they are adequately prepared, function properly, and are ready for use.

42. The complexity and high cost of instrumentation, diversity of materials, and potential for patient injury require that the nurse know what special handling is required, which cleaning and sterilization methods are appropriate, and how to determine whether an instrument is functioning properly and, therefore, safe for use in surgery.

Loaner Instruments

43. When the hospital does not own the instruments needed for a particular procedure, a "loaner set" of instruments can be borrowed from the manufacturer or from another facility. This is particularly true of orthopedic instruments used for joint surgery, where the healthcare facility purchases the implant but borrows the instrumentation necessary for the procedure. There may be a fee for this service.

Borrowing a "loaner set" is also common with instruments for a new procedure that is just being introduced.

44. All "loaner" instruments should be inspected, inventoried, cleaned, packaged, and sterilized in-house before use. The perioperative nurse provides for patient safety by ensuring that all instruments used have been processed according to facility standards.

45. The "loaner set" must be delivered to the healthcare facility with sufficient time before the procedure for it to be processed appropriately.

46. The perioperative nurse should never accept instruments for a procedure that have not been processed in the facility's SPD. Non-sterile instruments and sets that have been packaged and sterilized in another healthcare facility should be sent to the SPD where they will be inventoried, inspected, cleaned, packaged, and sterilized before use in surgery.

47. The exception to accepting instruments that have been processed elsewhere is when instruments have been processed by a company whose business is instrument processing and with which the healthcare facility has a contract. Such businesses have processes in place to ensure appropriate processing and aseptic transportation of instrumentation.

Section Questions

1. What types of patient injury can be related to instruments? [Refs 2–3]

2. How can such injuries be prevented? [Ref 7]

3. Which recent advance in surgery has led to the development of a whole new array of surgical instruments? [Ref 17]

4. Which characteristics of the 300 and 400 series of stainless steel make them ideal for surgical instruments? [Ref 21]

5. What is the purpose of heat-treating or tempering surgical instruments? [Ref 23]

6. What do passivation and polishing accomplish? [Refs 24–26]

7. Which joint type is the most frequently used on modern instruments? [Ref 27]

8. What is the purpose of the three different types of finishes found on surgical instruments? [Refs 29–31]

9. What advantages does titanium have over stainless steel? [Ref 33]

10. What are some of the naming patterns for surgical instruments? [Ref 35]

11. Who is responsible for the care and handling of surgical instruments? [Ref 39]

12. Name one easily managed cause of corrosion on stainless instruments. [Ref 40]

13. Why might a facility use a "loaner set" of instruments? [Ref 43]

14. How should loaner sets of instruments be managed? [Refs 44–45]

15. What is the exception to in-house processing of borrowed instruments? [Ref 47]

Categories of Instruments

48. Surgical instruments can be organized into five categories:

    - Cutting—such as scalpels, scissors, osteotomes, curettes, and rongeurs
    - Grasping—such as clamps, forceps, and needle holders
    - Retracting—such as hand-held and self-retaining retractors, and specula
    - Suctioning—such as suction tips
    - Miscellaneous instruments—such as cannulas, probes, dilators, and calipers

Cutting Instruments
Scalpels and Suture Needles

49. It is the scrub person's responsibility to ensure that cutting instruments, such as scalpels, scissors, curettes, and osteotomes, are sharp. Dull

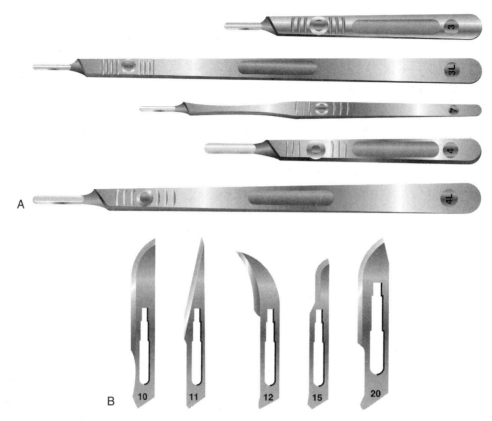

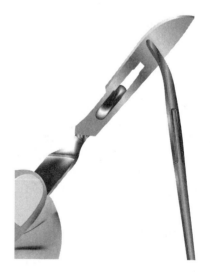

Figure 8-2 (A) Scalpel handles #3, #3 Long, and #7 handles accommodate the same blades and are more commonly used than the #4 and #4 Long handles that accommodate a larger blade. (B) Scalpel blades #10, #11, #12, and #15 fit the #3 and #7 handles. The larger #20 blade goes with the #4 handle.

instruments can cause patient injury, and replacing instruments can delay the procedure and increase the patient's anesthesia time.

50. Reusable scalpels are comprised of a handle and a disposable blade. The handle has a groove at the tip for attaching the blade. Blades are changed as needed during the procedure.

51. Scalpel handles are available in a variety of lengths and sizes appropriate for the procedure and location in which they will be used. A wide variety of scalpel blades is available, but a few are much more common than the rest (**Figure 8-2**).

52. Blades are commercially prepackaged and are sterile. They may have a rounded, tapered, or hooked cutting edge. Blades are delivered to the sterile field by the circulating nurse, and the scrub person contains them in a manner that will prevent accidental injury.

53. To prevent accidental injury when attaching or changing blades, the scrub person should use a needle holder to attach the blade to the

Figure 8-3 Attaching a scalpel blade.

knife handle. Blades must not be attached or removed from the handle by hand (**Figure 8-3**).

54. Scalpels and other sharp instruments of all kinds are passed using a hands-free technique

that minimizes the opportunity for accidental injury.

- The passing zone is designated by a magnetic pad, instrument mat, or receptacle for the item (**Figure 8-4**).
- Only one person touches the item at a time.
- Good communication between scrub person and surgeon facilitates passing and prevents injury. Verbalizing the transfer such as "blade ready" and "blade back" can increase transfer efficiency.

55. During the procedure, used needles and blades are collected in a device designed to aid in counting and safe disposal of sharps. At the end of the procedure, all sharps are sealed into the collection device, which is then discarded in a designated sharps container (**Figure 8-5**).

56. As a result of the 2000 Needlestick Safety and Prevention Act, the Occupational Safety and Health Administration (OSHA, 2011) amended the bloodborne pathogen standard to require the use of safer devices to protect healthcare workers from sharps injury. In response, many facilities have converted to safety products including shielded scalpel blades, needles with retractable covers, and blunt sutures.

57. Policies for safe handling of scalpels and other sharps may vary according to the institution; however, all facilities should have a sharps policy that is strictly enforced.

Scissors

58. Scissors are manufactured in many different sizes and styles specific to the tissue and depth for which they are used. The most common surgical scissors are Mayo scissors and Metzenbaum scissors. Both are round-tipped (blunt) scissors and are included in basic instrument sets for most surgical specialties (**Figure 8-6**).

59. Mayo scissors are sturdy, have either straight or curved blades, and are manufactured in a variety of lengths. Curved Mayo scissors are used to cut heavy, tough tissue. Straight Mayo scissors are used for cutting sutures and may be used to cut dressings or disposable drapes as needed.

60. Metzenbaum scissors, both straight and curved, are more delicate than Mayo scissors and are used to cut or dissect delicate tissue.

61. Most surgical scissors open and close in the same manner as household scissors. One difference is that, when holding any ringed surgical instrument, the fourth finger, instead of the third finger, is placed in the second ring. This leaves the first two fingers free to manipulate other objects (e.g., load suture, open sponges) while still holding the instrument.

62. Spring-action scissors are designed for more delicate surgeries, such as plastic, micro, or eye surgery. The jaws remain open until the thumb and forefinger press the spring together, closing the jaws. Releasing the pressure opens the jaws. Castroviejo scissors are a popular example of this type (**Figure 8-7**).

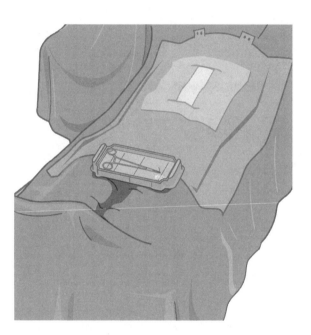

Figure 8-4 Safe zone or "no touch" zone.

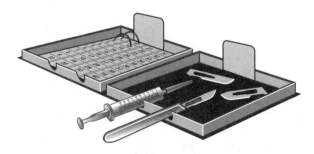

Figure 8-5 Sharps collection device.

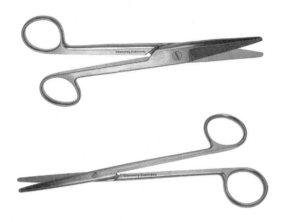

Figure 8-6 Mayo and Metzenbaum scissors.
Courtesy of Symmetry Surgical, Nashville, TN. Used with permission.

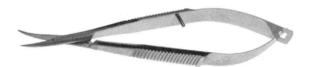

Figure 8-7 Castroviejo scissors. This same instrument design is used for needle holders for delicate suture.
Courtesy of Symmetry Surgical, Nashville, TN. Used with permission.

Other Sharp Instruments

63. Osteotomes, chisels, curettes, and rongeurs are used for cutting bone.

64. Periosteal elevators separate tissue from bone or from other tissue (**Figure 8-8**).

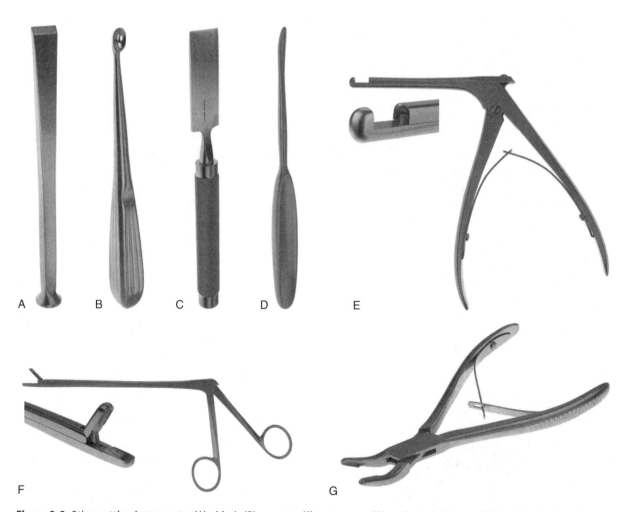

Figure 8-8 Other cutting instruments: (A) chisel, (B) currette, (C) osteotome, (D) periosteal elevator, (E) Spurling-Kerrison bone rongeur, (F) pituitary rongeur, (G) Langenbeck bone rongeur.
Courtesy of Symmetry Surgical, Nashville, TN. Used with permission.

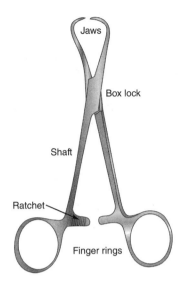

Figure 8-9 Clamp.

Clamps

65. Clamps are designed to hold tissue or other materials. They are manufactured in a wide variety of shapes and sizes, with tips that are straight, curved, or angled. Some clamps are fine and delicate; others are more substantial.

66. The overall design is similar for all clamps (**Figure 8-9**):

- Finger rings for holding the instrument
- A ratchet for locking the instrument in a closed position
- A shaft
- A joint (called a box lock) that joins the two halves of the instrument and permits opening and closing
- Distal tip or jaw (The design of the jaw determines the instrument's use.)

Hemostatic Clamps

67. Hemostatic clamps, commonly referred to as hemostats, are designed to control bleeding. The clamping jaws of the instrument have horizontal serrations. This design allows the clamp to compress the vessel with enough force to stop bleeding. The serrations also prevent the clamp from slipping off the tissue.

68. Common hemostats include the mosquito, Crile, Kelly, Pean, tonsil (Schnidt), and right angle or Mixter (**Figure 8-10**):

- Mosquitoes are small clamps that may be either curved or straight. They are most often used to clamp small bleeders in the superficial layers of tissue. Mosquitoes are sometimes called "snaps."
- Criles are curved and slightly longer and heavier than mosquitoes. Criles are more delicate than Kellys or Peans.
- Tonsil clamps are curved and longer than Criles. They are used where additional length is needed.
- Kellys and Peans are straight or curved and are heavier than Crile or tonsil clamps.
- The Mixter has a right-angle tip that can be passed under a vessel to capture a suture tie. Longer Mixters are useful for clamping and separating tissue in the abdominal cavity. Shorter Mixters are often used to separate tissue during surgery on vasculature that is not deep within the body.

69. The jaws of vascular clamps have opposing rows of fine serrations (DeBakey serrations) designed to occlude a vessel without crushing it. The jaws may be straight, curved, rounded, or angled.

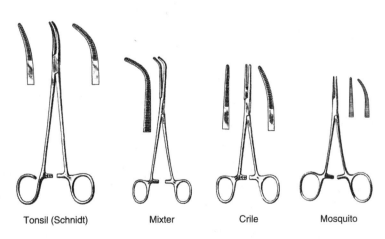

Tonsil (Schnidt)   Mixter   Crile   Mosquito

Figure 8-10 Hemostats.
Permission granted by Integra LifeSciences Corporation, Plainsboro, New Jersey, USA.

Occluding Clamps

70. Occluding clamps are used to clamp tissue, such as bowel or blood vessels, where prevention of leakage and minimization of tissue trauma are desired. The serrations on occluding clamps are vertical, close together, and arranged in multiple rows.

Grasping and Holding Clamps

71. Grasping or holding clamps have a variety of tip shapes. They are used for retracting tissue and to facilitate dissection and suturing. The surgeon can grasp the tissue with one hand and suture or dissect it with the other hand. Some grasping clamps are used to hold sponges, suture needles, or suture ties.

72. Common grasping clamps include the Allis, Babcock, Kocher (Ochsner), sponge forcep, towel clip, tenaculum, and needle holders (**Figure 8-11**).

73. The tips of an Allis clamp have multiple blunt teeth that do not crush or damage tissue. Allis clamps are used on delicate tissue.

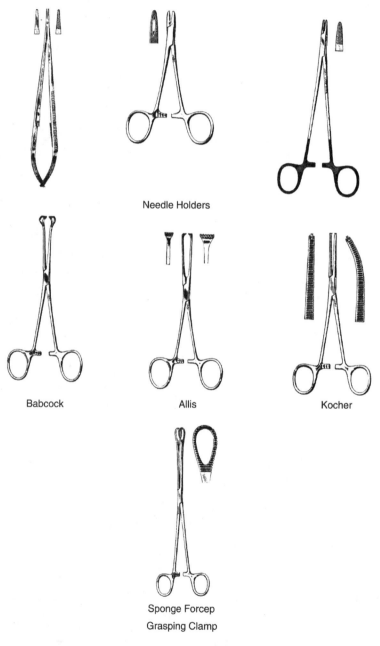

Needle Holders

Babcock   Allis   Kocher

Sponge Forcep
Grasping Clamp

Figure 8-11 Common needle holders grasping clamps.
Permission granted by Integra LifeSciences Corporation, Plainsboro, New Jersey, USA.

74. Babcock clamps have a curved and fenestrated tip with no teeth. A Babcock can be used to grip or enclose delicate structures such as a fallopian tube, a ureter, or bowel.

75. A Kocher clamp has transverse serrations and a single heavy tooth at its tip. It is useful for grasping tough tissue.

76. Sponge forceps (ring forceps) can be used to hold tissue, but most often are used to hold a folded gauze sponge (4×4 or RayTec) that can be used to blot or sponge fluids or blood or to retract tissue.

77. Towel clips are used to secure towels around the operative site and to hold drapes in place. Towel clips may have sharp tips that penetrate drapes or blunt tips that do not. When towel clips that penetrate the drapes are used, the points are considered contaminated; they cannot be removed and repositioned (**Figure 8-12**).

78. Needle holders are designed to hold a needle securely in place so that the needle does not rotate or slip. Needle holders may or may not have a locking ratchet. The surface of the jaws may be smooth, diamond-cut made from tungsten carbide, or cross-hatched (**Figure 8-13**). Tungsten carbide diamond-cut jaws are designed to prevent the needle from twisting and turning. Needle holders with

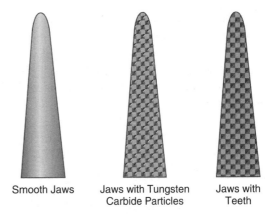

| Smooth Jaws | Jaws with Tungsten Carbide Particles | Jaws with Teeth |

Figure 8-13 Needle holder jaws.
Courtesy of Ethicon, Inc., Sommerville, NJ.

tungsten carbide jaws are identified by gold-plated ring handles.

79. Needle holders used for very fine sutures have a spring action rather than a ratchet action. The needle is held in place when the surgeon presses the spring together between the thumb and forefinger. When the pressure is released, the jaws open and the needle is released. Some spring-operated needle holders have a locking mechanism; most don't (Figure 8-7).

Forceps

80. Grasping and holding instruments that are not shaped as clamps are referred to as forceps or pickups (**Figure 8-14**). Forceps are similar to tweezers, with two arms and a spring action. They lift and hold tissue when the arms of the forceps are squeezed together, which

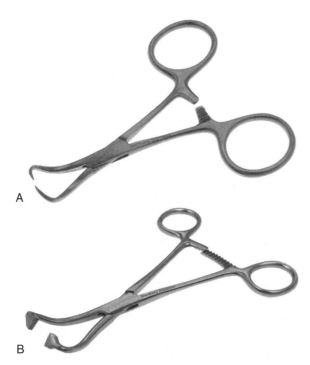

Figure 8-12 Towel clips: (A) Sharp tips, (B) Blunt tips.
Courtesy of Symmetry Surgical, Nashville, TN. Used with permission.

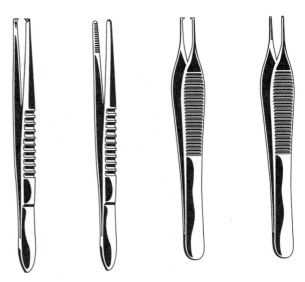

Figure 8-14 Tissue forceps with and without teeth.
Permission granted by Integra LifeSciences Corporation, Plainsboro, New Jersey, USA.

approximates the tips; releasing the pressure separates the tips.

81. The surgeon frequently holds forceps in one hand to grasp the tissue while cutting, coagulating, separating, or suturing tissue with the other hand.

82. Forceps vary in length and sturdiness, may have vertical or horizontal serrations, and may have one or more teeth at the tips.

83. Toothed forceps are used to hold thick tissue, such as skin that may require extra grip. Forceps without teeth hold more delicate tissue and cause minimal trauma.

Retractors

84. Retractors are designed to facilitate visualization of the operative field while preventing trauma to the surrounding tissue.

85. Retractors are available in many sizes and shapes. Some retractors require that the surgeon or assistant exert pressure to retract tissue from the operative site; other retractors are self-retaining.

86. Common non-self-retaining retractors include rakes, Richardsons, Deavers, Army-Navys, Parkers, and malleables (ribbons); (**Figure 8-15**). Slender, colored, radiopaque silicon bands (vessel loops) can be used to retract delicate structures.

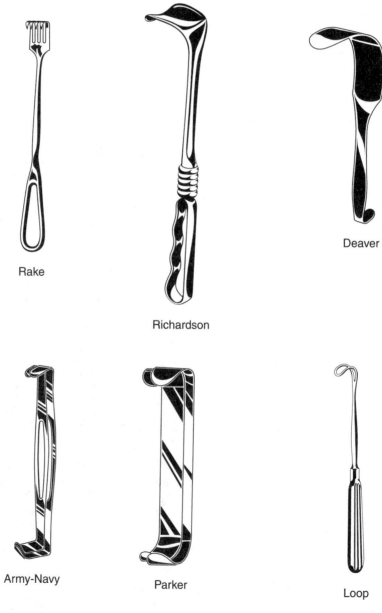

Rake

Richardson

Deaver

Army-Navy

Parker

Loop

Figure 8-15 Handheld retractors.
Permission granted by Integra LifeSciences Corporation, Plainsboro, New Jersey, USA.

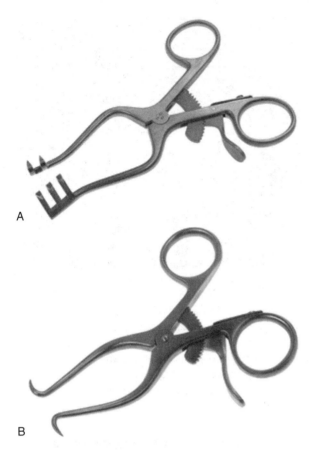

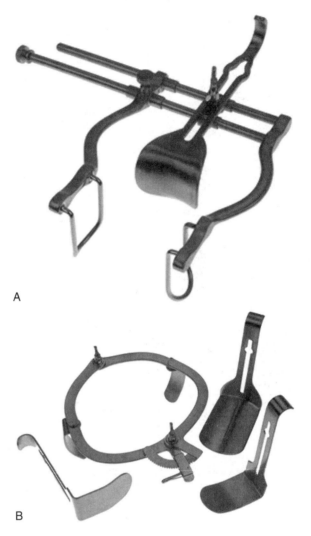

A

Figure 8-16 Self-retaining abdominal retractors:
(A) Weitlaner retractor, (B) Gelpi retractor.
Courtesy of Symmetry Surgical, Nashville, TN. Used with permission.

B

Figure 8-17 Self-retaining abdominal retractors with assorted blades: (A) Balfour abdominal retractor, (B) O'Sullivan-O'Connor abdominal retractor.
Courtesy of Symmetry Surgical, Nashville, TN. Used with permission.

87. Weitlaners and Gelpis are self-retaining retractors (**Figure 8-16**). A Balfour is an abdominal self-retaining retractor with a blade to hold back internal structures (**Figure 8-17**). Some self-retaining retractors, such as the Bookwalter and Thompson retractors, can be attached to the operating table and support blades of various lengths and configurations (**Figure 8-18**).

Suction

88. Suction instruments are used to remove blood and other fluids from the operative field.

89. Frazier, Yankauer, and Poole suction devices may be included in a basic instrument set (**Figure 8-19**).

90. A Frazier-tip suction is an angled tube that comes in a variety of diameters. A small-diameter Frazier suction is used where capillary bleeding and small amounts of fluid are

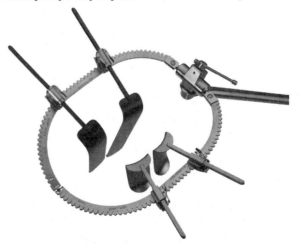

Figure 8-18 Bookwalter adjustable self-retaining retractor (attaches to the OR table).
Courtesy of Symmetry Surgical, Nashville, TN. Used with permission.

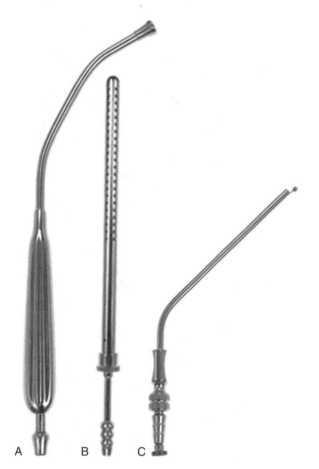

Figure 8-19 Suction cannulas: (A) Yankauer, (B) Poole, (C) Frazier (with Stylet).
Courtesy of Symmetry Surgical, Nashville, TN. Used with permission.

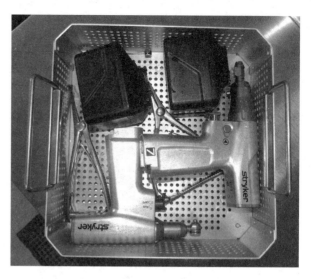

Figure 8-20 Drills.

encountered so as to maintain a dry field without the use of sponges. Some Frazier suction devices incorporate an active electrode into the tip so they may be used to coagulate tissue in addition to suctioning fluid.

91. A Yankauer suction is a slightly angled tube that is used in most general surgeries and in procedures involving the mouth and throat.

92. A Poole suction is a straight tube with an outer perforated shield that acts as a filter. It is useful where large amounts of blood or fluid collect and where the surgical area is deep, such as a body cavity.

Specialty Instrumentation

93. Thousands of instruments have been designed for specific surgical specialties. For example, each manufacturer of joint implants has developed a set of instruments specific to that implant.

94. Powered instruments, including drills and saws, have been customized for orthopedic, neuro, and ear, nose, and throat (ENT) surgery. Power sources for drills include electricity, compressed air or nitrogen, and batteries (**Figure 8-20**).

95. Some powered instruments can be steam sterilized; others must be processed with low-temperature sterilization. It is essential to know how each item is processed, because putting an expensive, heat-sensitive drill or saw in a steam sterilizer can be a costly mistake.

96. All powered instruments represent sophisticated construction with moving parts and attachments. Some powered items require oiling; others do not.

97. Powered instruments require meticulous cleaning as blood and debris gets into hard-to-clean places. It is essential to know what must be cleaned by hand and which items can tolerate automated processes.

Laparoscopic Instruments

98. The phenomenal growth in minimally invasive surgery has led to the development of a wide variety of rigid and flexible fiberoptic endoscopes and accessory instruments.

99. Rigid scopes have become commonplace in the operating room and are used in every surgical specialty. Laparoscopes, cystoscopes, hysteroscopes, and arthroscopes are the most widely used rigid endoscopes.

100. An increasing number of small-diameter semi-rigid and flexible fiberoptic endoscopes, such as sinus scopes, esophagoscopes, nasolaryngoscopes, ophthalmoendoscopes, ureteroscopes, and cholenephroscopes, are also available.

101. Large-diameter flexible fiberoptic endoscopes such as colonoscopes, gastroscopes, enteroscopes, duodenoscopes, and sigmoidoscopes are more commonly used in endoscopy units for diagnostic and gastrointestinal procedures.

102. Laparoscopic instrumentation typically includes several trocars with sleeves to create and maintain access to the surgical site, the scope to which a camera is attached, and a variety of accessory instruments to perform procedures. The entire procedure is viewed, not by direct visualization, but on a monitor.

103. Instruments to dissect, cut, grasp, cauterize, clip, suction, and suture tissue have been designed and adapted for minimally invasive surgery. The typical design includes a ring handle for holding the instrument; a long, small-diameter, insulated shaft inserted through a port into the patient; and a tip or jaw engineered for a specific purpose (**Figure 8-21**).

104. Laparoscopic instruments are complex and delicate and must be cleaned meticulously and inspected carefully. The long, narrow lumens of cannulated instruments must be kept free of debris, and bioburden cannot be allowed to dry on the intricate moving parts.

    With the advent of robotic surgery, another set of specialized instruments that are similar to laparoscopic instruments has been developed (**Figure 8-22**).

105. As surgical procedures become more sophisticated, the instrumentation required to implement new technology becomes more complex and specialized. The perioperative nurse must be committed to keeping abreast of the nursing responsibilities associated with rapidly advancing surgical technology.

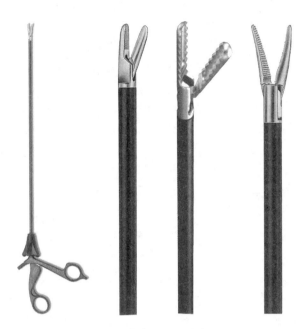

Figure 8-21 Laparoscopic instrumentation.
Courtesy of Aesculap, Inc, Center Valley, PA. Used with permission.

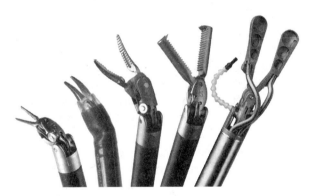

Figure 8-22 DaVinci robotic instruments.
© 2015 Intuitive Surgical, Inc. Used with permission.

Section Questions

1. Which negative outcomes can occur when cutting instruments are not sharp? [Ref 49]
2. How does the scrubbed person prevent injury when attaching or detaching a scalpel blade from the handle? [Ref 53]
3. Describe safe techniques for passing sharp instruments among scrubbed personnel. [Ref 54]
4. What are the primary functions of the two most commonly used surgical scissors? [Refs 58–60]

(continues)

Inspection

106. Instruments should be inspected by the scrubbed person just prior to surgery. Although time may permit only a cursory inspection, this check is sometimes sufficient to detect a defective instrument that could result in a delay in surgery or cause a patient injury.

107. During surgery, the surgeon may detect an instrument malfunction that is not immediately visible and can be observed only when the instrument is used. For instance, tissue scissors should not be tested on other materials. When this occurs, the instrument should be set aside and marked clearly for repair.

108. Inspection should include the following steps:
    - Clamps, scissors, and forceps are checked to ensure that tips are even and that they approximate properly. Tips should be in alignment and should not overlap.
    - To be in perfect alignment, the serrations on the jaws of the clamps must mesh perfectly. To test how well the serrations mesh, clamps are fully closed and held up to a light. If the serrations mesh perfectly, no light will be visible between the jaws. Misuse of clamps often results in misalignment.

- Instruments that feature a tooth or teeth at the tips are checked to ensure that they approximate and open freely. Tips that are not aligned properly will stick together. Release will be sluggish and can result in torn tissue.
- Ratchets and hinges must close easily and hold firmly. If the jaws of clamps spring open during use, they may be misaligned, the ratchet teeth may be worn, or the shanks may be bent or have insufficient tension. To test the ratchet, the instrument is closed on the first ratchet tooth and held by the box lock; the ratchet portion is then tapped against a solid surface. If the instrument springs open, the ratchets are faulty. A clamp that springs open when clamped on a blood vessel can cause injury to the patient.
- Joints and hinges should move easily. Stiff joints may indicate inadequate cleaning, a need for lubrication, or a defective instrument.
- Box locks are inspected for cracks and looseness. Excessive play in the box lock indicates an alignment problem. Clamps with loose box locks will not hold tissue securely. Cracked box locks are an indication of impending breakage. Broken instruments have the potential for causing patient injury.

- Scissor cutting edges must be smooth and sharp. Blades are inspected for burrs and chips. Scissor blades with burrs and chips will not cut cleanly and can cause trauma to tissue. Tips of Mayo and Metzenbaum scissors should cut through four layers of gauze with little resistance.

- Inspect the edges of sharp instruments, such as osteotomes, chisels, and rongeurs, for chips, nicks, or dents.

- Needle holders should hold a needle securely without slipping or rotation. Test this by securing a needle in the jaws and locking the instrument in the second ratchet tooth. If the needle can be easily moved by hand, the holder is worn and needs repair or replacement.

- Because rigid endoscopes may become damaged during repeated sterilization, the scrubbed person may do a quick check for clarity prior to surgery by holding the scope toward light and looking through the eyepiece, holding the scope far enough away from the eye so as not to risk contamination. A cloudy lens may indicate a leak in the lens seal with a subsequent accumulation of moisture inside. A partially blocked view or black spots in the field of vision may indicate a crack in one or more of the internal glass lenses or rods. More sophisticated tests that assess the resolution, clarity, and projected image of rigid endoscopes are typically conducted by SPD personnel just prior to packaging.

- Inspect flexible fiberoptic endoscopes for obvious external defects to the outer sheath. Rotate positioning controls to ensure they move smoothly and easily. Hold the lens to the light while observing the distal end for tiny black spots. Black spots indicate a broken fiber, and broken fibers result in decreased light transmission.

- Inspect fiberoptic cords for nicks. Attach a cord to a light source and observe the distal end for tiny black spots that indicate broken fibers that will result in diminished illumination.

- Connect the camera to a video monitor and observe the picture. The coupler and the controls should move easily.

- Determine that all parts of a multipart instrument are present and that instruments are assembled correctly. Loose pins and screws can cause an instrument to malfunction, and a part can be lost inside a patient.

- Inspect instruments with insulation to verify that all insulation is intact. Insulation cracks or flaws can cause a patient burn that could lead to serious injury such as peritonitis, or even death.

General Guidelines for Care and Cleaning at the Point of Use

109. Instrument processing begins at the point of use. It is the responsibility of personnel in the operating room, both scrub person and circulator, to use surgical instruments properly, to prepare them appropriately for postprocedure processing, and to communicate effectively with their partners in the SPD.

110. Instruments should be kept free of visible bioburden. During the procedure, instruments should be kept free of gross soil by wiping with a moistened sponge. Lumens are kept free of debris by irrigating with a syringe held below the surface of the water to prevent aerosolization of debris.

111. Blood and other debris allowed to dry in joints, lumens, serrations, and blades cause rusting and pitting, and can cause the instrument to malfunction.

112. Bioburden that remains on an instrument can prevent sterilant from contacting all surfaces and interfere with the sterilization process.

113. Dead organisms in organic debris can cause pyrogenic or foreign-body reactions (AAMI, 2011, p. 64). Improperly processed flexible endoscopes have been responsible for contaminated specimens and for patient infections.

114. Instruments ready to return to the SPD should have a minimum of visible soil, and should be sent as soon as possible after surgery. Instruments should be treated with an enzymatic solution, foam, or gel spray to prevent drying of debris; they should not be left soaking in water or saline. Saline is corrosive and can damage the instruments; biofilms form in water that has been sitting for a period of time.

115. Following a surgical procedure, instruments should be cleaned promptly. Instruments are washed and rinsed in water, not in saline. Prolonged exposure to blood and saline can cause corrosion and pitting of stainless steel.

116. All instruments should be handled according to the manufacturer's instructions. General guidelines for care and cleaning of instruments include the following points:

    • Instruments should be used only for the purpose for which they were designed. Misuse can result in improper alignment, dulling of sharp edges, and cracking of joints or tips.

    • Instruments should be handled gently and individually or in small lots.

    • During use, instruments may be kept clean by wiping and frequent rinsing.

    • Instruments should be placed carefully, not tossed, into basins or instrument trays. Entangled instruments can become misshapen or damaged.

    • All instruments with hinges and joints should be opened to expose box locks and serrations where blood and debris may be concealed.

    • Lighter, more delicate instruments should be placed on top of heavy, sturdier instruments.

    Delicate instruments can be damaged easily by the weight of heavier instruments.

    • Sharp instruments should be separated to avoid injury.

    • Multipart instruments should be disassembled and the parts kept together to prevent loss.

117. All instruments opened for a surgical procedure, whether or not they were actually used, are considered contaminated and are subjected to the same cleaning and decontamination process.

118. Some instrument sets, especially those intended for orthopedic surgery, are housed in specialty trays imprinted with a template inscribed with the name of each instrument and where in the set the instrument should be placed. The instruments fit snugly into the outlined slots. The template makes it easy for the scrubbed person to select the instruments that the surgeon requests, and it helps SPD personnel reassemble the set correctly.

Section Questions

1. When does the process of inspecting instruments occur? [Ref 106]

2. What should you look for when inspecting clamps, scissors, and forceps? [Ref 108]

3. What makes the teeth of forceps stick together? [Ref 108]

4. How can you test the ratchet of a clamp to be sure that it is functioning properly? [Ref 108]

5. How can you test the sharpness of Mayo and Metzenbaum scissors? [Ref 108]

6. How do you test a needle holder to see if it holds needles securely? [Ref 108]

7. What is the significance of a cloudy endoscope lens? [Ref 108]

8. What is the significance of a partially blocked view or black spots in the field of an endoscope lens? [Ref 108]

9. What do tiny black spots in a fiberoptic cord signify? [Ref 108]

10. What serious outcomes can faulty insulation cause? [Ref 108]

11. How are instruments kept clean during a surgical procedure? [Ref 110]

12. Why is wiping and rinsing debris immediately from instruments important? [Refs 111–112]

13. What are some adverse patient reactions to organic debris? [Ref 113]

14. How should instruments be treated to keep bioburden from drying on them before they arrive in the sterile processing department? [Ref 114]

15. What can happen to instruments that remain in contaminated water? [Ref 114]

16. Describe components of proper handling of instruments. [Ref 116]

(continues)

Section Questions (continued)

17. How are hinged instruments prepared for reprocessing? [Ref 116]

18. What does one do with instruments with more than one piece? [Ref 116]

19. Why should one segregate sharp instruments from the rest? [Ref 116]

20. How do you differentiate the instruments actually used on the procedure from those that remained unused on the back table? [Ref 117]

References

Association for the Advancement of Medical Instrumentation (AAMI). (2011). *Comprehensive guide to steam sterilization and sterility assurance in health care facilities* (ANSI/AAMI ST79:2011). Arlington, VA: Author.

Association of periOperative Registered Nurses (AORN). (2011). *Perioperative nursing data set*. Denver, CO: Author.

Occupational Safety and Health Administration (OSHA). (2011). *Bloodborne pathogens*. In: 1910.1030 (d)(4)(iii)(b). 56 Fed. Reg. 64004 (2011, December). Retrieved from https://www.osha.gov/pls/oshaweb/owadisp.show_document?p_table=STANDARDS&p_id=10051

Post-Test

Read each question carefully. Each question may have more than one correct answer.

1. What are adverse outcomes associated with the use of surgical instruments?
   a. Infection
   b. Foreign body reactions
   c. Blood clots
   d. Tearing of tissue

2. What is one difficulty in diagnosing patient reactions related to poorly processed surgical instrumentation?
   a. Patients rarely have reactions to poorly processed surgical instruments.
   b. If a reaction doesn't occur within 48 hours, it is not considered related to the surgical procedure.
   c. Timing of reactions often makes cause-and-effect relationships difficult to establish.
   d. Reactions occur so infrequently that they are not documented.

3. What changed the character of surgical instrumentation from ornate implements of various materials to precision metal instruments?
   a. The advent of anesthesia
   b. The introduction of instrument sterilization
   c. The development of titanium in Germany
   d. The acceptance of Lister's germ theory

4. The majority of surgical instruments are made of which material?
   a. Titanium
   b. Vitallium
   c. Stainless steel
   d. Plastic

5. Passivation is the process during instrument manufacture that
   a. puts an ebony finish on the instrument to reduce glare.
   b. hardens the metal and ensures that the instrument will retain its shape.
   c. removes spots and stains from the instrument.
   d. protects the surface and minimizes corrosion.

6. The most common type of hinge on surgical instruments is the
   a. box lock.
   b. semi-box.
   c. screw joint.
   d. screw lock.

7. Which of the instrument finishes best resists corrosion?
   a. Ebony
   b. Titanium
   c. Highly polished
   d. Satin, matte

8. What instrument finish is used for safety purposes in laser procedures?
   a. Series 400 stainless
   b. Titanium

    c. Ebony

    d. Matte, dull

9. Which material has a bluish tint and is stronger, lighter, and more corrosion resistant than stainless steel?

    a. Tungsten

    b. Titanium

    c. Carbonized steel

    d. Magnesium

10. Rake, hook, and ribbon retractors are examples of instruments named

    a. scientifically.

    b. for the inventor.

    c. by visual description.

    d. by function.

11. Nursing responsibilities related to surgical instrumentation include

    a. familiarity with all names by which an instrument can be called.

    b. the ability to determine whether an instrument has been adequately prepared for use.

    c. knowing the material from which each instrument on the sterile field is made.

    d. removing as much visible debris as possible before returning used instruments to the SPD.

12. Which of the following is one of the biggest culprits in instrument corrosion?

    a. Sterile water

    b. Alkaline detergent

    c. Dried blood

    d. Prep solution

13. When instruments for a procedure have been borrowed from the vendor or another facility, the perioperative nurse must ensure that the instruments

    a. are sterile when they arrive.

    b. arrive at the facility in time for the procedure.

    c. are accompanied by the vendor's representative in case questions about the instruments arise.

    d. have been inspected, inventoried, cleaned, packaged, and sterilized in-house.

14. What precautions protect the scrub person from injury when attaching a blade to the scalpel handle?

    a. The scrub person uses a needle holder to affix the blade to the handle.

    b. This is not a problem because scalpel blades and handles come preassembled.

    c. The scrub person must pinch the blade firmly above the notch before sliding onto the handle.

    d. The blade and the handle can be passed to the surgeon separately.

15. Which of the following is *not* a component of hands-free technique?

    a. One person touches the item at a time.

    b. The passing zone/safe zone is designated by a mat, pad, towel, or container.

    c. The instrument is placed in the surgeon's hand so that the sharp is clearly visible.

    d. Scrub person and surgeon communicate when passing sharps.

16. Which of the following is the most accurate description of Mayo or Metzenbaum scissors?

    a. Metzenbaum scissors are sturdy and used to cut suture.

    b. Straight Mayo scissors are used primarily for cutting tissue.

    c. Curved Metzenbaum scissors are delicate and used to dissect tissue.

    d. Curved Mayo scissors are primarily utility scissors used to cut suture.

17. The anatomy of a clamp comprises which of the following structures?

    a. Spring action joint

    b. Box lock

    c. Ratchet

    d. Finger rings

18. A "tonsil" hemostat

    a. is shorter than a Crile.

    b. is heavier than a Kelly.

    c. has a tooth at the end of the jaw.

    d. is longer than a Crile.

19. What differentiates vascular clamps from other hemostats?

    a. They have fine rows of serrations to occlude a vessel without crushing it.

    b. They are longer and sturdier than hemostats.

    c. The ratchets are more delicate to keep from crushing the vessel.

    d. They are always angled instead of curved or straight.

20. Babcock and Allis clamps have what characteristic(s) in common?

    a. They are vascular clamps.

    b. They are utility clamps used in many different ways.

    c. They are used on delicate tissues.

    d. They are heavy-duty clamps.

21. The significance of gold-plated finger rings on needle holders is

    a. to indicate that they have diamond-cut tungsten carbide inserts.

    b. to indicate that they are expensive and require special care.

    c. that they are heavier than regular instruments and can be used on tough tissue.

    d. that they can be used on very fine sutures.

22. Another name for grasping forceps is

    a. tweezers.

    b. clamp.

    c. retractor.

    d. pickups.

23. What is the purpose of a retractor?

    a. To hold the suture in place during wound closure

    b. To facilitate visualization of the operative field

    c. To give the surgical assistant something to do

    d. To make the incision larger without extending the incision

24. Which of the following is *not* a self-retaining retractor?

    a. Bookwalter

    b. Gelpi

    c. Richardson

    d. Weitlaner

25. Frazier, Yankauer, and Poole are three types of
    a. hemostatic clamps.
    b. retractors.
    c. needle holders.
    d. suction devices.

26. Which of the following is *not* a source of power for "powered surgical instruments"?
    a. CO_2
    b. Nitrogen
    c. Electricity
    d. Batteries

27. Can powered instruments be steam sterilized?
    a. Yes
    b. No
    c. Some can; some can't
    d. Only in a gravity displacement sterilizer

28. Cystoscopes, hysteroscopes, and arthroscopes are examples of
    a. jointed instruments.
    b. rigid endoscopes.
    c. flexible endoscopes.
    d. powered endoscopes.

29. The typical design of accessory instrumentation for minimally invasive surgical procedures includes the following elements:
    a. ring handle; long, small-diameter, insulated shaft; and tip or jaw.
    b. grip handle, long shaft, fiberoptic cable, and atraumatic tip.
    c. ring handle; long, large-diameter shaft; and insulated tip or jaw.
    d. grip handle, long insulated shaft, and fiberoptic tip or jaw.

30. As technology becomes more complex and specialized, the perioperative nurse must
    a. pick a specialty because there is too much to learn to master more than one specialty.
    b. get a degree in biomedical engineering.
    c. commit to continued education to keep abreast of the associated nursing responsibilities.
    d. spend more time in the sterile processing department in order to learn more about the equipment.

Competency Checklist:
Instrumentation—Care and Handling

Under "Observer's Initials," enter initials upon successful achievement of the competency. Enter N/A if the competency is not appropriate for the institution.

Name_____

	Observer's Initials	Date
1. Instrument inspection prior to procedure:	_____	_____
a. Tips approximate.	_____	_____
b. Serrations mesh.	_____	_____
c. Ratchets hold securely.		
d. Jaws open and close easily.	_____	_____
e. Cutting instruments are sharp.	_____	_____
f. Needle holders hold needle securely.	_____	_____
g. Scopes are clear.	_____	_____
h. Electrode insulation is intact.	_____	_____
i. Camera relays image to monitor.	_____	_____
2. Instruments handled properly during procedure:	_____	_____
a. Scalpel loaded and passed safely	_____	_____
b. Needle holder loaded and passed safely		
c. Sharp instruments handled and passed safely	_____	_____
d. Instruments handled carefully (placed, not tossed into basin and set)	_____	_____
e. Instruments kept clean during procedure (rinsed, wiped, irrigated)		
f. Instrument as free of visible soil as possible when ready for transport to decontamination area		
3. Transport of instruments from procedure room:	_____	_____
a. Instruments contained/covered in preparation for transport to the decontamination area	_____	_____
b. Instruments awaiting washing are moistened with enzymatic instrument spray	_____	_____
c. Instruments used only as intended (e.g., does not open medication vial with a Kocher clamp)	_____	_____

Observer's Signature   Initials   Date

_____

Orientee's Signature

_____

9

Wound Management: Wound Closure

LEARNER OBJECTIVES

1. Identify potential patient injuries related to wound healing.
2. Identify desired patient outcomes related to wound healing.
3. Differentiate among healing by first, second, and third intention.
4. Describe three stages of wound healing.
5. Contrast the characteristics of monofilament and multifilament suture material.
6. Describe criteria for the selection of absorbable and nonabsorbable suture material.
7. Interpret the information on suture boxes and individual packages.
8. Match suture and needle characteristics with their intended use.
9. Explain the purpose of surgical wound drains.
10. Describe the nursing responsibilities related to wound closure.

LESSON OUTLINE

Nursing Diagnoses

1. Patients undergoing surgery are at risk for compromised or interrupted wound healing and infection. Interrupted wound healing

includes *dehiscence*, the partial or complete separation of the wound edges after wound closure, and *evisceration*, the actual protrusion of the abdominal viscera through the incision.

2. Both wound dehiscence and evisceration are relatively uncommon, but they are associated with a risk of mortality. Other adverse outcomes include prolonged length of stay, subsequent surgeries, and incisional herniation (Agency for Healthcare Research and Quality [AHRQ], 2014).

3. Many factors determine the patient's risk for injury related to wound closure.

   • Dehiscence or evisceration that occurs on days 1 to 3 postoperatively is usually the result of inadequate wound closure.

   • Occurrences after the third postoperative day are often the result of excessive vomiting or coughing, infection, distention, or dehydration.

   • Patients with preexisting conditions, such as obesity, diabetes, malignancy, immunocompromise, dehydration, or malnourishment with hypoproteinemia, may experience delayed or complicated wound healing, which usually accounts for wound separation that occurs 2 or more weeks postoperatively.

4. Aseptic technique, suture materials, and surgical technique also influence wound healing. The majority of surgical wound infections are initiated along or adjacent to suture lines (Berry & Kohn, 2013, p. 553).

5. A break in aseptic technique and poor surgical technique can contribute to wound infection. Suture materials vary in their ability to avoid infection.

Desired Patient Outcomes/Criteria

6. The desired outcomes for the patient who undergoes surgery are freedom from injury and infection related to wound closure.

7. Evaluation criteria include absence of the following conditions:

   • Dehiscence or evisceration

   • Excessive scar formation

   • Wound-site infection, including abscess, serous drainage, cellulitis, fever 72 hours postoperatively, redness, and pain or swelling 72 hours postoperatively

Surgical Wound Classification

8. Wound classification is an assessment of the degree of contamination of a surgical wound at the time of the operation. Although specific rate predictions vary, evidence demonstrates that surgical site infection (SSI) rates increase as wounds progress from clean to dirty.

9. The wound classification system is also an important predictor of postoperative outcomes. One study of more than 15,000 cases found that wound classification was a significant predictor of overall complications, reoperation, and mortality (Mioton, Jordan, Hanwright, Bilimoria, & Kim, 2013).

10. Surgical wound classifications used by the Centers for Disease Control and Prevention (CDC) were introduced by the National Academy of Sciences in 1964 (**Table 9-1**).

    • Class I: clean

    • Class II: clean contaminated

    • Class III: contaminated

    • Class IV: dirty or infected

11. *Clean wound* (Class I):

    • The gastrointestinal (GI), genitourinary, and respiratory tracts are not entered.

    • No inflammation is encountered.

    • There has been no break in aseptic technique.

12. Examples of clean surgical procedures include hernia repair, carpal tunnel repair, total joint replacement, and cataract extraction.

13. The majority of surgical wounds are Class I. Most are elective surgeries that are not predisposed to postoperative infection.

14. Class I wounds are closed primarily and usually do not have a drain or are drained with a closed drainage system. The wound edges are brought together, and healing occurs with minimal edema or discharge with no localized infection.

Table 9-1	Surgical Wound Classification

I. Clean:
- Uninfected, no inflammation
- Result of non-penetrating, blunt trauma
- No involvement of respiratory, gastrointestinal, genitourinary, or urinary tracts
- Primary wound closure
- If drained, used closed drainage system

Examples: Ex lap, mastectomy, neck dissection, thyroid, vascular, hernia, splenectomy

II. Clean-contaminated:
- Procedure enters respiratory, gastrointestinal, genitourinary, or urinary tracts under controlled conditions with no unusual contamination
- Laparoscopic procedures
- Presence of inflammation
- Minor break in surgical technique

Examples: Cholecystectomy, small bowel resection, Whipple, liver transplant, gastric surgery, bronchoscopy, colon surgery

III. Contaminated:
- Open, fresh, accidental wounds
- Major break in sterile technique
- Gross Spillage from gastrointestinal tract
- Acute nonpurulent inflammation

Examples: Inflamed appendectomy, bile spillage in cholecystectomy, diverticulitis, rectal surgery, penetrating wounds

IV. Dirty:
- Old traumatic wounds, devitalized tissue
- Existing infection or perforation
- Microorganisms present BEFORE procedure

Examples: Abscess Incision & Drainage, perforated bowel, peritonitis, wound debridement, positive cultures pre-op, fresh trauma with environmental contamination

Modified from Michigan Apps for Surgical Trainees. (2012). Surgical wound classifications. Retrieved from http://www.med.umich.edu/surgery/mast/r_surgwoundclass.html.

15. *Clean contaminated wound* (Class II):
    - The GI, genitourinary, or respiratory tract is entered under planned, controlled circumstances.
    - Surgeries involve the biliary tract, appendix, vagina, and oropharynx provided there is no major break in aseptic technique, no spillage occurs, and no infection is present.
    - The wound is nontraumatic.
    - Inflammation may be present.
    - A minor break in aseptic technique may have occurred.

16. Examples of clean contaminated procedures include cholecystectomy, cystoscopy, hysterectomy, bronchoscopy, and intestinal resection when done under controlled circumstances.

17. *Contaminated wound* (Class III):
    - Gross contamination without obvious infection
    - Incisions with acute, nonpurulent inflammation or gross spillage from the GI tract
    - A major break in aseptic technique
    - Open, fresh accidental wounds

18. Examples of contaminated procedures include gunshot wounds, colon resection with GI spillage, and rectal procedures.

19. *Dirty or infected wound* (Class IV):
    - Old traumatic wound with dead tissue
    - Infection present

20. Examples of dirty or infected procedures include colon resection for ruptured diverticulitis, appendectomy for ruptured appendix, and amputation of a gangrenous appendage.

Wound Healing

Intention

21. Surgical wounds may heal by primary, secondary, or tertiary intention.

22. The preferred method of wound healing is by primary intention. Tissue is handled gently with minimal tissue damage; all layers of the wound are approximated, obliterating dead space; and the wound edges are brought together. The wound generally heals quickly with minimal scarring (**Figure 9-1A**).

23. Wounds that heal by secondary intention cannot be sutured at the time of surgery. The wound is left open to granulate. An example of secondary intention is a soft tissue ulcer left to heal from the bottom upward. Granulation tissue is characterized by a red, beefy appearance; it forms in the wound and gradually fills in the defect. The wound heals slowly, leaving a depressed scar slightly smaller than the original wound. Because the wound is left open, there is a greater risk for infection than if the wound were closed and healing by primary intention (Figure 9-1B).

24. Wounds that heal by tertiary intention or delayed primary closure are not sutured until several days after the initial surgery. Extensive tissue loss from injury or debridement of dirty or infected tissue may result in a wound that cannot be closed at the time of the procedure. The open wound is packed with gauze that is typically changed twice a day. When there is no sign of wound infection, usually within 3 to 5 days, and granulation tissue has begun to form, the wound edges are approximated. Wounds healing by third intention have the highest probability of infection because they usually begin as Class III wounds at best.

Stages

25. Wound healing is generally divided into three overlapping stages: inflammatory, proliferation, and maturation.

26. The first phase—the *inflammatory stage*—begins when the incision is made and extends through the fourth or fifth postoperative day. The "inflammatory stage" should not to be confused with an "inflammatory response" that includes redness, swelling, and pain.

27. The inflammatory stage is characterized by hemostasis and phagocytosis. Platelets form a clot, fibrin is deposited in the clot, and new blood vessels develop across the sutured wound. A thin layer of epithelial cells bridge and seal the wound.

28. The inflammatory stage is followed by the *proliferation stage*, in which the epithelial cells are regenerated, collagen is synthesized, and more new blood vessels form. The new highly vascular tissue is referred to as granulation tissue.

29. The proliferation stage generally lasts 3 to 20 days. Toward the end of this stage, the wound begins to take on a raised pinkish scar and will have gained enough strength to permit suture removal.

30. The final stage of wound healing is the *maturation or remodeling stage*, which can last more than a year. Collagen continues to be

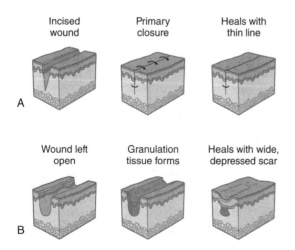

Figure 9-1 Healing by primary and secondary intention:
(A) Primary intention (B) Secondary intention.

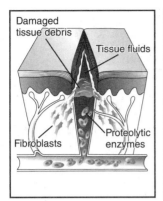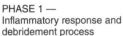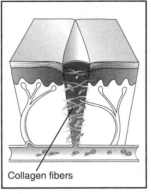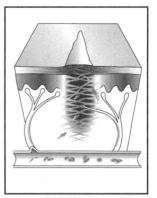

PHASE 1 —
Inflammatory response and
debridement process

PHASE 2 —
Collagen formation
(scar tissue)

PHASE 3 —
Sufficient collagen laid down

Figure 9-2 Phases of wound healing.
Courtesy of Ethicon, Inc., Sommerville, NJ.

deposited and remodeled, the wound shrinks and contracts, and the thick reddish scar matures to a thin white line (**Figure 9-2**).

31. Tissue edges generally knit together within 48 hours but initially have little tensile strength. Collagen deposition and remodeling contribute to increased tensile strength, reaching 20% within 3 weeks. Peak tensile strength of a wound occurs approximately 60 days after injury. A healed wound only reaches approximately 80% of the tensile strength of unwounded skin (Simon, Romo, & Al Moustran, 2014). Wound healing will take longer in patients who are immunocompromised, taking steroids, or are otherwise debilitated. While the wound is regaining tensile strength, it needs the extrinsic support of sutures to keep it together (Dunn, 2015, p. 2).

Section Questions

1. What risk for adverse outcomes related to a surgical incision do all patients face? [Ref 1]
2. Contrast wound dehiscence with wound evisceration. [Ref 1]
3. What other adverse outcomes are associated with wound dehiscence or evisceration? [Ref 2]
4. Discuss the various causes of wound dehiscence, evisceration, and infection. [Refs 3–5]
5. What are the evaluation criteria for desired outcomes for patients who undergo surgery? [Ref 7]
6. What are the criteria for Class I (*clean*) wounds? [Ref 11]
7. List some procedures that are considered *clean* cases. [Ref 12]
8. What are some of the characteristics of *clean* cases? [Refs 13–14]
9. What are the criteria for Class II (*clean contaminated*) wounds? [Ref 15]
10. List some procedures that are considered *clean contaminated* cases. [Ref 16]
11. What criteria indicate that a wound is *contaminated* (Class III)? [Ref 17]
12. Identify some surgical procedures that are considered *contaminated* cases. [Ref 18]
13. Which wounds make up Class IV (*dirty*)? [Ref 19]

(continues)

Section Questions (continued)

14. List some surgical procedures that are considered *dirty* cases. [Ref 20]

15. Describe healing by primary intention. [Ref 22]

16. Describe the process of healing by secondary intention. [Ref 23]

17. Why is there a greater risk for infection with healing by secondary intention than by primary intention? [Ref 23]

18. What types of wounds heal by tertiary intention? [Ref 24]

19. What characterizes the inflammatory stage of wound healing? [Ref 27]

20. Physiologically, what occurs in the wound during the first phase of wound healing? [Ref 27]

21. What happens in the wound during the proliferation stage? [Ref 28]

22. What is granulation tissue? [Ref 28]

23. During which phase are the sutures removed from the wound? [Ref 29]

24. What is the primary physiologic activity that occurs during *maturation* or *remodeling?* [Ref 30]

25. What patient conditions retard wound healing? [Ref 31]

Suture Material

32. The noun *suture* refers to a strand of material used to tie (ligate) a blood vessel (occlude the lumen) or a stitch or row of stitches holding together the edges of a wound or surgical incision.

33. The verb *suture* refers to sewing tissue together. The process of *suturing* refers to approximating tissue edges and holding them in anatomical alignment with suture material until healing takes place.

34. Desired characteristics of all sutures include:

    • Sterility

    • Pliability and ease of handling and knotting

    • Consistent tensile strength appropriate to the suture size

    • Ability to maintain the tissue layers in approximation during the healing process

    • Minimal reactivity in tissue

35. Tensile strength, expressed in pounds, is the amount of tension or "pull" that a suture can withstand before it breaks. Tensile strength determines the amount of wound support that the suture provides during the healing process. The tensile strength of any suture material should be as strong as the tensile strength (ability to withstand stress) of the tissue in which it is placed. As the diameter of suture material decreases, tensile strength decreases (**Figure 9-3**).

36. Suture materials must be sterile when they are placed inside the patient's body. This requires packaging that permits sterile presentation to the field.

37. Suture material should be pliable and it should elicit minimal drag, meaning the suture material will slide easily through tissue. The suture must tie easily and hold a knot securely.

38. Because suture material is a foreign body, some tissue reaction is inevitable. The foreign-body reaction will persist until the suture is absorbed by the body, encapsulated, or removed. Suture selection includes material that offers the least potential for tissue reaction.

39. Many factors influence the surgeon's choice of suture. These factors include:

    • The surgeon's familiarity with the product

    • Physical and biological characteristics of the suture material

    • Suture coatings

    • Healing characteristics of the tissue in which the suture will be placed

    • Presence of infection or contamination

    • Patient characteristics such as age, weight, and state of health

    • Expected postoperative course of the patient

40. Although suture selection is the surgeon's responsibility, the perioperative nurse must be familiar with suture material, its unique characteristics, and its appropriate uses in

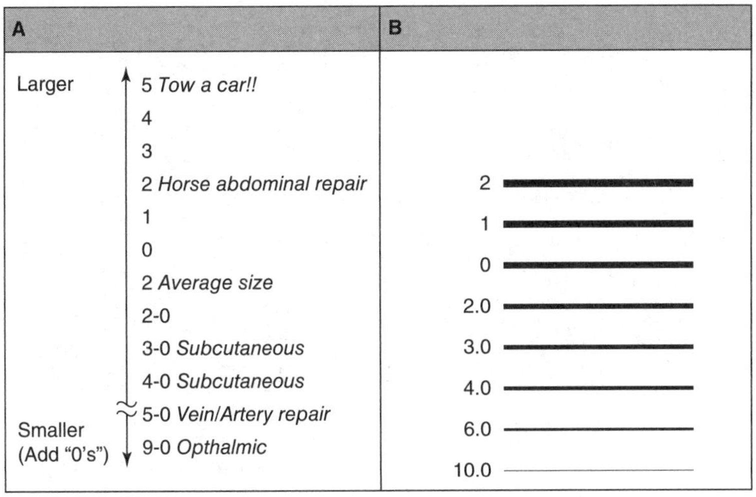

Figure 9-3 Suture size: the more zeros, the smaller in diameter the suture becomes.

order to plan for surgical procedures and to respond to unanticipated events, such as surgical complications, emergencies, and suture substitutions.

Classification of Suture Material

41. Standards and classification of sutures are set by the United States Pharmacopeia (USP).

42. Suture classifications include:
    - Monofilament or multifilament
    - Absorbable or nonabsorbable
    - Coated or uncoated
    - Sutures may also be:
    - Natural or synthetic
    - Dyed or undyed

Monofilament and Multifilament Sutures

43. Monofilament sutures are comprised of a single strand of material. These sutures incur little resistance (drag) as they are drawn through tissue and as they are tied.

44. Knots made with monofilament suture have a tendency to loosen. Additional throws are needed to secure the knot.

45. Monofilament sutures do not harbor bacteria and, therefore, reduce the potential for a suture-line infection.

46. Multifilament sutures comprise several strands of material that are twisted or braided together. They handle and tie securely and provide greater tensile strength than monofilament sutures.

47. Multifilament sutures exhibit more drag as they are pulled through tissue. Knots in multifilament sutures are secure and don't require additional throws.

48. Multifilament sutures have a certain amount of capillarity—a process that allows tissue fluid to be absorbed into the suture and travel along the strand. Any microorganisms contained in tissue fluid can be carried along the strand into the wound and cause an infection.

49. Multifilament sutures may be coated to improve their handling characteristics and to reduce capillarity.

Section Questions

1. Identify the desirable characteristics of all sutures. [Ref 34]
2. How does the tensile strength of suture affect wound healing? [Ref 35]
3. What does it mean for a suture to have "minimal drag"? [Ref 37]

(continues)

Section Questions (continued)

4. Why is some tissue reaction to suture inevitable? [Ref 38]

5. What factors influence the surgeon's choice of suture? [Ref 39]

6. Why is it important for the nurse to know the unique characteristics of different suture options? [Ref 40]

7. Differentiate monofilament from multifilament suture. [Refs 43, 46]

8. Which suture (monofilament or multifilament) requires extra throws to keep the knot from loosening? [Ref 44]

9. What benefit do multifilament sutures have over monofilament? [Ref 47]

10. What is the challenge posed by the capillarity of multifilament sutures? [Ref 48]

Absorbable Suture

50. Absorbable suture is considered temporary, because it is assimilated by the body during the healing process. The assimilation time varies with the type of suture material and patient factors that may accelerate absorption. As the suture is absorbed, its tensile strength decreases.

51. Absorbable suture is made of material that is digested by body enzymes or is hydrolyzed (broken down by water in tissue fluids).

52. Absorbable suture may be either natural or synthetic. Natural absorbable sutures consist of highly purified collagen and are made from the submucosal layer of sheep intestine or the serosa layer of beef.

53. The most common natural absorbable suture is plain or chromic surgical gut.

54. Plain surgical gut is natural suture with limited use. Its tensile strength decreases rapidly; hence, the suture provides support for the wound for only 7 to 10 days. Plain gut suture is used primarily to ligate superficial blood vessels and to suture the subcutaneous tissue layer where tensile strength is not an issue.

55. Surgical gut that has been treated with a chromium salt solution is referred to as chromic gut. Chromatization makes the gut more resistant to absorption.

56. Chromic gut provides more support for healing tissues than plain gut. It retains tensile strength for 10 to 14 days and is absorbed in approximately 90 days.

57. Plain gut, chromic gut, and collagen sutures are digested by body enzymes through phagocytosis, which results in varying degrees of inflammatory reaction.

58. The rate of decline in tensile strength and absorption of surgical gut is influenced by the type of tissue in which the suture is used, the condition of the tissue, and the state of health of the patient. If the patient is anemic, malnourished, protein deficient, debilitated, or has an infection, the rate of absorption and the loss of tensile strength may be accelerated.

59. Surgical gut sutures are packaged in a conditioning fluid of alcohol and water that prevents drying and keeps the suture pliable. Surgical gut should be handled only when moist; therefore, it should be used immediately upon removal from the package. Gut suture that is removed from the package and allowed to dry will lose its pliability. Moistening it with sterile saline just prior to use will restore pliability. Gut suture should not be immersed or permitted to remain in saline or water, because excessive moisture will reduce tensile strength.

60. Synthetic absorbable sutures are made from synthetic polymers of lactic and glycolic acid and polyester. They are absorbed through hydrolysis, which causes the polymer chain to break down. Hydrolysis results in less tissue reaction than enzymatic suture absorption.

61. Synthetic suture's absorption time and loss of tensile strength are predictable, and it is affected only minimally by the presence of infection, the type of tissue, or the patient's state of health.

62. The tensile strength of synthetic absorbable sutures is greater than that of natural materials and varies from several weeks to several months. For some sutures, a 25% tensile strength remains after 6 weeks; for others, all tensile strength is lost in 2 weeks.

63. The selection of suture must be based on knowledge of its tensile strength, the rate of degradation of the suture material, and the time required for wound healing.

64. Synthetic absorbable sutures that provide the longest wound support times are appropriate

for patients who heal slowly, such as the elderly; patients with acquired immunodeficiency syndrome (AIDS); or those receiving radiation therapy.

65. Synthetic absorbable sutures are packed dry and should not be immersed in solutions, because fluids can reduce tensile strength.

66. Examples of synthetic absorbable sutures include Dexon (polyglycolic acid), Vicryl (polyglactin 910), PDS (polydioxanone), Maxon (polyglyconate), Monocryl (poliglecaprone), Panacryl (lactide and glycolide), and Biosyn (synthetic polyester).

67. Absorbable suture coated with the antibacterial agent triclosan (Vicryl Plus, PDS Plus, Monocryl Plus) is also available. This suture is useful in preventing bacterial colonization.

Nonabsorbable Suture

68. Nonabsorbable suture is made of either natural or synthetic material, is not assimilated by the body, and is considered permanent once it is placed in tissue.

69. Silk and cotton are natural nonabsorbable sutures. Cotton is used rarely because it is more reactive than other alternatives. It is made from cotton fibers that have been combed, aligned, and twisted into a multifilament strand. Moisture enhances the tensile strength of cotton.

70. Surgical silk is a natural material made from thread spun by silkworms. The silk strands are twisted or braided and are usually dyed black. Silk suture also comes undyed.

71. Silk is one of the most widely used nonabsorbable sutures, often used in the GI tract. It is pliable and holds a knot securely.

72. Because it is braided, silk has capillarity and is treated to resist absorption of body fluids.

73. Silk loses its tensile strength within 1 year after implantation and cannot be used where very long-term support is needed, such as to secure a heart valve in place.

74. Silk is not totally nonabsorbable and may dissolve after several years. On occasion, a silk suture will migrate to the wound surface—a process referred to as "spitting."

75. Nylon, polyester, polyethylene, polybutester, and polypropylene are some of the synthetic polymers used to manufacture synthetic nonabsorbable sutures. Synthetic fibers cause less tissue irritation, retain their strength longer, and have a higher tensile strength than natural fibers.

76. Nylon suture (e.g., Ethilon, Dermalon, Nurolon, and Surgilon) has high tensile strength and is inert in the body. It is smooth and slides easily through tissue. Additional throws in the knot and square ties are necessary to provide knot security.

77. Nylon is often used for skin closure and, because it can be manufactured into very fine strands, is suitable for ophthalmic surgery, microsurgery, and neurosurgery.

78. Nylon suture used on the face and neck is removed in 2 to 5 days. On other skin areas, suture removal is typically within 8 days.

79. Polypropylene suture (e.g., Prolene, Pronova, Surgilene, Surgidac) is an inert monofilament, has good tensile strength, and slides smoothly through tissue. It is available in a variety of sizes, including very fine strands.

80. Polypropylene suture is frequently used in cardiovascular surgery and other surgeries where prolonged healing is anticipated. Additional throws and square ties are necessary to ensure knot security.

81. Polypropylene suture should be gently stretched before use to eliminate memory and prevent kinking.

82. Polypropylene suture (blue) is also used as an easier-to-see alternative to Nylon (black) for skin closure on dark skin and scalp closures for dark-haired patients.

83. Polyester suture (e.g., Dacron, Mersilene, Ethibond, Tevdek, Bondek, and Ti-Cron) is closely braided, is available in a variety of sizes, and is usually coated with a specially designed lubricant to reduce drag as the suture passes through tissue. Polyester suture is often used in cardiac surgery and neurosurgery.

84. Polybutester suture (Novafil) is a monofilament suture with more flexibility and elasticity than other synthetic polymers, is more easily stretched, and may produce more compliant anastomoses.

85. Stainless steel suture has the highest tensile strength and is the most inert of all sutures. It is particularly useful where strong permanent wound security is needed, such as for approximating the sternum following cardiovascular surgery. Metallic suture is difficult to handle and requires an exacting suture technique. It has very limited application.

Section Questions

1. How does absorption affect the tensile strength of suture? [Ref 50]

2. By which mechanisms is suture absorbed by the body? [Ref 51]

3. Of which material is the most common natural absorbable suture made? [Ref 53]

4. How does chromatization address the limitations of plain surgical gut? [Ref 55]

5. What causes the inflammatory response to plain and chromic surgical gut? [Ref 57]

6. What patient factors affect the decline of the tensile strength of suture? [Ref 58]

7. Why are surgical gut sutures packaged in fluid? [Ref 59]

8. Why do synthetic absorbable sutures result in less tissue reaction than chromic and plain gut? [Ref 60]

9. What benefits do synthetic absorbable materials have over natural material? [Ref 61–62]

10. Which types of patients benefit from synthetic absorbable sutures that provide the longest wound support times? [Ref 64]

11. Why are synthetic absorbable sutures packed dry? [Ref 65]

12. Of what benefit is a triclosan coating on absorbable suture? [Ref 67]

13. Of which materials are natural, nonabsorbable sutures made? [Ref 69]

14. Why is cotton suture infrequently used? [Ref 69]

15. Why is silk not used where long-term support is required? [Ref 73]

16. What does the term "spitting" mean when referring to sutures? [Ref 74]

17. Which advantages do synthetic nonabsorbable materials have over silk and cotton? [Ref 75]

18. Why is nylon often used for skin closure? [Ref 77]

19. Describe the benefits of the various synthetic nonabsorbable materials. [Refs 79–84]

20. What is the primary benefit of stainless steel suture? [Ref 85]

Suture Selection: Considerations

86. Many factors influence suture selection, such as expected length of time for healing, presence of contamination in the wound, desired cosmetic results, and surgeon preference.

87. Absorbable sutures are used in tissue that heals rapidly. Typical applications include subcutaneous fat, stomach, submucosal layer of the colon, bladder, and biliary tract.

88. Nonabsorbable suture is used where extended wound support is needed, such as with fascia and tendons. It is also routinely used in vascular, cardiac, and neurosurgery.

89. When further tissue growth is expected, as in pediatric patients, absorbable suture with long-lasting tensile strength, such as polydioxanone (PDS II), is used.

90. Nonabsorbable suture that will be removed is used in ophthalmic surgery, for skin closure, and when temporary additional wound support is needed.

91. In some cases, retention sutures are used to provide temporary additional abdominal wound support, such as to support the primary suture line in abdominal wound closure in an obese patient. Retention sutures are nonabsorbable materials placed approximately 2 inches beyond the edge of the primary suture line and passed through all layers of the abdominal wall. Once it is ascertained that the primary wound has healed sufficiently, the retention sutures are removed (**Figure 9-4**).

Suture Package Information

92. Sutures are supplied sterile from the manufacturer in a double envelope package. The inner sterile package contains the sterile suture(s). The outer package is a peel package designed to permit aseptic delivery of the inner suture package to the sterile field.

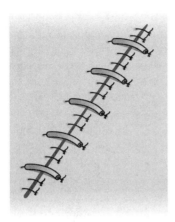

Figure 9-4 Retention suture bolster.

93. Information required by the USP is printed on each suture package:
    - Type of material
    - Trade name and generic name
    - Product number

- Size, length, and color
- Braided or monofilament
- Coating material (if used)
- Absorbable or nonabsorbable
- Number of needles in the package if more than one
- Needle description
- Manufacturer, date manufactured, expiration date, and a statement of compliance with USP standards (**Figure 9-5**)

94. Sutures are supplied in boxes containing multiple packages. They are commercially sterilized with ethylene oxide or ionizing radiation.

95. The suture manufacturer does not supply reprocessing guidelines; therefore, sutures are not intended to be resterilized. Product integrity cannot be guaranteed using hospital sterilization processes and cycles, and use characteristics of resterilized suture are not predictable. Using reprocessed sutures could jeopardize patient safety.

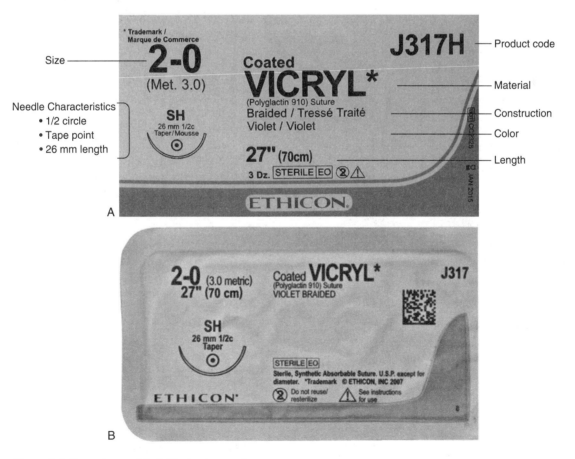

Figure 9-5 Suture box and individual suture package.
Courtesy of Ethicon, Inc., Sommerville, NJ.

Surgical Needles

Needle Characteristics

96. Surgical needles are designed to carry suture material through tissue with minimal trauma. They are precision-made to provide some flexibility without breaking. Surgical needles come in different sizes and have different curvatures and point designs.

97. The three basic parts of the needle are the point, shaft or body, and attachment (**Figure 9-6**).

98. Needle points may be tapered, cutting, or blunt.

99. Tapered needles are used in tissue that offers little resistance to the needle as it passes through, such as peritoneum or intestine. A taper-point needle is designed with the shaft gradually tapering to a sharp point so as to introduce the needle into the tissue through the smallest possible hole (Figure 9-7).

100. A cutting-point needle is designed with a razor-sharp tip and is used for tissue that is difficult to penetrate, such as skin or tendon. (Figure 9-7).

101. The point of a cutting needle is not round, but has sharp edges that extend along the shaft. Variations of the cutting needle are used according to surgical preference in selected tissue.

102. Blunt-tip needles have a rounded end and are used in friable tissue, such as the liver or kidney, when neither piercing nor cutting is appropriate. Blunt needles are also used for safety purposes to reduce risk of exposure to blood-borne pathogens. They are especially useful for suturing in a deep cavity where visualization is difficult, as in gynecological surgery.

103. Most suture needles have ¼, ⅜, ½, and ⅝ circle curvature (**Figure 9-8**), although straight (Keith) needles may be available for specific applications. The selection of needle shape and size is determined by the size and properties of the suture material, the type and location of tissues being sutured, and the surgeon's preference.

Needle Attachment

104. The vast majority of suture comes attached to a needle. The suture and needle are attached during manufacture with a process called *swaging* that incorporates the suture firmly into the hollow end of the needle. This suture is called atraumatic because needle and suture pass through the tissue through the same-diameter hole (**Figure 9-9A**).

105. Free needles are used rarely today, but may be available for special circumstances when a surgeon wants to double-arm (place a needle on the other end of) a suture, or if a surgeon wants a specific, otherwise unavailable, suture/needle combination. The eye of a free needle can be a closed oval or a French eye, slotted speed up needle threading by pushing the suture into the eye (Figure 9-9B, 9-9C). Free needles are more traumatic because two strands of suture must pass through the tissue at the same time.

106. A modification of the permanently swaged suture is the controlled-release suture, sometimes referred to as a "pop-off." In this type of attachment, the needle and suture are one continuous unit; however, they are easily separated with a light tug. Controlled-release sutures facilitate rapid, interrupted suturing techniques.

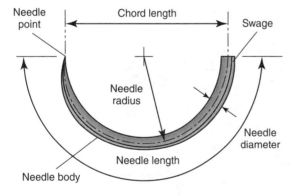

Figure 9-6 Anatomy of a suture needle.
Courtesy of Ethicon, Inc., Sommerville, NJ.

POINT/BODY SHAPE	APPLICATIONS	
TAPERCUT Surgical Needle 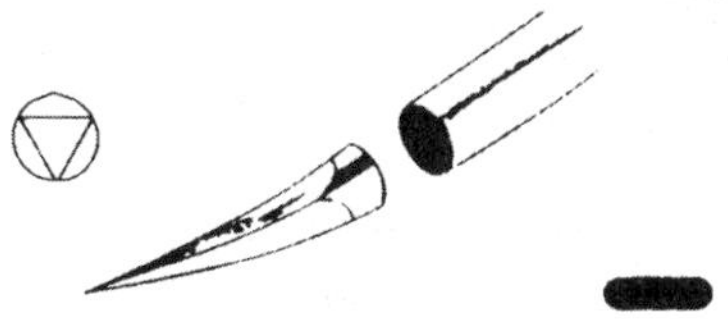	bronchus calcified tissue fascia ligament nasal cavity oral cavity ovary perichondrium periosteum	pharynx tendon trachea uterus vessels (sclerotic)
Taper 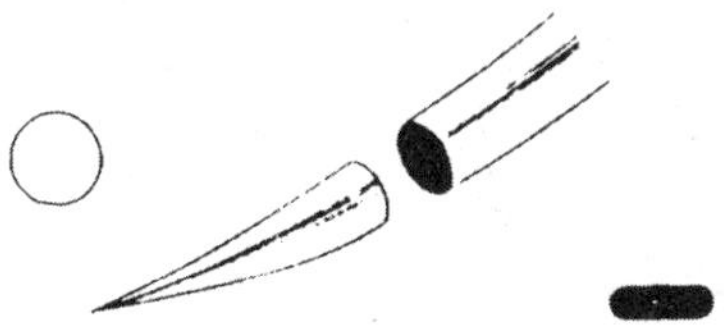	aponeurosis biliary tract dura fascia gastrointestinal tract muscle myocardium nerve peritoneum	pleura subcutaneous fat urogenital tract vessels
Blunt 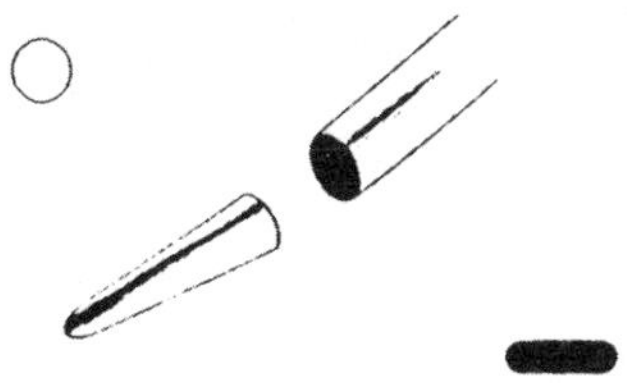	blunt dissection (friable tissue) fascia intestine kidney liver spleen cervix (ligating incompetent cervix)	
CS ULTIMA Ophthalmic Needle 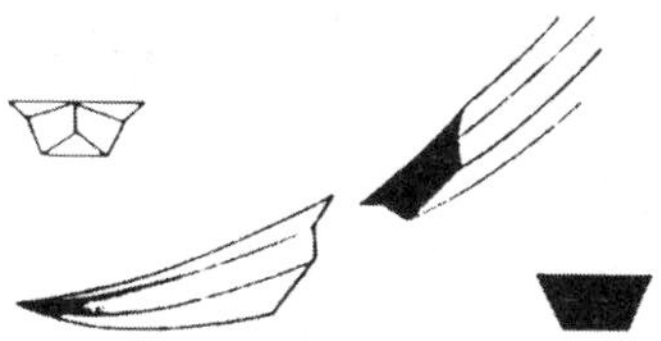	eye (primary application)	
PC PRIME Needle 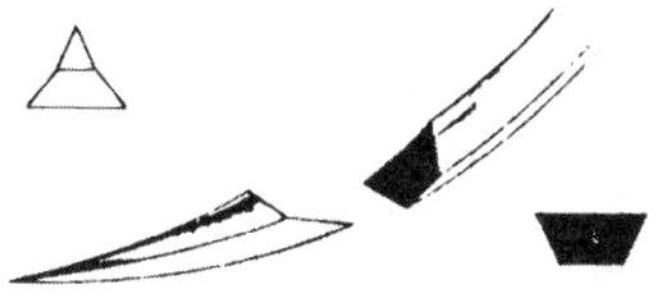	skin (plastic or cosmetic)	

Figure 9-7 Needle points and body shapes with typical applications.
Courtesy of Ethicon, Inc., Sommerville, NJ.

POINT/BODY SHAPE	APPLICATIONS
Conventional Cutting 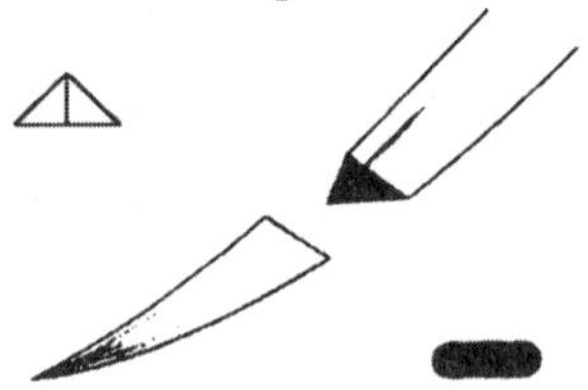	ligament nasal cavity oral cavity pharynx skin tendon
Reverse Cutting 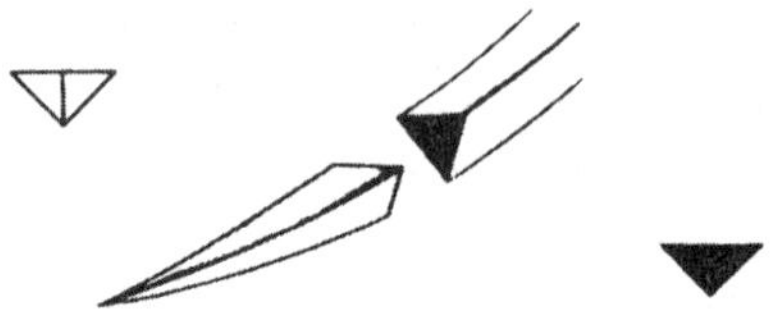	fascia ligament nasal cavity oral mucosa pharynx skin tendon sheath
MICRO-POINT Reverse Cutting Needle 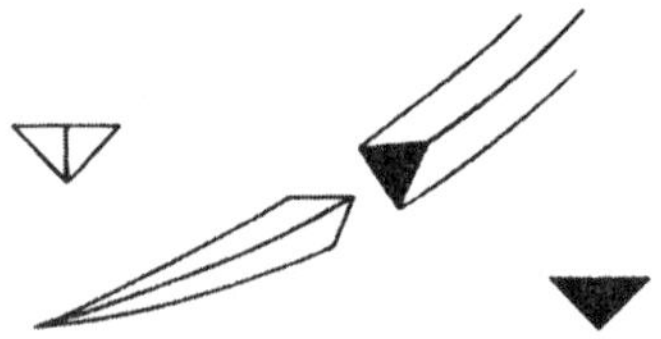	eye
Precision Point Cutting 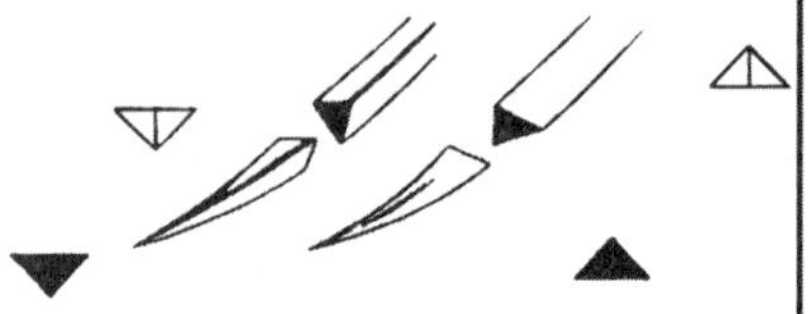	skin (plastic or cosmetic)
Side-cutting Spatula 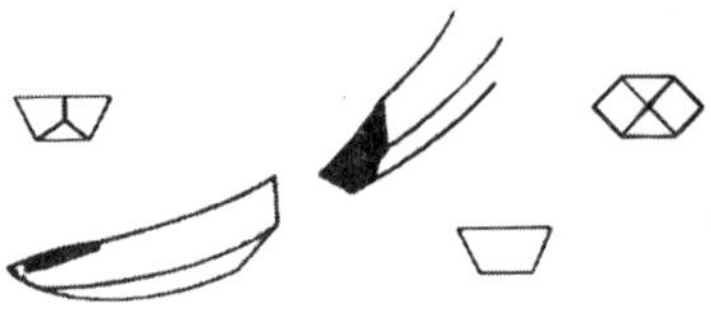	eye (primary application) microsurgery ophthalmic (reconstructive)

Figure 9-7 (Continued) Needle points and body shapes with typical applications.
Courtesy of Ethicon, Inc., Sommerville, NJ.

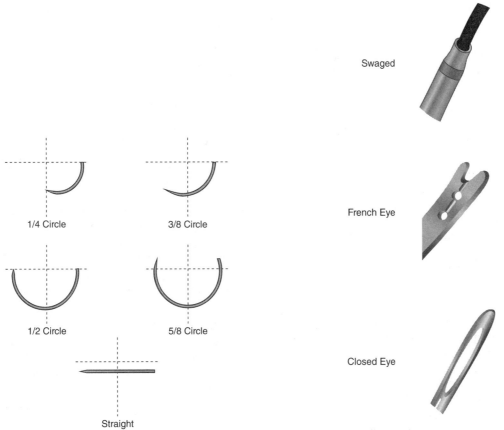

1/4 Circle

3/8 Circle

1/2 Circle

5/8 Circle

Straight

Figure 9-8 Needle shapes.

Swaged

French Eye

Closed Eye

Figure 9-9 Needle attachments.
Courtesy of Ethicon, Inc., Sommerville, NJ.

Section Questions

1. What are some factors that influence suture selection? [Ref 86]

2. Contrast the use of absorbable with nonabsorbable suture. [Refs 87–88]

3. What is a retention suture? [Ref 91]

4. What is the purpose of supplying suture in a package within a package? [Ref 92]

5. What information is provided on the suture package? [Ref 93]

6. What directions are given by the manufacturer for reprocessing suture? [Ref 95]

7. Name the three parts of a surgical needle. [Ref 97]

8. Explain the need for having suture with cutting needles and suture with taper needles. [Refs 99–100]

9. What is the purpose of a blunt needle? [Ref 102]

10. What factors affect the choice of surgical needle? [Ref 103]

11. Describe a swaged suture. [Ref 104]

12. Why are swaged sutures considered atraumatic? [Ref 104]

13. What is a "double-armed" suture? [Ref 105]

14. Describe a pop-off suture. [Ref 106]

15. When are pop-off sutures useful? [Ref 106]

Other Wound-Closure Devices

Stapling Devices

107. Stapling devices are available for approximation of internal tissues, for fascia, and for skin closure. Staples are made of stainless steel or titanium. Individual stapling devices are designed for stapling specific tissue and are not interchangeable. For example, skin staples are not used on fascia (**Figure 9-10**).

108. Staples can be applied individually, such as skin or fascia staplers with clips or staples that are delivered one at a time. Stapling devices used in intestinal and thoracic surgery deliver multiple staples simultaneously.

Miscellaneous Closures

109. Efficient devices have been developed for challenging closures. One example is the sternal closure following a median sternotomy. The traditional approach to closing the sternum is stainless steel sutures (**Figure 9-11A**). Instead

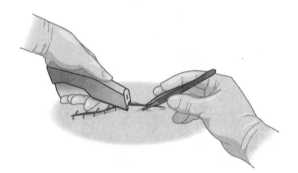

Figure 9-10 Skin staples.

of tying a knot, the suture ends are twisted tightly and folded to bury the sharp points. If the patient is thin, the suture might be felt under the skin, and in some cases can produce significant discomfort.

110. An alternative to sutures, a device much like a zip tie, has been developed to hold the sternum securely with no protrusion to cause discomfort (**Figure 9-11B**).

111. The sternum can also be closed with hardware designed specifically for that purpose (**Figure 9-11C**).

112. Barbed suture is an innovation for obtaining a secure tissue closure. The suture is available in both absorbable and nonabsorbable strands to accommodate different tissues. The barbs are evenly spaced facing in the same direction, providing a secure closure by gripping the tissue at numerous points, spreading tension across the wound.

113. Strands are either double armed or have a fixation loop at one end (**Figure 9-12**). With a double-armed suture, closure begins in the middle of the wound; with a fixation loop, closure begins at one end of the wound and progresses to the other.

Skin Tapes and Skin Adhesives

114. Adhesive skin tapes (Steri-Strips, Proxi-Strips) are used to approximate surgical incision wound edges (**Figure 9-13**). When they are used in conjunction with subcuticular sutures to hold incision edges in place, skin sutures or staples are not necessary, and the healed incision line has no suture tracks.

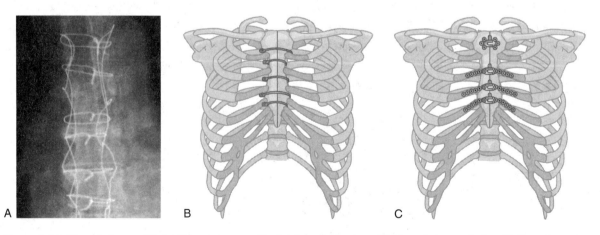

A   B   C

Figure 9-11 Sternal closure: (A) Traditional closure with stainless steel suture (B) Sternal closure device (C) Sternal closure with hardware.

Photo reproduced from Aykut, K., Albayrak, G., Kavala, A., Guzeloglu, M., Karaarslan, K., Hazan, E. Early repair of sternal instability prevents mediastinitis. World Journal of Cardiovascular Surgery, 4(2). DOI:10.4236/wjcs.2014.42003.

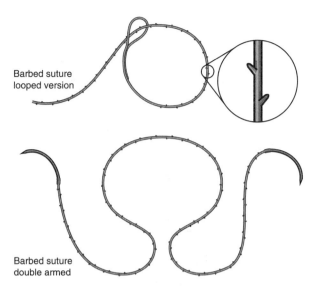

Barbed suture
looped version

Barbed suture
double armed

Figure 9-12 Barbed suture.

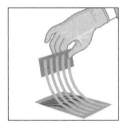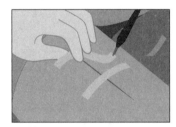

Figure 9-13 Adhesive skin tapes.

115. Skin tapes may also be used as a complement to suture or staple closures. They are often used to reinforce a wound after skin staples or sutures have been removed.

116. Skin tapes are available in widths of ⅛, ¼, and ½ inch and in lengths from 1½ to 4 inches.

117. Skin adhesives (Dermabond, Indermil) are used to glue skin edges together. These materials are useful where cosmetic considerations are important, because they leave no suture tracks along the healed incision line.

118. Skin adhesives are also used to seal a sutured incision to prevent entry of microorganisms and are particularly useful in traumatic surgery where risk of infection is greatest.

Surgical Mesh

119. In addition to suture, knitted mesh made from polyester or polypropylene is sometimes used to reinforce tissue and provide support during

and after wound healing. Mesh is particularly useful in hernia repair where a defect in the fascia exists.

Drains

120. Drains are used primarily to obliterate dead space where tissue might not have been adequately approximated, to remove foreign or harmful materials such as infected or necrotic tissue, or when hemostasis is uncertain. A drain is used when a wound is anticipated to produce fluid sufficient to place undue stress on closure.

121. The three types of drains are passive, active, and sump. Passive drains function through gravity and capillary action. Active drains employ negative pressure. Sump drains are double-lumen devices that may be attached to either continuous or intermittent low suction.

122. The simplest drain is a passive drain (e.g., Penrose drain)—a simple lumen drain made from rubber or silicone. Fluid in the wound follows the path of the drain and empties because of gravity or capillary action into a surgical dressing where drainage is captured. Two important disadvantages of the Penrose drain are that it provides a pathway for microorganisms to migrate from the surrounding environment into the wound, and wound drainage cannot be accurately measured.

123. Commonly used active drains are the Hemovac and the Jackson-Pratt (**Figure 9-14**). Drainage flows from inside the wound through tubing that exits adjacent to the incision site and is attached to a closed reservoir. The reservoir is collapsed before being attached to the drain, creating negative pressure that directs drainage out of the wound and into the reservoir.

124. The reservoir may be emptied and negative pressure reinstated to collect additional drainage. Unlike the Penrose drain, Hemovac and Jackson-Pratt drains permit accurate measurement of drainage. They are also closed systems that provide less of a pathway for microorganisms to migrate into the wound.

125. Sump drains are double-lumened devices. One lumen provides for the passage of filtered air into the wound, and the other lumen permits passage of drainage material from the

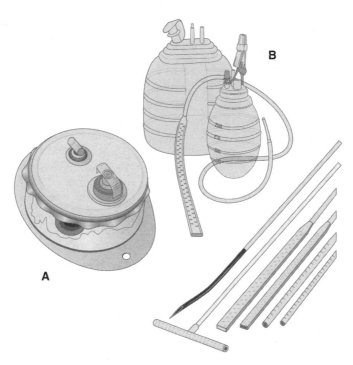

Figure 9-14 Drains: (A) Hemoval (B) Jackson Pratt.

wound. In the presence of copious drainage, the sump pump may be connected to external suction.

Dressings

126. Most surgical incisions are closed primarily and covered with a sterile surgical dressing. Typically, a nonadherent dressing that will not stick to the wound and cause trauma (Telfa) is applied first, followed by a gauze dressing and tape to hold it in place. In the case of a large wound or one in which some additional absorbency is needed, the gauze layer will be covered with an absorbent pad.

127. A clean wound with minimal drainage might be covered with a nonadherent dressing (Telfa), followed by a thin, transparent, semipermeable dressing that is oxygen permeable but serves as a barrier to bacteria and water (Tegaderm, OpSite).

128. A variety of other types of dressings are available, such as mesh nonadherent dressings, dressings impregnated with petrolatum (Vaseline gauze), and dressings impregnated with an antimicrobial.

129. In recent years, there has been an increase in development and use of dressings containing silver. Because of silver's antimicrobial properties, these dressings are particularly useful for infected wounds or wounds at risk for infection.

Nursing Responsibilities Related to Wound Management

130. The selection and use of wound-closure material and devices is primarily the surgeon's responsibility, but knowledge and understanding of suture and needle characteristics can help prevent patient injury. For example, use of a cutting needle in a vascular procedure, where a tapered point is desired and anticipated, can cause trauma to the patient and result in additional bleeding; similarly, use of an absorbable suture where permanent wound support is desired can result in wound separation. Knowledge of suture characteristics will facilitate the appropriate choice of an alternative suture when the requested suture is not available.

131. The more knowledgeable the nurse is regarding wound closure materials and devices, the less likely that inappropriate materials and devices that can compromise patient safety will be utilized. The nurse who understands sutures, drains, and dressings will be able to

anticipate the surgeon's needs and assist in keeping surgery time to a minimum.

132. Prior to the procedure, the circulating nurse and the scrubbed person should review the surgeon's preference card for the intended procedure to determine the types of sutures that will be needed. Familiarity with the procedure and the surgeon's routine will assist the nurse to determine the approximate number of sutures of each type that will be needed.

133. To minimize waste, the nurse should consult with the surgeon prior to the procedure to ascertain whether any changes in suture are anticipated. Because suture cannot be resterilized, an excess of suture should not be delivered to the sterile field. An adequate supply of the suture to be used during the procedure should be available to be delivered to the field when it is needed.

134. Multipack suture should be selected when a large number of the same sutures will be needed. If selected appropriately, multipack sutures can prevent waste and save time required to open individual packets.

135. On occasion, a suture packet that is not opened is returned to stock and placed into the wrong box. Before delivering suture to the sterile field, the nurse should read the label on the packet to prevent error and waste.

136. The following are additional responsibilities related to suture:
    - Both the circulating nurse and the scrubbed person should:
        - Handle needles and sutures in a safe and effective manner, promoting safety for the surgical team and the patient
        - Count sutures according to suture package information and verify this number upon opening the package
    - The scrubbed person should:
        - Arrange suture packets on the back table in the order in which they will be used
        - Prepare one or two sutures for immediate use (i.e., load them on needle holders; keep the remainder in the package until needed)
        - Place loaded needle holders so as to prevent accidental exposure
        - To prevent recoil, grasp the suture just below the needle and at the end and tug gently prior to passing them to the surgeon. Be careful not to tug at the point of needle attachment.
        - Pass suture so as to prevent accidental exposure
        - Place used needles on appropriate collection pad
        - Close the needle collection pad and deposit it into a sharps container

Section Questions

1. What are stapling devices? [Ref 107]
2. For what purpose(s) are devices that deliver multiple staples at a time used? [Ref 108]
3. Describe an innovation in closing the sternum following a median sternotomy. [Refs 110–111]
4. How does barbed suture enhance wound closure? [Ref 112]
5. How can adhesive skin tapes (Steri-Strips) be used in wound closure? [Refs 114–115]
6. What are two applications for skin adhesives? [Refs 117–118]
7. What is the value of using mesh in a surgical procedure? [Ref 119]
8. What is the primary function of a surgical drain? [Ref 120]
9. Describe how a passive drain functions. [Ref 122]
10. Identify two disadvantages of the passive drain. [Ref 122]
11. How does an active drain differ from a sump drain? [Refs 123, 125]
12. Explain how an active drain works. [Refs 123–124]

(continues)

Section Questions (continued)

13. What are two advantages of active drains? [Ref 124]

14. Typically, what forms the first layer of the dressing for a surgical incision? [Ref 126]

15. Describe the benefit of transparent semipermeable dressings. [Ref 127]

16. What is the benefit of a dressing impregnated with silver? [Ref 129]

17. How can the nurse's knowledge of wound-closure materials affect patient safety? [Refs 130–131]

18. What are some ways in which the nurse can minimize wasted sutures? [Ref 133]

19. When are multipack sutures most useful? [Ref 134]

20. What must the scrubbed person remember when pulling on sutures to prevent recoil? [Ref 136]

References

Agency for Healthcare Research and Quality (AHRQ). (2014). PSI-14: Postoperative wound dehiscence in *Quality Indicators Toolkit*. Retrieved from http://www.qualityindicators.ahrq.gov/Downloads/Modules/PSI/V44/TechSpecs/PSI%2014%20Postoperative%20Wound%20Dehiscence%20Rate.pdf

Phillips, N., & Berry, E. (Eds). (2013). *Berry & Kohn's operating room technique* (12th ed.). St. Louis, Mo.: Elsevier.

Dunn, D. L. (Ed.). (2015). *Wound closure manual*. Somerville, NJ: Ethicon, Inc. Retrieved from http://surgery.uthscsa.edu/pediatric/training/woundclosuremanual.pdf

Mioton, L., Jordan, S., Hanwright, P., Bilimoria, K.,& Kim, J. (2013). The relationship between preoperative wound classification and postoperative infection: A multi-institutional analysis of 15,289 patients. *Archives of Plastic Surgery, 40*(5), 522–529. Retrieved from http://synapse.koreamed.org/DOIx.php?id=10.5999/aps.2013.40.5.522

Simon, P., Romo, T., & Al Moustran, H. (2014). Skin wound healing. Retrieved from http://emedicine.medscape.com/article/884594-overview#a5

Suggested Reading

Mangram, A., Horan, T., Pearson, M., Silver, L. C., & Jarvis, W. R. (1999). Guideline for prevention of surgical site infection. *Infection Control and Hospital Epidemiology, 20*(4), 247–278.

Post-Test

Read each question carefully. Each question may have more than one correct answer.

1. Which statement(s) is/are true?

    a. Wound dehiscence is actual protrusion of the abdominal viscera through the incision.

    b. Wound dehiscence and evisceration are associated with other adverse outcomes of surgery.

    c. Inadequate wound closure accounts for most instances of dehiscence or evisceration that occur 1–3 days postoperatively.

    d. Obesity and diabetes are risk factors for wound separation.

2. Which statement(s) is/are true?

    a. Wound healing is influenced by choice of suture and surgical technique.

    b. Dehydration and malnutrition are risk factors for delayed or complicated wound healing.

    c. A break in aseptic technique can lead to infection.

    d. Suture materials vary in their ability to prevent infection.

3. The wound classification system

    a. is an important predictor of postoperative complications.

    b. is an assessment of the degree of contamination at the time of the operation.

    c. places most surgical wounds in Class II.

    d. indicates that Class I wounds are more predisposed to infection than Class II wounds.

4. Clean contaminated (Class II) wounds include

    a. wounds without inflammation.

    b. wounds involving the gastrointestinal, respiratory, and genitourinary tracts.

    c. a major break in aseptic technique.

    d. open, fresh accidental wounds.

5. Wound healing by primary intention

    a. is the preferred method of wound healing.

    b. means the wound edges are approximated at the time of surgery.

    c. requires development of granulation tissue for healing.

    d. produces a wound that heals quickly with minimal scarring.

6. Wound healing by secondary intention

    a. means the wound is sutured loosely at the time of surgery because the wound edges cannot be approximated effectively.

    b. heals from the inside or bottom upward.

    c. produces minimal scarring.

    d. is more prone to infection than healing by primary intention.

7. Wounds that heal by tertiary intention

    a. are not sutured at the time of surgery.

    b. heal by forming granulation tissue characterized by red, beefy-looking tissue.

    c. are usually wounds with extensive tissue loss.

    d. are generally packed with gauze for 3–5 days.

8. Which statement(s) is/are true about wound healing?

   a. The inflammatory stage is characterized by hemostasis and phagocytosis.

   b. The proliferation stage produces granulation tissue.

   c. Platelets form a clot in the proliferation stage.

   d. Maturation can take more than a year to transform a reddish, thick scar into a thin white line.

9. Which statement(s) is/are true about sutures?

   a. As a noun, "suture" refers to a strand of material used to ligate a vessel or close a wound.

   b. Desired characteristics of sutures include sterility, pliability, consistent tensile strength, and minimal tissue reactivity.

   c. Sutures come in packages that can be delivered to the field in sterile condition.

   d. A suture is a foreign body that can create a tissue reaction.

10. Which statement(s) is/are true about sutures?

    a. Monofilament sutures drag as they are drawn through tissue.

    b. Knots tied with monofilament sutures have a tendency to loosen.

    c. Multifilament sutures provide greater tensile strength.

    d. Multifilament sutures can promote infection when fluids are carried along the strand to the wound.

11. Natural absorbable suture

    a. is purified collagen that retains its tensile strength for 90 days.

    b. is digested by body enzymes or is hydrolyzed.

    c. is used to ligate superficial blood vessels and approximate the subcutaneous tissue layer.

    d. should be soaked in water once the package is opened to prevent drying and increase tensile strength.

12. Synthetic absorbable gut suture

    a. is digested by the body's enzymes.

    b. has less tensile strength than natural absorbable suture.

    c. should be immersed in solution to increase its tensile strength.

    d. provides the longest wound support and is appropriate for patients who heal slowly.

13. Which statement(s) is/are true about silk?

    a. Silk cannot be used for long-term support.

    b. Silk can "spit" or migrate to the wound surface.

    c. Silk is treated to resist absorption of body fluids because of its capillarity.

    d. Silk is pliable and holds a knot securely.

14. Which statement(s) is/are true about nonabsorbable suture?

    a. Synthetic fibers cause less tissue reaction than silk.

    b. Synthetic fibers have higher tensile strength than silk.

    c. Nylon slides easily through tissue and makes knots easily and securely.

    d. Prolene is a frequently used nonabsorbable suture for cardiovascular surgery and other surgeries where prolonged healing is anticipated.

15. Which statement(s) is/are true about suture selection?

    a. Wound contamination can influence the selection of suture.

    b. Tensile strength is an important factor in choosing suture for pediatric patients.

    c. Absorbable suture is used in tissues that heal rapidly.

    d. Retention sutures are used to support a suture line in an obese patient.

16. Which statement(s) is/are true about surgical needles?

   a. The three parts of a surgical needle are the point, the shaft, and the attachment.

   b. Tapered needles are used on tissue that offers significant resistance.

   c. Blunt needles are used on friable tissue.

   d. Cutting needles are used on skin and tendon.

17. Which statement(s) is (are) true about surgical needles?

   a. When the suture is attached to the needle during manufacturing, it is called swaged or atraumatic.

   b. Controlled-release suture is threaded onto the needle by the scrubbed person.

   c. Free needles cause tissue trauma, because two strands are pulled through the tissue instead of one.

   d. A French-eyed needle comes with suture attached.

18. Which statement(s) is/are true?

   a. Skin stapling devices can deliver staples one at a time or multiple sets of staples simultaneously.

   b. Barbed suture grips tissue at numerous points to increase security of the closure.

   c. Skin tapes may be used as a complement to sutures or staples or to reinforce a wound after sutures or staples have been removed.

   d. Skin adhesives are used when the wound requires additional support.

19. Which statement(s) is/are true about drains?

   a. Drains are used primarily to obliterate dead space and remove harmful material, and when hemostasis is uncertain.

   b. A Hemovac drain is passive, using gravity or capillary action to remove fluid from the wound.

   c. Active drains have a reservoir that can be collapsed to create negative pressure that draws fluid from the wound into the reservoir.

   d. Single-lumen sump drains are connected to external suction.

20. Which statement(s) is/are true about nursing responsibilities?

   a. A nurse who is knowledgeable can prevent injury such as might result from using a cutting needle inappropriately or an absorbable suture where a permanent suture is needed.

   b. Nurses who have a good understanding of sutures, drains, and dressings can minimize surgery time and reduce waste by delivering only the supplies that are needed to the field.

   c. Knowledgeable nurses will reduce surgical time and waste by selecting multipacks when sutures are used in large numbers.

   d. The knowledgeable nurse will handle needles and sutures in a safe and effective manner, promoting safety for both the surgical team and the patient.

Competency Checklist:
Prevention of Injury—Wound Management

Under "Observer's Initials," enter initials upon successful achievement of the competency. Enter N/A if the competency is not appropriate for the institution.

Name_____

	Observer's Initials	Date
1. Sutures selected according to preference card and anticipated need	_____	_____
2. Sutures counted correctly	_____	_____
3. Package contents verified when opened	_____	_____
4. Sutures arranged on back table in order of anticipated use		
5. Sutures and staples loaded in anticipation of need	_____	_____
6. Loaded sutures placed on the Mayo/back table in a manner that avoids accidental exposure (needlestick)	_____	_____
7. Suture with memory (e.g., Prolene) pulled gently (without exerting pull on needle attachment) before being passed to the surgeon to prevent rebound	_____	_____
8. Suture passed in safe manner (e.g., sharp announced)	_____	_____
9. Needles removed from the suture in a safe manner	_____	_____
10. Needles placed carefully on a magnetic needle mat or other appropriate receptacle	_____	_____
11. Needles deposited in sharps box following procedure	_____	_____

Observer's Signature   Initials   Date

_____

Orientee's Signature

_____

10

Anesthesia and Medication Safety

LEARNER OBJECTIVES

1. Identify potential patient injuries related to anesthesia.
2. Identify desired patient outcomes related to anesthesia.
3. Discuss the role of the perioperative nurse during the administration of anesthesia.
4. Describe assessment factors related to the selection of anesthetic agents and techniques.
5. Describe malignant hyperthermia and its treatment.
6. Describe four patient monitoring devices and the rationale for their use.
7. Differentiate between depolarizing and nondepolarizing neuromuscular blocking agents.
8. Describe techniques of general anesthesia, regional anesthesia, and moderate sedation/analgesia.
9. Match commonly used anesthetic agents with their actions.
10. Discuss the role of the perioperative nurse regarding medication administration and safety.

LESSON OUTLINE

I. Overview
   A. Nursing Diagnoses and Desired Patient Outcomes
   B. Anesthesia Providers
   C. Nursing Responsibilities

II. Preanesthesia
   A. Assessment Data
   B. Patient Preparation/Teaching

III. Selection of Anesthetic Agents and Technique
   A. Anesthesia Techniques
   B. Preparation/Premedication

IV. Monitoring
   A. Pulse Oximetry
   B. Blood Pressure
   C. Temperature
   D. Capnography

V. General Anesthesia
   A. Inhalation Agents
   B. Anesthesia Machine
   C. Intravenous Agents
      i. Dissociative Induction Agents
      ii. Narcotics
      iii. Tranquilizers/Benzodiazepines
      iv. Neuromuscular Blockers (Muscle Relaxants)

Overview

1. Little more than 100 years ago, anesthesia for surgical procedures was limited to a crude open-drop administration of ether. Depth of anesthesia and physiologic response were inconsistent and poorly controlled. The risk of complication was high. Before the 1970s, the death rate associated with complications from anesthesia was approximately 357 per 1 million. By the early 2000s, the rate had dropped to 34 per 1 million (Bainbridge et al., 2012).

2. Factors responsible for transforming the delivery of anesthesia into a highly refined process include (ASA, 2012b):
   - Development of sophisticated anesthesia and airway management techniques
   - Anesthetic agents
   - Improved preanesthesia assessment
   - Technologically advanced monitoring devices

3. Although the death rate associated with anesthesia is extremely low, the risk of complications related to compromised ventilation, perfusion, and cardiac output, and altered hypothalamic thermoregulation persists.

Nursing Diagnoses and Desired Patient Outcomes

4. Nursing diagnosis: high risk for injury related to anesthesia (e.g., untoward drug reaction or interaction, ineffective airway, decreased cardiac output, electrolyte or fluid imbalance, ineffective breathing pattern, alteration in thought process, and ineffective thermoregulation or hypothermia).

5. The type of anesthesia, anesthetic agents, the surgical procedure, and the patient's preanesthesia physiologic condition all influence the degree of risk for complications.

6. Desired outcomes: successful recovery and a return to the preanesthesia physiologic state, including normothermia, unimpeded air exchange, adequate ventilation, maintenance of cardiac output and fluid volume, electrolyte and fluid balance, absence of allergic reaction, and unimpaired thought processes.

7. The timeframe for achieving the desired outcomes varies with the procedure, anesthetic agents, and anesthesia technique (i.e., local, regional, or general).

8. The most common of the scoring systems used to assess a patient's recovery from general anesthesia is the Aldrete system. Evaluation criteria include patient activity, respiration, circulation, and oxygen saturation. Discharge from the postanesthesia care unit (PACU) depends upon the score the patient achieves on each criterion (**Exhibit 10-1**).

9. The "passing" score varies with facility policy and where the patient will go when discharged from PACU. A patient going to a unit with continued nursing care might not require as high a score as a patient who will be going home.

Anesthesia Providers

10. Anesthesia providers include the following:
    - Anesthesiologist—medical doctor with postgraduate training in anesthesia
    - Certified registered nurse anesthetist (CRNA)—advanced practice registered nurse with clinical experience in critical care, who has graduated from a 2- to 3-year postgraduate program and has passed the national certification exam. Sixteen states allow CRNAs to practice independently; the remaining 34 states require supervision by a physician.

Exhibit 10-1 Aldrete Score

Activity	Able to move four extremities voluntarily on command	2
	Able to move two extremities voluntarily on command	1
	Able to move no extremities voluntarily on command	0
Respiration	Able to breathe deeply and cough freely	2
	Dyspnea or limited breathing	1
	Apneic	0
Circulation	BP 1 20 of preanesthetic level	2
	BP 1 20–49 of preanesthetic level	1
	BP 1 50 of preanesthetic level	0
Consciousness	Fully awake	2
	Arousable on calling	1
	Not responding	0
O_2 Saturation	Able to maintain O_2 saturation > 92% on room air	2
	Needs O_2 inhalation to maintain O_2 saturation > 90%	1
	O_2 saturation < 90% even with O_2 supplement	0

Reproduced from Alrdete, A.J., and Wright, A. Anesthesiology News,18 (11): 17, 1992. In Litwack, K. (Ed.), Post anesthesia care nursing. St. Louis: Mosby Year Book, Inc., 1995.

- Anesthesiologist assistant (AA)—individual with a bachelor's degree who has completed an accredited AA program. AAs are considered physician extenders and practice under the supervision of an anesthesiologist. In 2015, AAs were licensed to practice in 14 states and the District of Columbia, and had delegated authority to practice in Michigan and Texas.

11. Preoperatively, the anesthesia provider will perform a patient assessment, and, collaboratively with the surgeon and patient, will determine the anesthesia technique for the surgical procedure.

12. The anesthesia provider and the circulating nurse visit with the patient prior to the procedure. The perioperative nurse provides and reinforces information regarding the surgical experience, preparation for anesthesia, and procedure-specific postoperative instructions.

13. Goal #2 in The Joint Commission's (TJC, 2015) National Patient Safety Goals is to "improve the effectiveness of communication among caregivers." Patient safety is dependent upon every caregiver having the information needed to make the best patient care decisions. The anesthesia provider and circulating nurse share pertinent patient data from their preoperative assessments to be sure that all relevant information is communicated to the surgical team.

14. The anesthesia provider monitors the patient during the perioperative period, interprets monitoring data, and administers medications, fluids, and oxygen to maintain the patient's physiologic stability.

15. During procedures where the patient receives moderate sedation/analgesia and an anesthesia provider is not present, the perioperative nurse assumes even more responsibility for patient monitoring.

Nursing Responsibilities

16. The anesthesia provider and the circulating nurse both document relevant times related to the procedure (e.g., time in the room, time of induction, time of incision). It is essential that the documentation of these times be consistent in all of the various patient records.

17. The anesthesia provider participates actively in the "time-out," and usually contributes information related to the administration of prophylactic antibiotics.

18. Because anesthesia providers are responsible for the patient's airway and vascular access, they direct the rest of the team during patient positioning and transfer from one surface to another.

19. The circulating nurse will assist the anesthesia provider intraoperatively, particularly during induction and extubation, and during transfer of the patient to the PACU.

20. The circulating nurse accompanies the anesthesia provider and the patient to the PACU and gives a hand-off report to the PACU nurse that includes information necessary to prepare for the patient's admission to PACU and the patient's recovery from anesthesia.

21. The hand-off report to the PACU nurse should include at least the following information:
    - Patient name, age, and sex
    - Surgical procedure
    - Surgeon and anesthesiologist/CRNA/AA
    - Anesthetic agents/technique
    - Intraoperative medications
    - Estimated blood loss
    - Fluid and blood administration
    - Urine output
    - Response to surgery/anesthesia
    - Lab results
    - Chronic and acute health history
    - Drug allergies
    - Concerns, possible problems, and desired patient outcomes not met
    - Discharge plan

22. The perioperative nurse may assist both the anesthesia provider and the PACU nurse in stabilizing the patient.

23. In some facilities, particularly in ambulatory settings and small rural facilities, the perioperative nurse continues to provide patient care through the recovery period. Many larger facilities, due to staffing variances, facility policy, and/or limited resources, require their perioperative nurses to demonstrate competence in postanesthesia care as well as preoperative and intraoperative nursing.

24. Even where the perioperative nurse's responsibilities do not include postanesthesia care, he or she must demonstrate competence in the use of monitoring equipment and in the interpretation of the data. The perioperative nurse must also be familiar with anesthetic agents and techniques to anticipate patient events, implement nursing interventions quickly, and assist the anesthesia provider.

25. Postoperatively, the anesthesia provider evaluates the patient's readiness for discharge and writes a discharge order.

Preanesthesia

Assessment Data

26. Historically, in preparation for surgery and anesthesia, patients had an assessment by both the surgeon and the anesthesia provider several days prior to surgery. Diagnostic testing was ordered based on the patient's medical and surgical history, the results of the physical examination, and the intended surgical procedure. Testing may have included a chest X-ray; electrocardiogram (ECG, or EKG); blood chemistry panel, including a clotting profile; urinalysis; and other tests specific to the patient's health status.

27. The trend today is toward minimal preoperative testing, and a healthy patient may require no laboratory or diagnostic procedures. There is a lack of evidence showing that routine laboratory testing affects patient outcomes. Most diagnostic testing today is patient and procedure specific.

28. With the continuing transition from inpatient to ambulatory surgery, the patient might not be seen by the anesthesia provider or perioperative nurse until the day of surgery. Preoperative instructions are usually provided by the nurse who is present at the time that the decision for surgery is made. Instructions may also be reinforced by telephone a day or so prior to surgery.

29. Preoperative diagnostic requirements vary according to facility policy and anesthesia provider preference.

30. American Society of Anesthesiologists (ASA) guidelines and facility policy may mandate an ECG and chest X-ray for patients with risk factors and/or over a certain age who will undergo general anesthesia or moderate sedation/analgesia.

31. During preoperative assessment, the perioperative nurse reviews the patient's chart and assessment data and assesses the patient's readiness for surgery, plans for the patient's intraoperative care, and identifies data pertinent to anesthesia such as comorbidities, history of asthma, previous surgeries, experiences related to anesthetics, and complications.

32. Family history of experiences with anesthetics can be suggestive of possible adverse reactions, such as malignant hyperthermia, that can be prevented.

33. Drug allergies and information about the patient's current medications, including herbal medications, is essential to prevent the use of anesthesia medications that might react unfavorably with current medications or cause an allergic reaction. Allergies to contrast dyes, iodine solutions, adhesive tape, food allergies, and sensitivity to latex are relevant.

34. It is important to know if the patient has a history of substance abuse, because drug and alcohol use can alter the effect of anesthesia medications.

35. Patients on a beta-blocker should have been instructed to take their beta-blocker medication prior to arrival. The beta-blocker should be administered within 24 hours of surgery or discharge from the PACU (Centers for Medicare and Medicaid Services [CMS] Core Measure; Surgical Core Improvement Project [SCIP], 2015).

36. Patients who will be intubated should be assessed for cracked lips, lacerations in or around the mouth, and loose or chipped teeth. Dentures should be removed prior to general anesthesia, because they can become dislodged and interfere with intubation and anesthetic delivery.

37. Mouth and tongue jewelry can interfere with or become dislodged during intubation.

38. Patients who smoke have been documented to experience more difficulty with wound healing, pulmonary and cardiac complications, an increased need for postoperative intensive care, and longer periods of hospitalization than nonsmokers. Smokers have also been documented to need increased anesthetic dosages and greater amounts of postoperative pain medication. Avoiding smoking for as few as 12 hours prior to surgery has been shown to measurably reduce the negative effects of smoking. Smokers should be encouraged to stop smoking as early as possible prior to surgery.

39. Check to ensure that any diagnostic tests ordered were actually performed and that the results are present in the chart. Ensure that all team members are aware of any abnormalities in the test results.

40. Many facilities have policies that require confirmation of pregnancy on all female patients of child-bearing age. Confirming pregnancy status may necessitate a urine pregnancy test.

41. The patient's physical status is classified according to the ASA's classification system. Patients may be assigned a physical status (PS) from 1 to 5 as follows (ASA, 2014):

    - PS 1: a normal healthy patient. Example: healthy, nonsmoking, no more than minimal alcohol use

    - PS 2: mild systemic disease. Example: current smoker, social alcohol drinker, pregnancy, obesity (body mass index [BMI]≥ 40), well-controlled diabetes or hypertension, mild lung disease

    - PS 3: severe systemic disease. Example: one or more moderate to severe diseases: poorly controlled diabetes, hypertension, chronic obstructive pulmonary disease (COPD), morbid obesity (BMI ≥40), active hepatitis, alcohol dependence or abuse, implanted pacemaker, cerebrovascular accident (CVA, or stroke), transient ischemic attack (TIA), or coronary artery disease (CAD)/stents

    - PS 4: severe systemic disease that is a constant threat to life. Example: recent (within 3 months) myocardial infarction (MI), CVA, TIA, or CAD/stents, ongoing cardiac ischemia or severe valve dysfunction, severe reduction of ejection fraction, sepsis, disseminated intravascular coagulation (DIC), acute respiratory distress (ARD), or end-stage renal disease (ESRD) not undergoing regularly scheduled dialysis

    - PS 5: moribund and not expected to survive without the operation. Example: ruptured abdominal/thoracic aneurysm, massive trauma, intracranial bleed with mass effect, ischemic bowel in the face of significant cardiac pathology or multiple organ/system dysfunction

- PS 6: declared brain-dead patient whose organs are being removed for donor purposes
- The addition of "E" denotes emergency surgery. Emergency: when delay in treatment of the patient would lead to a significant increase in the threat to life or body part

42. The ASA classification system is useful in determining the anesthesia technique to be used. For example:

- Some facility policies do not permit PS 3 patients to undergo surgery under general anesthesia as an ambulatory surgery patient.
- PS 3 and higher patients must have an anesthesiologist, a CRNA, or an AA present during surgery even when the anesthesia technique is limited to moderate sedation/analgesia.

Patient Preparation/Teaching

43. Ideally, patient teaching is initiated at the time the decision is made to have surgery.

44. Instruction on preoperative routines, expected outcomes of surgery, and day-of-surgery instructions may be given by the nurse in the surgeon's office or in the clinic.

45. Teaching should continue during the presurgical examination or diagnostic workup. In some facilities, a preanesthesia clinic nurse or a PACU nurse initiates preoperative teaching in preparation for anesthesia and reinforces the instructions with a phone call the night before surgery.

46. Surgical patients already in the hospital may be instructed by the nurse on the patient's unit.

47. In any case, the circulating nurse should verify that the patient has complied with instructions for the day of surgery and reinforce the teaching done during the preoperative period.

48. Preanesthesia instructions are individualized based on the intended surgical procedure, the patient's condition, and the anesthesia technique planned. Instructions should include the following:

- Preoperative shower or enema (if indicated).
- Medications to be taken on the day of surgery, both routine and single-dose medications. On occasion, specific medications will be ordered for the patient to take prior to surgery, and other medications that the patient routinely takes will be held.

- Food and liquid intake depend upon the anesthesia technique planned.
  - Traditionally, patients receiving general anesthesia have been instructed to take nothing by mouth (NPO) for 6 to 8 hours prior to surgery. For the patient who is admitted on the day of surgery, typical instructions are "NPO after midnight."
  - With the loss of a protective airway reflex under general anesthesia, a patient who vomits or regurgitates as little as 0.4 mL of acid from the stomach with a pH of 2.5 is at high risk for aspiration pneumonitis, which can occur as a result of food and liquid intake too close to surgery.
  - Expectations of the surgical experience: length of surgery, expected recovery time, postoperative anesthesia care and routines.

49. The following summary of minimum fasting recommendations is limited to healthy patients of all ages (ASA, 2011a):

- Clear liquids: 2 hours
- Human milk: 4 hours
- Infant formula: 6 hours
- Nonhuman milk: 6 hours
- Light meal: 6 hours
- Fried or fatty foods: 8 hours

50. These guidelines do not apply to the following patients:

- Patients who undergo procedures with no anesthesia or only local anesthesia when upper airway protective reflexes are not impaired, and when no risk factors for pulmonary aspiration are apparent
- Women in labor

51. These guidelines may not apply to, or may need to be modified for, the following patients:

- Patients with coexisting diseases or conditions that can affect gastric emptying or fluid volume (e.g., pregnancy, obesity, diabetes, hiatal hernia, gastroesophageal reflux disease, ileus or bowel obstruction, emergency care, enteral tube feeding)
- Patients in whom airway management might be difficult

52. Anesthesiologists and other anesthesia providers recognize that these conditions can increase the likelihood of regurgitation and pulmonary aspiration. Additional or alternative preventive strategies may be appropriate for such patients (ASA, 2011a).

Section Questions

1. What developments helped to increase the safety of anesthesia administration? [Ref 2]
2. Which risks of injury are associated with complications of anesthesia? [Ref 4]
3. Which factors affect the patient's risk for complications of anesthesia? [Ref 5]
4. List the desired outcomes for the patient who undergoes anesthesia. [Ref 6]
5. Which factors affect the timeframe for achieving desired outcomes? [Ref 7]
6. Which four parameters are assessed in the Aldrete score? [Ref 8]
7. Identify and describe three anesthesia providers. [Ref 10]
8. How is the anesthetic technique for each patient determined? [Ref 11]
9. Discuss the importance of communicating among caregivers. [Ref 13]
10. What are the components of the anesthesia provider's role in the operating room? [Ref 14]
11. What is important about the times documented by the anesthesia provider and the circulating nurse? [Ref 16]
12. Why is it important for the anesthesia provider to direct the patient's transfer from one surface to another? [Ref 18]
13. Which types of patient information should be included in hand-off communication? [Ref 21]
14. What is the current trend in preoperative testing? [Ref 27]
15. Which types of information gathered preoperatively might alert the anesthesiologist to possible adverse reactions to anesthesia? [Refs 31–32]
16. What allergy information can impact decisions related to anesthesia? [Ref 33]
17. Why is documentation of drug and alcohol abuse important? [Ref 34]
18. What is the SCIP protocol related to beta-blockers? [Ref 35]
19. What are some important assessment details related to the mouth that might affect anesthesia delivery? [Refs 36–37]
20. How does smoking affect the response to surgery and anesthesia? [Ref 38]
21. Describe the criteria for ASA classifications PS1 though PS6. [Ref 41]
22. When should teaching begin for the surgical patient? [Ref 43]
23. What determines the specific preoperative instructions the patient should receive? [Ref 48]
24. What information is included in preanesthesia instructions? [Ref 48]
25. What patient conditions might require modification of food and liquid intake guidelines? [Ref 51]

Selection of Anesthetic Agents and Technique

53. Anesthesia medications are designed to induce amnesia, analgesia, and muscle relaxation.

54. Many factors influence the selection of anesthetic agents and technique. Each patient is unique, and the assessment will determine those drugs that best meet the surgical requirements and provide for the patient's well-being. Factors that are considered include the following:

- Age
- Medical history
- Current physical status and emotional or mental status (extreme anxiety, mental retardation, communication issues)
- Intended surgical procedure and expected length of recovery from anesthesia

- Patient preference
- Surgeon preference/requirements
- Anesthesia provider preference and expertise
- Patient's previous anesthesia/recovery experience
- Elective versus emergent surgery
- Considerations for postoperative pain management

Anesthesia Techniques

55. Anesthesia may administered by general, regional, local, or moderate sedation/conscious sedation techniques.

56. General anesthesia depresses the central nervous system. The patient is unconscious and reflexes are obtunded. The patient's physiologic status is controlled by the anesthesia provider.

57. Characteristics of general anesthesia include amnesia, analgesia, and muscle relaxation.

58. The effects of regional anesthesia are limited to a region of the body, such as a limb or the lower half of the body.

59. Regional anesthesia can be divided into central and peripheral techniques:

- Central techniques include neuraxial blocks (epidural anesthesia, spinal anesthesia).
- Peripheral techniques include plexus blocks (e.g., brachial plexus blocks) and single nerve blocks.

60. Regional anesthesia may be administered as a single injection or by inserting a catheter through which medication is administered over a prolonged period (e.g., epidural, continuous peripheral nerve block).

61. An intravenous regional block (Bier block) involves isolating the vasculature of a limb with a double tourniquet and injecting a local anesthetic such as lidocaine (Xylocaine), bupivacaine (Marcaine), chloroprocaine (Nesacaine), or tetracaine (Pontocaine) directly into the vein. The patient is awake but does not feel pain over the anesthetized region. Additional medications may be administered to reduce anxiety and provide sedation.

62. Local anesthesia is actually a form of regional anesthesia; however, only a small, localized area is infiltrated using an anesthetic such as lidocaine (Xylocaine) or bupivacaine (Marcaine). This infiltration is often performed by the surgeon on the field rather than by the anesthesia provider.

63. Moderate sedation/analgesia is also called conscious sedation, anesthesia standby, or local standby. It is most often used for healthy patients having minor procedures and managed by a perioperative nurse under the supervision of the surgeon.

64. The patient's condition, ASA classification, the procedure, or facility policy may indicate the need for an anesthesia provider to be present. The anesthesia technique is then termed monitored anesthesia care (MAC).

65. When an anesthesia provider is not present, facility policy, in conjunction with the state's nurse practice act, determines whether the nurse, the surgeon, or both are responsible for the administration of intravenous (IV) drugs.

66. If a perioperative nurse assumes responsibility for administering conscious sedation, the nurse should have no competing responsibilities. In no case should the circulating nurse be responsible for conscious sedation.

Preparation/Premedication

67. Protocols related to preoperative medication vary among facilities and anesthesia providers. Current practices support the evaluation of each patient's needs prior to ordering and administering medications, rather than relying on standard medication protocols.

68. Today, it is not unusual for the patient to receive no preoperative medication. This is particularly true for ambulatory surgery patients, for whom preoperative medication may prolong recovery and delay discharge. In addition, residual effects of medication cannot be monitored after discharge.

69. Goals of preoperative medication may include one or more of the following:

- Reduction of anxiety
- Sedation
- Analgesia
- Amnesia
- Prevention of nausea and vomiting
- Reduction in gastric volume and acidity
- Facilitation of induction
- Reduction of risk of allergic reaction
- Decrease of secretions
- Prevention of infection

70. Oral preoperative medications are usually given 60 to 90 minutes prior to surgery, and IV agents 30 to 60 minutes prior to surgery. Some agents—such as metoclopramide (Reglan), which is used to promote gastric emptying and lower stomach pH—are given 15 to 30 minutes before induction.

71. Benzodiazepines, such as midazolam (Versed), diazepam (Valium), and lorazepam (Ativan), reduce anxiety and provide sedation and moderate to significant amnesia. Diazepam is given less frequently because of its relatively long duration of action.

72. Barbiturates, such as secobarbital (Seconal) and pentobarbital (Nembutal), provide sedation with minimal cardiac or respiratory depression.

73. H_2-receptor blocking agents, such as ranitidine (Zantac, Glaxo), cimetidine (Tagamet), and famotidine (Pepcid), raise gastric pH and reduce the risk of and complications from aspiration. Nonparticulate antacids, such as sodium citrate (Bicitra), also raise gastric pH.

74. Dopamine antagonists, such as metoclopramide (Reglan), increase gastric emptying. Agents that raise pH or increase gastric emptying are particularly useful for patients at high risk for aspiration.

75. Conditions that suggest high risk for aspiration include the following:
    - Morbid obesity
    - Old age
    - Pregnancy
    - History of hiatal hernia with reflux
    - Uncertain NPO status coupled with the need for emergency surgery
    - History of diabetes with gastroparesis
    - History of partial bowel obstruction
    - History of peptic ulcer disease

76. Anticholinergic agents, such as atropine, scopolamine, and glycopyrrolate (Robinul), decrease oral and tracheobronchial secretions and prevent bradycardia, which can occur during parasympathetic stimulation or with certain anesthetic agents during induction. These agents are also antiemetics and reduce the likelihood of postoperative nausea.

77. Anticholinergics are useful for:
    - Patients who exhibit excessive salivation problems that put them at risk for aspiration

    - Toddlers and young children, who have a tendency to increase salivation up to tenfold when oral mucous membranes are stimulated (Litwack, 1995, p. 118)

78. Patients who are given anticholinergics may complain of a very dry mouth. A moistened gauze pad to wet the patient's lips and tongue will decrease the patient's discomfort.

79. Antiemetic agents, such as ondansetron (Zofran), a serotonin 5-HT$_3$ receptor antagonist; diphenhydramine (Benadryl); and the scopolamine patch (Transderm-Scop) are given to prevent nausea and vomiting. These medications are particularly useful for patients who report a history of nausea and vomiting after anesthesia and surgery. In 2001, the U.S. Food and Drug Administration (FDA) required droperidol (Inapsine) to carry a warning label related to "sudden cardiac death"; this change in the labeling has resulted in less frequent administration of this drug.

80. In an effort to reduce postoperative complications, a number of organizations have developed initiatives to prevent surgical site infection (SSI). SCIP (2015) is a national quality partnership committed to improving the safety of surgical care through the reduction of postoperative complications.

81. One of the SCIP's (2015) process and outcome measures, based on multiple research studies, is the administration of a prophylactic antibiotic within 1 hour prior to the surgical incision to reduce the incidence of SSI. Cefazolin (Ancef, Kefzol), cefoxitin (Mefoxin), and cefotetan (Cefotan), are used frequently. Vancomycin requires an hour for infusion and must be started before the 1-hour window.

82. The following factors determine when an antibiotic should be administered and which antibiotic is appropriate:
    - Probable risk of infection if a prophylactic agent is not administered
    - Probable contaminating flora associated with the operative site
    - Activity of the agent relative to the majority of pathogens likely to contaminate the operative site

83. Although the decision to administer an antibiotic preoperatively and the choice of antibiotic are made by the surgeon and/or

anesthesia provider, institutional policy may assign responsibility for administration of the agent to the perioperative nurse.

84. Narcotics, such as meperidine (Demerol), fentanyl (Sublimaze), alfentanil (Alfenta), sufentanil (Sufenta), remifentanil (Ultiva), hydromorphone (Dilaudid), and morphine, provide relief from pain.

85. Patients who have received narcotics must be observed closely for adequate ventilation. *All* narcotics are associated with dose-related respiratory depression and can cause nausea and vomiting. In fact, narcotic analgesics such as morphine, which dramatically decrease gastrointestinal (GI) motility, can lead to constipation and GI tract obstruction or ileus.

86. It is not uncommon for patients who anticipate general anesthesia to mistakenly believe that their premedication should put them to sleep. If patients are anxious because they are still awake, reassure them that they will be given additional anesthetic agents for surgery, will be asleep during the procedure, and will not feel pain.

87. The period just prior to surgery may be the most stressful for the patient and is a time when the presence of a nurse is crucial to alleviate anxiety.

88. In the preoperative period, patients are sometimes fearful of the unknown, of having to relinquish control, or of never awakening from anesthesia. Perioperative nurses need to listen to the patient, remain close by, and provide emotional support and reassurance.

Section Questions

1. Describe the effect of anesthesia medications on the patient. [Ref 53]

2. What factors influence the selection of anesthetic agents and technique? [Ref 54]

3. List the variety of anesthesia techniques available for patients undergoing surgical procedures. [Ref 55]

4. Describe the effects of general anesthesia. [Refs 56–57]

5. Describe regional anesthesia. [Refs 58–61]

6. Who is responsible for the administration of local anesthesia? [Ref 62]

7. Differentiate between moderate sedation/anesthesia and MAC. [Refs 63–64]

8. What factors determine whether a nurse can administer IV drugs? [Ref 65]

9. State one important criterion related to the nurse responsible for administering conscious sedation. [Ref 66]

10. Identify the goals of medications given prior to surgery. [Ref 69]

11. What differentiates diazepam (Valium) from other benzodiazepines? [Ref 71]

12. How do barbiturates affect cardiac and respiratory depression? [Ref 72]

13. Which drugs can be given to reduce the risk of complications from aspiration? [Refs 73–74]

14. List conditions that place patients at high risk for aspiration. [Ref 75]

15. Why are anticholinergic agents particularly important for toddlers and young children? [Ref 77]

16. Which types of drugs are given to prevent nausea and vomiting? [Ref 79]

17. Describe the SCIP protocol related to preoperative antibiotics to reduce the incidence of SSIs? [Ref 81]

18. How does the administration of vancomycin differ from the administration of other antibiotics? [Ref 81]

19. Which factors determine when an antibiotic should be administered and which antibiotic is appropriate? [Ref 82]

20. What information and support are appropriate for patients who are anxious or fearful about anesthesia and surgery? [Refs 86–88]

Monitoring

89. Patient monitoring during anesthesia detects physiologic changes in response to both the anesthesia and the surgical procedure. Ongoing monitoring is critical and provides the basis for appropriate and timely interventions that maintain satisfactory physiologic status.

90. The ASA has established standards for basic intraoperative monitoring (ASA, 2011a). Qualified anesthesia personnel should be present in the room throughout the delivery of all general anesthetics, regional anesthetics, and monitored anesthesia care. During all anesthetics, the patient's oxygenation, ventilation, circulation, and temperature should be continually evaluated.

91. With general anesthesia, end-tidal carbon dioxide concentration, oxygen concentration, end-tidal anesthetic gas concentration, and core body temperature are also monitored.

92. Monitoring devices may be invasive or noninvasive (devices that do not penetrate a body orifice).

93. Noninvasive monitors include ECG electrodes, blood pressure cuffs, and pulse oximeters and capnometers.

94. Invasive monitors (e.g., arterial lines, esophageal thermometer, and central venous catheters) are introduced beneath the skin or mucosa or enter a body cavity.

95. The choice of monitoring device is determined by the intended procedure, the patient's history and state of health, the anesthesia provider, the surgeon's judgment, and anticipated postoperative management.

96. Healthy patients undergoing simple surgical procedures usually require only noninvasive monitoring. Patients with complex health problems and those having complex and extensive surgical procedures will require extensive monitoring with a combination of invasive and noninvasive monitors. Examples include:

    - Cardiac surgery

    - When repeated blood samples will be required

    - When wide variations in blood pressure are anticipated

97. The perioperative nurse must be familiar with monitoring equipment and be able to recognize normal and abnormal physiologic responses, administer oxygen, and anticipate and assist in pharmacologic and emergency interventions.

98. During moderate sedation when the entire responsibility for monitoring rests with the perioperative nurse, monitoring is especially critical. In many facilities, supplementary monitoring competency requirements must be met before the perioperative nurse is permitted to monitor a patient independently.

99. A precordial stethoscope taped to the patient's chest or a stethoscope placed within the patient's esophagus facilitates continuous monitoring of cardiac rate and rhythm and breath sounds. The esophageal stethoscope also has a temperature sensor to continually monitor the patient's core temperature.

100. ECG monitoring detects changes in cardiac rate and rhythm, dysrhythmias, and myocardial ischemia.

101. Early detection and identification of cardiac irregularities permit timely and specific interventions that can prevent further complications.

102. Myocardial ischemia in the perioperative period may lead to myocardial infarction postoperatively.

103. ECG leads should be placed on clean, dry skin surfaces, and their adherence should be checked.

Pulse Oximetry

104. Pulse oximetry measures the oxygen saturation of arterial hemoglobin, an indicator of the oxygen transfer at the alveolar-capillary level.

105. A pulse oximeter has a photodetector with a light source on one side and a receptor on the other that is placed on a finger, toe, or ear lobe. Two different wavelengths (red and infrared light) are transmitted through the tissue to the receptor to measure the optical density of light passing through the tissue. Optical density is influenced by the amount of oxygen in the hemoglobin. The absorption of light for each color indicates the ratio of saturated blood to unsaturated blood. The photosensor should fit comfortably enough to prevent localized tissue ischemia.

106. Oxygen saturation readings should be near 100%. Readings of less than 90% are generally indicative of significant hypoxemia. Hypoxemia may lead to cardiac arrest.

107. Pulse oximetry facilitates prompt recognition of pending hypoxemia, and the anesthesia provider (or the perioperative nursing administering conscious sedation) can respond promptly by administering oxygen and ensuring that the airway is patent.

108. Satisfactory oxygen saturation readings from pulse oximetry are not a guarantee that tissues are being adequately perfused with oxygen. Other factors such as hemoglobin level must also be considered because hemoglobin carries oxygen. Even when the hemoglobin is saturated with oxygen, there may be insufficient hemoglobin to maintain appropriate tissue oxygen levels.

109. Ventilation should be assessed even when pulse oximetry readings are normal. Hypoventilation for an extended period will result in an accumulation of carbon dioxide in the blood that will cause respiratory acidosis, leading to a decrease in oxygen saturation. The onset of respiratory acidosis can occur more rapidly than a decrease in oxygen saturation. It is possible for a patient on 100% oxygen to have a normal oxygen level but be suffering from respiratory acidosis.

110. Improved pulse oximetry technology has diminished the impact of nail polish and acrylic nails on oximetry readings.

111. Several factors can interfere with the accuracy of pulse oximetry readings:

    - Bright lights—cover the photodetector with a towel or place it under the drapes

    - Intravascular dyes, such as methylene blue, which have caused dose-dependent decreases in measurements (Clifton, 2003)

112. Conditions causing vasoconstriction, such as Raynaud's disease, severe peripheral vascular disease, and hypotension, can also prevent an accurate pulse oximetry reading (Valdez-Lowe et al., 2009).

Blood Pressure

113. Blood pressure monitoring is a measure of the pressure in the heart during contraction and relaxation. Automatic monitors are incorporated into the anesthesia machine. They measure blood pressure and cardiac rate and display rhythm, and they can be set to take readings at predetermined intervals.

114. Cuffs should be situated to avoid compressing IV lines when activated. The cuff should be periodically inspected to ensure that it deflates adequately between readings, because extended inflation periods may lead to neurological injury.

Temperature

115. General anesthesia depresses the hypothalamus, preventing the patient from compensating for changes in ambient temperature. If the operating room is cold, the anesthetized patient can become hypothermic.

116. Nursing interventions should include those directed toward maintaining the patient's body temperature within normal limits.

117. Unintended hypothermia—defined as a core body temperature less than 36°C/96.8°F—is a relatively common occurrence in the unwarmed surgical patient (Hart et al., 2011).

118. Factors contributing to hypothermia include the low temperature setting in the operating room, evaporation of surgical skin preparation, exposure of body tissues in open procedures, infusion of cool fluids, and the effects of anesthetic drugs (Adriani & Moriber, 2013).

119. Maintaining normal body temperature during the perioperative period has a positive impact on patient outcomes and patient satisfaction.

120. Unintended hypothermia can lead to decreased resistance to infection, discomfort and stress on the body, shivering which increases oxygen consumption, increased duration of action of medications, increased length of hospital stay, and an increased risk of morbid cardiac events (Adriani & Moriber, 2013).

121. Even mild hypothermia significantly increases blood loss and the relative risk for transfusion. Maintaining perioperative normothermia reduces blood loss and transfusion requirement that is clinically significant (Rajagopalan et al., 2008).

122. Intraoperative hypothermia correlates with increased rates of SSIs. Patient temperature less than 35°C doubles the risk for postoperative SSI (Seaman et al., 2012).

123. Patients at greatest risk for unplanned hypothermia include infants, young children, the elderly, and patients with endocrine disorders. The length and type of surgical procedure also affect the risk for hypothermia.

124. Forced-air warming blankets are more effective in maintaining normothermia than warm blankets, warmed irrigating fluids, and head coverings such as towels or stockinettes.

125. Regardless of the length of the procedure, a forced-air warming blanket is recommended, beginning in the preoperative period and continuing throughout the intraoperative and recovery periods. Blanket accessories have been designed to cover any area of the body not immediately involved in the surgical procedure.

126. The system should be used strictly in accordance with the manufacturer's instructions. The air hose should never be used without being connected to the warming blanket provided with the device. The hose end has a dangerously high air temperature and the blanket serves to disperse this heat. Using the air unit without a blanket can result in serious burns (Association of periOperative Registered Nurses [AORN], 2015, p. 485; Wu, 2013).

127. The most significant change in patient temperature occurs during the first hour of surgery. Even with preoperative warming, there is a drop in body temperature during the first hour of surgery (AORN, 2015, p. 479).

128. The patient's temperature should be monitored when a procedure is expected to last more than 30 minutes. Monitoring approaches can include an external patch thermometer or a more accurate internal esophageal or rectal probe.

129. For infants, a head covering made from stockinette and Webril to wrap the arms and legs can help to maintain normal body temperature.

130. In addition to using a warming blanket, the temperature of the room may be raised to prevent hypothermia. This consideration is particularly important for burn patients, trauma patients, and babies. In some facilities, raising the room temperature may require a call to the maintenance department; make the request as soon as possible so the room can be warmed before the patient is brought in.

131. Warm fluids and IV solutions strictly according to the manufacturer's instructions for temperature, time limits, and whether the item can be rewarmed if not used. Monitor warming cabinet temperatures to ensure they remain within the range identified in the manufacturer's instructions for use (IFU).

132. Administer IV solutions and especially blood products, such as packed red blood cells (PRBCs) and fresh frozen plasma (FFP), through a fluid-warming device.

Capnography

133. Capnography monitors the inhaled and exhaled concentration or partial pressure of carbon dioxide in the respiratory gases. Capnography is useful for detecting acute changes in metabolic function that indicate the possibility of hypothermia or malignant hyperthermia. It is useful in detecting hypoventilation, esophageal intubation, and a disconnected circuit.

134. Carbon dioxide absorbs infrared radiation. When a beam of infrared light is passed across the gas to a sensor, the carbon dioxide absorbs the light and changes the voltage in the circuit, which is then displayed on a graph.

135. Most capnography units provide a digital display of end-tidal CO_2 and a waveform readout of expired CO_2 partial pressure versus time.

Section Questions

1. Why is monitoring essential during the administration of anesthesia? [Ref 89]

2. Describe the ASA's standards for basic intraoperative monitoring of patients receiving anesthesia. [Ref 90]

3. What additional parameters are monitored with general anesthesia? [Ref 91]

4. Identify invasive and noninvasive approaches to patient monitoring. [Refs 92–94]

5. What determines the choice of monitoring devices for a surgical patient? [Ref 95]

6. Cite examples of procedures where invasive monitoring is appropriate. [Ref 96]

7. Explain why a perioperative nurse must have knowledge of monitoring equipment and the ability to interpret data. [Ref 97]

8. What does an esophageal stethoscope monitor in addition to cardiac rate, rhythm, and breath sounds? [Ref 99]

(continues)

Section Questions (continued)

9. What is the benefit of identifying myocardial ischemia in the perioperative period? [Refs 101–102]

10. How does a pulse oximeter work? [Ref 105]

11. What is the implication of oxygen saturations less than 90%? [Ref 106]

12. Why is the oxygen saturation of arterial hemoglobin measured? [Ref 107]

13. Which other factors must be measured to ensure that tissues are adequately perfused with oxygen? [Ref 108]

14. Why is it necessary to assess ventilation even when pulse oximetry readings are normal? [Ref 109]

15. What factors can interfere with accurate pulse oximetry readings? [Refs 111–112]

16. How do anesthetic agents affect the patient's temperature? [Ref 115]

17. Identify factors that lead to unintended hypothermia. [Ref 118]

18. What impact does unintended hypothermia have on the patient? [Refs 120–122]

19. Which patient populations are at greatest risk for unplanned hypothermia? [Ref 123]

20. Discuss the relative value of forced-air warming for the patient. [Ref 124]

21. Discuss nursing responsibilities related to the use of forced-air warming. [Refs 125–126]

22. What are some approaches to preventing hypothermia in infants? [Ref 129]

23. What is one challenge that might be associated with increasing the temperature in the operating room? [Ref 130]

24. What are some implications for warming of IV fluids and blood products? [Refs 131–132]

25. What conditions can be detected via capnography? [Ref 133]

General Anesthesia

136. Effects of general anesthesia include amnesia (loss of memory), hypnosis (loss of consciousness), analgesia (absence of the sense of pain), and skeletal muscle relaxation. It is customary to administer a variety of agents to produce the various desired responses.

137. General anesthesia is delivered with inhalation agents and intravenous medications.

Inhalation Agents

138. Nitrous oxide (N_2O), isoflurane (Forane), desflurane (Suprane), and sevoflurane (Ultane) are the most commonly used inhalation anesthetic agents. They enter the system by inhalation and are removed by lung ventilation (**Table 10-1**).

139. Nitrous oxide is a sweet-smelling gas that acts rapidly but lacks potency. It is nonirritating and produces few aftereffects; recovery is rapid.

140. In combination with oxygen alone, nitrous oxide is sufficient only for minor procedures that do not produce intense pain. For major procedures, nitrous oxide can be used with other agents to potentiate the anesthetic state.

141. Nitrous oxide diffuses readily into gas-filled spaces such as the stomach, colon, and lungs. Avoid nitrous oxide in cases where expansion in these areas would be a problem (e.g., bowel obstruction, pneumothorax). Because it causes expansion in the stomach, nitrous oxide is associated with postoperative nausea and vomiting.

142. The concentration of nitrous oxide must be monitored carefully to prevent it from becoming too high, because this can lead to hypoxia.

143. Isoflurane, desflurane, and sevoflurane are volatile anesthetic agents that are liquid at room temperature, but evaporate easily. Volatile anesthetics pass through a vaporizer on the anesthesia machine and are inhaled by the patient.

Table 10-1	Inhalation Agents		
Agent	**Use**	**Advantages**	**Disadvantages**
Oxygen	Sustain life	Rapid induction and recovery; few aftereffects; nonirritating to respiratory tract	Poor relaxation, insufficient potency for general surgery, hypoxia a potential hazard
Sevoflurane	Maintenance of anesthesia; may be used for induction	Most rapid induction and emergence; no ether smell; easy to breathe; protects heart against myocardial irritability	Metabolizes to inorganic fluoride; raises fluoride level in patients with renal disease—unknown consequences; mild and transient chills, fever, nausea; contraindicated in patients susceptible to malignant hyperthermia
Desflurane (Suprane)	Maintenance for short period	Rapid emergence, good relaxation	Irritating to respiratory tract; can cause transient increase in heart rate and blood pressure
Isoflurane (Forane)	Maintenance of anesthesia; may be used for induction	Inexpensive; minimal aftereffects, obtunds laryngeal and pharyngeal reflexes; good relaxation, potentiates all muscle relaxants; protects heart against catecholamine-induced arrhythmias; cardiovascular system remains stable	Profound respiratory depressant; longest induction and recovery times; slow induction and emergence times

144. Desflurane provides excellent relaxation and offers the most rapid onset and emergence. It is not taken up by fatty tissue as rapidly as the other agents, which allows for faster emergence from anesthesia.

145. A transient increase in cardiac rate and blood pressure may occur on induction.

146. Due to desflurane's rapid induction and emergence, it is especially useful for ambulatory surgery procedures.

147. Desflurane is also the agent of choice for obese patients because of its low fat solubility.

148. Because of its pungent odor, which can cause gagging and laryngospasm, desflurane is not recommended for an inhalation induction, a technique often used for children that delivers only anesthetic agents by mask. Intravenous induction uses IV medications to induce a loss of consciousness prior to administration of an inhalation agent.

149. Sevoflurane has a moderate rate of induction and emergence. It acts more slowly than desflurane but much more rapidly than isoflurane.

150. Sevoflurane is not irritating to the respiratory tract and does not irritate the myocardium. It is the induction inhalation agent of choice for children and is also appropriate for ambulatory procedures.

151. The use of isoflurane has declined and has largely been replaced by desflurane and sevoflurane, because isoflurane has the longest induction and emergence times of the commonly used agents.

152. Isoflurane provides excellent relaxation and potentiates muscle relaxants. Isoflurane does not destabilize the cardiovascular system, and electrocardiographic abnormalities are not associated with isoflurane inhalation. Isoflurane does not sensitize the myocardium to catecholamines; therefore, epinephrine may be used for local vasoconstriction.

153. Isoflurane causes peripheral vasodilation. Hypotension is common at induction; however, blood pressure rapidly returns to normal.

Anesthesia Machine

154. Today's anesthesia machines provide accurate concentrations of volatile anesthetic agents and oxygen, and they provide mechanical ventilator, suction, and monitoring devices for blood pressure, ECG, inspired oxygen, and end-tidal carbon dioxide.

155. The vaporizer transforms volatile anesthetic agents from liquid into gas for delivery to the patient. End-tidal measuring of the inhalational agents and gases is commonly available.

156. Oxygen, nitrous oxide, and air are supplied through hoses from a central source within the healthcare facility or from cylinders attached to the machine. For safety purposes, the hoses and cylinders are color coded and their fittings are not interchangeable. Throughout the United States, oxygen cylinders and hoses are green, nitrous oxide is blue, and air is yellow. (*Note*: Compressed nitrogen used for pneumatic equipment comes in black tanks.)

157. Oxygen and other anesthetic inhalation agents are mixed and directed to and from the patient through a *breathing circuit*—disposable corrugated rubber or plastic tubes joined with a built-in Y connector that is attached to a face mask or an endotracheal tube for delivering the anesthetic. Anesthetic gases are carried to the patient through a one-way valve in one tube, and expired gases are returned through the other tube.

158. Flow meters attached to the machine are also color coded and indicate the amount of flow of nitrous oxide, air, and oxygen being delivered to the patient. The anesthesia provider selects the ratio of gases to deliver to the patient.

159. The delivery system includes a reservoir bag that functions much like an Ambu bag that can be manually compressed to force oxygen and inhalation agents into the lungs.

160. Expired gases from the patient pass through an absorber that removes the carbon dioxide.

161. The machine has a shutoff device that prevents nitrous oxide from being delivered if oxygen is not also delivered at a concentration of at least 21%.

162. There is an oxygen flush valve that delivers 100% oxygen to the patient.

163. The machine has an alarm system that indicates when the patient is experiencing apnea or the breathing circuit has become detached from the machine.

164. The disposable anesthesia carbon dioxide absorber is a soda lime canister that removes carbon dioxide from exhaled gases. The canister must be changed regularly.

165. Oxygen is added to the filtered exhaled gases, which are then returned to the patient (termed *rebreathing*).

166. Trace anesthesia gases are removed from the atmosphere by a scavenger system on the anesthesia machine that vents them to outside air. High concentrations of nitrous oxide and other anesthetic gases in the operating room air would present a serious health hazard to operating-room staff. Nausea, dizziness, headaches, fatigue, irritability, drowsiness, decreased mental performance, reduced fertility, and miscarriages, as well as neurological, renal, and liver disease, have been associated with exposure to these gases (Occupational Safety and Health Administration [OSHA], 2000, 2015).

167. The National Institute for Occupational Safety and Health (NIOSH) set limits for exposure to waste anesthetic gases and vapors in 1977. The NIOSH guidelines limit worker exposure to 25 parts per million (ppm) of nitrous oxide over an 8-hour, time-weighted average (NIOSH, 2015).

168. Anesthetic gases should be shut off except when they are being delivered to the patient. Routine testing of anesthesia equipment for leaks can help prevent overexposure to waste gases.

169. The level of waste anesthetic gases is periodically tested to determine the facility's compliance with NIOSH recommendations. The perioperative nurse should be aware of limits and of testing results.

Section Questions

1. How does general anesthesia affect the patient? [Ref 136]
2. In which two ways can general anesthesia be administered? [Ref 137]
3. Describe nitrous oxide (N_2O). [Refs 139–141]

(continues)

Intravenous Agents

170. Intravenous agents, introduced directly into the circulatory system, usually through a peripheral vein in the arm or hand, are most often used as a supplement to inhalation agents.

171. Unlike inhalation agents, which can be easily removed from the system by ventilating the lungs, most intravenous agents must be metabolized by the liver or kidneys to be eliminated/excreted from the body.

172. Barbiturates for induction of anesthesia were introduced in 1935 with thiopental sodium (pentothal). Sodium pentothal, sodium thiamylal (Surital), and methohexital sodium (Brevital) are used rarely, if at all, today.

173. Barbiturates are short-acting agents that result in a rapid progression from sedation to loss of consciousness; however, barbiturates do not provide analgesia.

174. They are also potent respiratory depressants; induction followed by transient apnea can be expected, which requires oxygen to support the patient's ventilation. Barbiturates also depress the cardiovascular system, and a degree of hypotension can be expected.

175. The nonbarbiturate drug propofol (Diprivan), a hypnotic-sedative agent, has become the most popular medication for producing a rapid induction.

176. Propofol is also used for sedation for short procedures such as colonoscopy, esophagogastroduodenoscopy (EGD), and pain therapies.

177. Propofol is delivered in a milky-white, intralipid emulsion that has been known to support microbial growth; therefore, handling of propofol requires strict aseptic technique. Administration should begin promptly and be completed within 6 hours after the container is opened. After 6 hours, the product should be discarded, and the lines should be flushed or discarded (Trissell, 2014).

178. The patient may experience pain upon injection, because propofol is a potent vein irritant. Discomfort can be reduced by prior injection of 1–2 mL of lidocaine, or 20 mg of lidocaine can be mixed in 200 mg propofol at the provider's discretion.

179. Recovery from propofol is more rapid than with barbiturates. This drug produces minimal aftereffects and fewer incidences of postoperative nausea and vomiting. It is often used in ambulatory surgery settings.

180. Etomidate (Amidate) is a nonbarbiturate induction agent that has minimal effects on myocardial function, cardiac output, and peripheral or pulmonary circulation. It is a short-acting agent and is generally utilized for patients with a positive cardiac history and patients who cannot tolerate dramatic changes in blood pressure.

181. Etomidate does not provide analgesia.

Dissociative Induction Agents

182. Ketamine hydrochloride (Ketalar) is a dissociative agent that produces a catatonic state and provides amnesia and analgesia. The patient will breathe unassisted, may move, and may appear to be awake even after reaching an anesthetized state. Surgery can be performed without patient response.

183. Ketamine is rapidly metabolized, and patients emerge quickly from its effects.

184. Ketamine may be given either intravenously (IV) or intramuscularly (IM).

185. Ketamine is useful for diagnostic procedures and procedures where it is desirable to have the patient breathe unassisted. It is sometimes used for children who undergo short procedures that do not require muscle relaxation.

186. Because ketamine often produces a dramatic increase in oral secretions, an antisialagogue is often used in conjunction with it.

187. Because ketamine is a dissociative agent, patients may experience hallucinations postoperatively. This aftereffect is more common in adults and may be minimized when diazepam or midazolam is given. The patient should recover in a quiet, darkened area.

Narcotics

188. Narcotics may be used preoperatively as a premedication or intraoperatively during anesthesia induction and maintenance.

189. Narcotics used intraoperatively include fentanyl (Sublimaze), sufentanil (Sufenta), alfentanil (Alfenta), morphine, hydromorphone (Dilaudid), and remifentanil (Ultiva). Fentanyl is 100 times more potent than morphine, and sufentanil is 5–10 times more potent than fentanyl.

190. Small doses of narcotics are used intraoperatively as adjuncts to other drugs and to provide pain relief in the early postoperative period.

191. Narcotics provide profound analgesia and can be particularly valuable in cardiac surgery, because sternotomy is especially painful/stimulating.

192. Narcotics are respiratory depressants, and patients who have received high doses of narcotics intraoperatively must be monitored closely to ensure that they are breathing adequately. A patient who has received a high dose of narcotic intraoperatively may appear to be awake and alert postoperatively but may suddenly begin to hypoventilate and lose consciousness.

193. The narcotic meperidine hydrochloride (Demerol) is used in the PACU to control shivering. This drug requires caution when used with patients taking monoamine oxidase (MAO) inhibitor drugs (phenelzine, selegiline, and tranylcypromine), because it may result in hypertensive crisis, hyperpyrexia, and cardiovascular system collapse, which could be fatal.

194. Demerol is used infrequently for purposes other than for shivering unless the patient has unmanageable adverse reactions to other first-line opioids.

195. Naloxone (Narcan) is an opiate antagonist that competitively binds to the opioid receptors. If the patient is apneic, it is recommended that 0.4 mg or 1 ampule of naloxone be administered IV or IM with careful monitoring. If the patient is not apneic but has a falling O_2 saturation, it is recommended that naloxone be titrated into effect.

196. In the apneic patient, it is important to support the airway, and the first drug of choice to administer is oxygen. The patient may renarcotize because the half-life of naloxone is only approximately 20 minutes—the half-life of most narcotics is longer.

197. Complications of naloxone administration include pulmonary edema and hypertension. Additionally, the patient is essentially forced into a rapid "withdrawal" and will experience pain, diaphoresis, nausea, and vomiting, similar to what an opioid addict would experience with withdrawal.

Tranquilizers/Benzodiazepines

198. Tranquilizers are used for induction and as adjuncts to other anesthetic agents; in combination with tranquilizers, lower doses of other agents can be administered.

199. Tranquilizers commonly used intraoperatively include diazepam (Valium) and midazolam (Versed).

200. Diazepam produces amnesia and reduces anxiety.

201. Midazolam is an excellent amnestic and also provides significant anxiolysis.

202. Flumazenil (Romazicon) is used to reverse the effects of benzodiazepines. It reverses sedation and respiratory depression without producing cardiovascular effects. Patients whose anesthesia is reversed in this manner must be closely monitored, because flumazenil may lose its effect sooner than the underlying benzodiazepine, and hypoventilation can recur.

Neuromuscular Blockers (Muscle Relaxants)

203. Muscle relaxants commonly used intraoperatively include succinylcholine (Anectine), cisatracuriumbesylate (Nimbex), rocuronium bromide (Zemuron), and vecuronium bromide (Norcuron) (**Table 10-2**).

204. The two primary indications for neuromuscular blockers are:

    - To relax the jaw and larynx to facilitate controlled breathing and tracheal intubation
    - To increase muscle relaxation to permit ease of tissue handling during surgery

205. Muscle relaxants vary in their onset and duration. Any of the agents can be used for intubation, but the length of time to achieve prime "intubating conditions" depends on the onset of the particular drug.

206. Neuromuscular blockers paralyze the neuromuscular junction and block impulses from motor nerves to skeletal muscle. The patient becomes paralyzed. Neuromuscular blockers may be either depolarizing or nondepolarizing.

207. Succinylcholine is a depolarizing muscle relaxant. When it reaches the neuromuscular junction, it acts like acetylcholine, producing a depolarization of the membrane at the motor end plate. The depolarization causes a muscle contraction that is followed by a neuromuscular block. The drug prevents repolarization, and the muscle remains relaxed and paralyzed. The muscle contractions are sometimes obvious and appear similar to twitching. This twitching, referred to as *fasciculation*, progresses in cephalocaudal sequence as the drug circulates through the patient's body.

208. Succinylcholine produces paralysis within seconds and is used for intubation. Because of its rapid onset of action, it is valuable in emergency situations where rapid intubation is required.

209. Succinylcholine will cause an increase in plasma potassium levels because the acetylcholine receptor is propped open, allowing ongoing flow of potassium ions into the extracellular fluid. This increase is transient in normal patients.

210. Conditions that make patients susceptible to succinylcholine-induced hyperkalemia include burns, closed head injury, acidosis, Guillain-Barré syndrome, cerebral stroke, drowning, severe intraabdominal sepsis, massive trauma, myopathy, and tetanus.

211. Succinylcholine is a known triggering agent for malignant hyperthermia.

212. Nondepolarizing muscle relaxants block the action of acetylcholine at the neuromuscular junction but do not cause depolarization at the motor end plate, so fasciculation does not occur.

213. Nondepolarizing agents have a slower onset than depolarizing agents, and their effect or duration of action is dose dependent.

214. Vecuronium, rocuronium, and cisatracurium are considered "intermediate-acting" neuromuscular blocking agents (NMBs), whose standard weight-based dose lasts approximately 45 minutes.

215. Pavulon is considered a long-acting agent and is mainly used in cardiac surgery or when the patient is not expected to be extubated at the end of the case.

216. The anesthesia provider continually monitors the patient to determine the degree of paralysis present. A nerve stimulator applied to a peripheral nerve, such as the ulnar nerve or a branch of the facial nerve, can be used to determine the degree of paralysis by observing for contractions resulting from nerve stimulation.

217. The anticholinergic or "reversal agents" pyridostigmine (Regonol) and neostigmine (Prostigmin) reverse the action of nondepolarizing agents. These two drugs are always used in combination with atropine sulfate or glycopyrrolate

Table 10-2	Muscle Relaxants		
Agent	**Use**	**Advantages**	**Disadvantages**
Depolarizing Muscle Relaxant—Rapid Onset, Short Duration			
Succinylcholine (Anectine, Quelicin)	Intubation Short procedures	Rapid onset; brief duration	Can cause muscle fasciculation, postoperative myalgia; requires refrigeration, contraindicated in patients with recent burn, muscle trauma, or recurrent neuromuscular disorder; can trigger malignant hyperthermia; prolonged effect in patients with serum cholinesterase deficiency
Nondepolarizing Muscle Relaxants—Intermediate Onset, Intermediate Duration			
Atracurium (Tracrium)	Intubation Maintenance of paralysis	Transient and generally minimal cardiovascular effects	Not currently available in the US; requires refrigeration; histamine release; facial flushing; transient hypotension and reflex tachycardia
Vecuronium (Norcuron)	Intubation Maintenance of paralysis	No significant cardiovascular effects; no release of histamine	Must be mixed
Rocuronium (Zemuron)	Intubation Maintenance of paralysis	Provides excellent intubating conditions; rapid onset	May increase heart rate; eliminated via liver, contraindicated in patients with hepatic disease, contraindicated for rapid intubation for cesarean sections
Cisatracurium (Nimbex)	Intubation Maintenance of paralysis	Does not require renal or hepatic elimination (uses Hoffman/enzymatic elimination) so can use in kidney or liver failure. No histamine release so cardiovascularly stable	Requires refrigeration
Nondepolarizing Muscle Relaxants—Delayed Onset, Longer Duration			
Tubocurarine (curare)	Maintenance of paralysis		Strong histamine release; automatic blockade can cause hypotension
Pancuronium (Pavulon)	Maintenance of paralysis	Long duration	Can cause hypertension and increased heart rate

(Robinul) to counteract the potentially profound muscarinic effects (bradycardia and salivation) of the anticholinesterases.

218. Even if the patient has been "reversed" and demonstrates a normal twitch response to the nerve stimulator, 75–85% of the receptors at the neuromuscular junction could still be occupied (inducing paralysis).

219. Administration of the reversal agent does not make the muscle paralysis magically disappear; patients may still be weak and require extra time to breathe on their own.

Section Questions

1. How are intravenous anesthetic agents removed from the patient's system? [Ref 171]
2. Which characteristics of barbiturates made them appropriate for induction? [Ref 173]
3. Which precaution is taken before administering barbiturates? [Ref 174]
4. Besides respiratory depression, which other system is affected by barbiturates? [Ref 174]
5. Describe propofol (Diprivan). [Refs 175–177]
6. Why must propofol be used within 6 hours of preparation using strict aseptic technique? [Ref 177]
7. Which characteristics of propofol make it appropriate for ambulatory surgery? [Ref 179]
8. Which characteristics of etomidate (Amidate) make it appropriate for patients with a positive cardiac history? [Ref 180]
9. What is the effect of ketamine on patients? [Ref 182]
10. Under what circumstances would ketamine be chosen as an anesthetic agent? [Ref 185]
11. What is an antisialagogue? [Ref 186]
12. Which interventions address the potential for hallucinations sometimes experienced with ketamine? [Ref 187]
13. For what purpose are narcotics used intraoperatively? [Refs 190–191]
14. What must be monitored closely in postoperative patients who have received high doses of narcotics? [Ref 192]
15. What effect can meperidine (Demerol), which is used in the PACU to control shivering, have on patients who take MAO inhibitor drugs? [Ref 193]
16. How does naloxone (Narcan) counter the adverse effects of opiates, such as apnea? [Ref 195]
17. How can a patient re-narcotize following administration of Narcan? [Ref 196]
18. Describe complications possible with use of Narcan. [Ref 197]
19. How do tranquilizers affect other anesthetic agents? [Ref 198]
20. What are two effects of diazepam? [Ref 200]
21. Describe two effects of midazolam. [Ref 201]
22. When flumazenil (Romazicon) is used to reverse sedation and respiratory depression, why must patients be closely monitored? [Ref 202]
23. What are two primary indications for neuromuscular blockers? [Ref 204]
24. Explain the difference between depolarizing and nondepolarizing neuromuscular blockers. [Refs 207, 212]
25. Explain the fasciculation ("twitching") that sometimes accompanies the use of a depolarizing muscle relaxant such as succinylcholine. [Ref 207]
26. Which characteristics of succinylcholine make it valuable in emergency situations? [Ref 208]
27. What conditions make patients susceptible to succinylcholine-induced hyperkalemia? [Ref 210]
28. Succinylcholine is a triggering agent for which specific adverse outcome associated with anesthesia? [Ref 211]
29. Which has a slower onset of action, depolarizing or nondepolarizing agents? [Ref 213]
30. What are three "intermediate-acting" neuromuscular blocking agents? [Ref 214]
31. Identify two situations in which the "long-acting" neuromuscular blocker Pavulon is used. [Ref 215]
32. How does the anesthesia provider use a nerve stimulator to assess the amount of paralysis present? [Ref 216]
33. What drug is always used in conjunction with pyridostigmine and neostigmine to counteract profound muscarinic effects? [Ref 217]
34. What are *muscarinic effects?* [Ref 217]
35. Explain the need for careful monitoring after an anticholinergic has been used. [Refs 218–219]

Stages of Anesthesia

220. In 1720, when ether was the primary anesthetic agent, Arthur Guedel integrated the four stages of anesthesia with their signs and symptoms into a system that was used to estimate the depth of anesthesia by observing the patient's physiologic changes and reflex responses. The system applied to patients who were not premedicated and who breathed spontaneously.

221. With today's sophisticated anesthetic agents, the patient passes so quickly from one stage to another, that the individual stages have little relevance, except with mask induction in children. Even then the inhalation agents work so quickly that it is easy to miss the transition from one stage to another.

222. Stages of anesthesia:

- Stage I: Relaxation—from administration of anesthesia to loss of consciousness. Patient response: dizziness, drowsiness, exaggerated hearing, and a decreased sense of pain.

- Stage II: Excitement—from loss of consciousness to onset of regular breathing. Patient response: irregular breathing, increased muscle tone and involuntary motor activity, and thrashing and struggling activity (susceptible to auditory and tactile stimulation).

- Stage III: Surgical anesthesia—from onset of regular breathing to cessation of respiration. Patient response: regular thoracoabdominal breathing, a relaxed jaw, a loss of pain and auditory sensation, and loss of eyelid reflex.

- Stage IV: Danger—from cessation of respiration to circulatory failure and death. Patient response: fixed and dilated pupils, rapid and thready pulse, and paralyzed respiratory muscles. The patient should never be at this depth of anesthesia.

Recovery from anesthesia occurs in reverse order (Stage IV to Stage I). During emergence, which often takes place at the same time as the dressing is being applied, it is important to understand that stimulating the patient by touching them near the head or neck, pressing on the abdomen, or moving an extremity can trigger laryngospasm. The nurse should maintain good communication with the anesthesia provider to determine the right time to place dressings and move the patient.

Preparation for Anesthesia: Nursing Responsibilities

223. As much as possible, the room should be ready and preparations for surgery completed before the patient is brought into the operating-room suite and transferred to the operating bed.

224. Once the patient is in the room, the circulating nurse must focus attention on providing emotional support, ensuring patient dignity, instituting safety measures, and assisting the anesthesia provider.

225. Induction covers the time from administration of the first anesthetic drug until the patient is stabilized at the desired level of anesthesia.

226. Prior to anesthesia induction, there should be a working suction with catheter in place within easy reach of the anesthesia provider. Suction is incorporated into the anesthesia machine. Ensure that it is functioning and that a tonsil/Yankauer suction cannula is available.

227. Prior to induction, confirm that the safety strap, electrocardiographic leads, blood pressure cuff, and intravenous line are in place.

228. Maintain the patient's dignity and privacy during induction. Adjust the patient's gown to ensure privacy; close the operating-room doors; cover the windows, if necessary; and keep unnecessary personnel from the room.

229. Induction represents a critical time during the administration of anesthesia. It is essential for patient safety that the perioperative nurse be present and available to assist the anesthesia provider with suctioning and intubation and, if necessary, to restrain the patient (particularly children).

230. Just prior to induction, patients often become anxious. Remain at the patient's side, speak calmly, explain the process, and answer any questions; be reassuring. Nonverbal support, such as making eye contact and holding the patient's hand, can be the most supportive interventions in preparation for induction.

231. Ensure that everyone in the room is quiet and still to avoid stimulating the patient or interrupting the calming effect of the preoperative medication. Scrub personnel should arrange instruments and supplies quietly; door should remain closed; the patient should not overhear any conversation related to "blades," "needles," "mosquitoes," and so forth, which can be frightening. Conversation during the intraoperative period should be kept to a minimum and must always be respectful of the patient's dignity.

232. Hearing is the most difficult sense to anesthetize, and it is the last sensation lost before unconsciousness.

233. In young children, who may not tolerate the placement of an intravenous line, and in patients with a tracheostomy tube, induction is usually begun with an inhalation agent administered by mask.

234. The circulating nurse also assists the anesthesia provider in positioning the patient properly for intubation.

235. Some patients' anatomy makes them a "difficult intubation," in which case blankets or a positioning device may be necessary to achieve the "sniffing" position (a position that maximizes laryngoscopy). The nurse might also need to call for additional airway equipment (e.g., a fiber-optic scope or airway cart).

Sequence for General Anesthesia: Nursing Responsibilities

236. The typical sequence for general anesthesia in patients who have an intravenous line:
    - The patient breathes 100% oxygen for a few minutes via mask. The oxygenation serves as a safety margin in the event of an airway obstruction or brief period of apnea during insertion of the endotracheal tube.
    - A narcotic and/or a benzodiazepine is injected and ventilation is monitored.
    - Propofol, etomidate, or a barbiturate is injected to produce sleep. Sleep will usually occur within 1 or 2 minutes. The anesthesia provider may assess depth of sleep by stroking the eyelashes, which are very sensitive to touch.
    - With the mask over the patient's nose and mouth, the anesthesia provider ventilates the patient and observes the chest rise. If the chest does not rise, the head and mandible are repositioned until a patent airway is established.
    - When a patent airway is confirmed, a paralyzing dose of muscle relaxant facilitates intubation. (Muscle relaxants with a longer onset may be injected before the patient is asleep, because the effect will not occur until after the patient falls asleep.)
    - The anesthesia provider visualizes the vocal cords with a laryngoscope and passes an endotracheal tube into the trachea (intubation). The perioperative nurse might assist with intubation by pulling gently on the corner of the patient's mouth to increase visualization of the vocal cords and facilitate placement of the endotracheal tube.
    - The perioperative nurse might also pass the endotracheal tube to the anesthesia provider so he or she does not have to look up to pick up the tube.
    - The tube is inserted directly through the larynx into the trachea. The cuff is inflated with a 10-mL syringe to prevent secretions from entering the trachea and lungs. A cuffed endotracheal tube is considered a "secured" airway, because it prevents gastric contents from entering the trachea.

237. The anesthesia provider will confirm correct endotracheal tube placement:
    - Observe fog in the clear endotracheal tube.
    - Observe the patient for bilateral chest excursion without epigastric enlargement.
    - Listen for bilateral breath sounds.
    - Identify carbon dioxide expiration through end-tidal monitoring. CO_2 waveform capnography is the gold standard for the confirmation of tube placement within the trachea.

238. After appropriate positioning to ensure the tube is not past the carina or the bifurcation into the right and left main-stem bronchi, the anesthesia provider will secure the tube in place with tape, then connect it to the breathing circuit. Inhalation agents are delivered automatically according to parameters set by the anesthesia provider.

239. Depending on the procedure and the necessity for paralysis, the patient will either be ventilated or will breathe spontaneously.

240. For short procedures and procedures where paralysis is not necessary, the patient is usually not intubated. A combination of inhalation agents will be administered via a mask or laryngeal mask airway (LMA).

    • The mask is strapped or held over the patient's nose and mouth and connected via anesthesia tubing to the anesthesia machine. The patient may breathe spontaneously, or breathing and delivery of anesthetic agents may be accomplished manually by compressing a reservoir bag on the anesthesia machine. This is also referred to as "bagging" the patient.

    • The LMA is a device that provides good airway management without intubation. It is inserted into the patient's mouth, positioned securely over the larynx, and inflated to keep it securely in place. The patient is connected to the anesthesia machine via an anesthesia circuit. The patient may breathe spontaneously or be mechanically ventilated. An LMA is not a "secured airway," because it does not have a cuff that prevents gastric contents from entering the trachea (**Figure 10-1** and **Figure 10-2**).

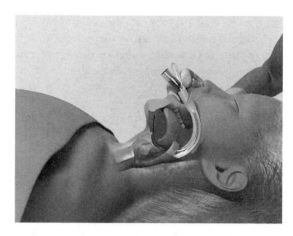

Figure 10-2 Laryngeal mask airway in place.
Image courtesy of LMA North America, Inc., San Diego, CA.

Rapid-Sequence Intubation

241. Regional anesthesia is the technique of choice for patients at high risk for aspiration. However, when regional anesthesia is not appropriate, rapid-sequence intubation is the best alternative.

242. When a barbiturate or hypnotic is given at the start of induction, it will quickly reach the patient's brain, causing apnea. The patient's pharyngeal muscles and tongue relax, and airway obstruction can occur. If a clear airway is not maintained, the patient will attempt to breathe as the drug washes out of the brain. The abdominal muscles may strain and pull the diaphragm down, compressing the stomach and causing the patient to regurgitate. If the patient regurgitates and attempts to breathe, he or she can aspirate gastric contents into the lungs, resulting in aspiration pneumonia.

243. Aspiration of stomach contents can be fatal. The perioperative nurse's first priority is to remain at the patient's side at the head of the table, prepared to assist the anesthesia provider until intubation is complete and assistance is no longer needed. A suction with a Yankauer catheter tip, a nasogastric tube, an emesis basin, and a towel should be immediately available in case the patient aspirates.

244. Patients at high risk for aspiration include those who have not been NPO for the required period of time, such as the patient who ate before becoming ill, the trauma victim

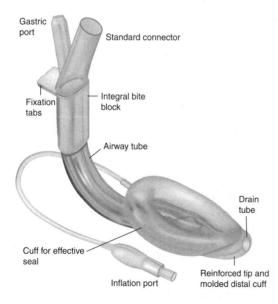

Gastric port
Standard connector
Fixation tabs
Integral bite block
Airway tube
Drain tube
Cuff for effective seal
Reinforced tip and molded distal cuff
Inflation port

Figure 10-1 Laryngeal mask airway (LMA).
Image courtesy of LMA North America, Inc., San Diego, CA.

with blood or food in the stomach, and the patient with a hiatal hernia.

245. Rapid-sequence intubation results in rapid unconsciousness (induction) and neuromuscular blockade (paralysis).

- The patient is preoxygenated with 100% oxygen for 3–5 minutes to allow for apnea during tracheal intubation.

- A fast-acting hypnotic agent is administered along with a rapid-acting neuromuscular blocking drug.

- Cricoid pressure is applied to decrease the chance of stomach contents entering the larynx.

   - The perioperative nurse may be asked to assist by firmly pressing the cricoid cartilage posteriorly with the index finger or thumb and forefinger. This maneuver, called the Sellick maneuver (developed in 1961 by Brian Sellick), compresses the esophagus between the cricoid cartilage and the vertebral column, aids in visualization of the tracheal lumen for intubation, and occludes the esophagus to prevent regurgitation (Sellick, 1961) (**Figure 10-3**).

   - It is not unusual to be asked to move the trachea left or right to help with visualization.

   - The nurse should not release the pressure until the anesthesia provider indicates that the endotracheal tube is in place and inflated, and placement has been verified.

246. Once the cuff is inflated, the endotracheal (ET) tube is connected to the anesthesia machine.

Nursing Responsibilities

247. Following the induction of anesthesia and positioning for the surgical procedure, the perioperative nurse should scan the patient from head to foot to ensure that the body alignment is maintained and padding is adequate to prevent pressure damage. This is a critical review—once the patient is draped, it's difficult to assess and adjust the patient's position.

248. Before positioning or repositioning the patient, the perioperative nurse should confer with the anesthesia provider to determine that the patient can be moved without compromise to the airway or ventilation, and that he or she is

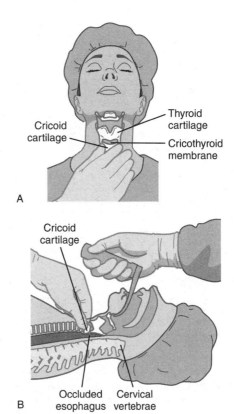

Figure 10-3 Sellick maneuver.

ready to assist in repositioning by guiding and securing the patient's head to prevent accidental extubation or disconnection from the ventilator.

249. If the patient is moved or repositioned during the procedure, another check is required to ensure a safe and proper position.

250. During the surgical procedure, the perioperative nurse helps the anesthesia provider assess fluid balance by monitoring fluid output and replacement, blood loss, blood and blood product replacement, and the amount of irrigating solution used.

251. Emergence from anesthesia, particularly during extubation, is a critical period when the perioperative nurse must be at the patient's side and immediately available to assist the anesthesia provider.

252. Extubation can initiate bronchospasm or laryngospasm reflex. The airway may become obstructed, and vomiting can occur. Airway management and adequate ventilation are priorities. Prior to extubation, the perioperative nurse should confirm that a suction catheter is within reach of the anesthesia provider and that suction is turned on and working.

Section Questions

1. Describe the patient response in each of the four stages of anesthesia. [Ref 222]
2. Once the patient enters the operating room, what is the circulating nurse's primary focus? [Ref 224]
3. What is the timeframe associated with the *induction* period? [Ref 225]
4. What patient safety precautions does the nurse confirm prior to induction? [Ref 227]
5. How can the nurse promote privacy for the patient during induction? [Ref 228]
6. What can the nurse due to allay the patient's anxiety? [Refs 230–231]
7. Why is it important to monitor the quality of conversation in the operating room, even after the patient is anesthetized? [Refs 231–232]
8. Describe the typical sequence for inducing the patient having general anesthesia. [Ref 236]
9. How can the nurse assist the anesthesia provider with insertion of the endotracheal tube? [Ref 236]
10. What is the purpose of the cuff on the endotracheal tube? [Ref 236]
11. How does the anesthesia provider confirm the correct placement of the endotracheal tube? [Ref 237]
12. Under which circumstances might the patient not be intubated? [Ref 240]
13. What is the reason for doing a rapid-sequence intubation? [Ref 241]
14. Why must we avoid aspiration of stomach contents? [Ref 243]
15. What patient populations are at high risk for aspiration? [Ref 244]
16. Describe the Sellick maneuver and the purpose for using it. [Ref 245 & Figure 10-3]
17. What is the purpose of scanning the patient from head to toe immediately after positioning? [Ref 247]
18. Why should the nurse confer with the anesthesia provider before positioning or repositioning the patient? [Ref 248]
19. What challenging situations can occur during extubation? [Ref 252]
20. What are two priorities during extubation? [Ref 252]

Unintended Intraoperative Awareness

253. Unintended intraoperative awareness occurs in approximately one patient per 1,000 receiving general anesthesia. The duration and severity vary, though instances of severe awareness are highly unusual (American Association of Nurse Anesthetists [AANA], 2015). The patient may recall surroundings, an event, pressure, or even pain.

254. Age, sex, ASA physical status, and drug resistance or tolerance may be associated with intraoperative awareness, as are certain procedures for which deep anesthesia might be contraindicated (e.g., C-section, cardiac surgery, trauma) and anesthesia techniques such as rapid-sequence induction (ASA, 2006). Sensitivity and response to anesthesia vary with age. Women have a pharmacogenetic predisposition to awaken faster than men from general anesthesia (Gan, 1999).

255. Devices such as the bispectral analysis monitor (BIS) assess depth of anesthesia on a scale of 0 to 100. A value in the range of 50 indicates an acceptable depth of anesthesia. Values in the higher ranges may give warning of impending arousal (The Joint Commission [TJC], 2004).

256. A patient who exhibits anxiety about unintended awareness should be assured that the phenomenon is rare. The anesthesia provider can discuss techniques and tools for monitoring depth of anesthesia.

Malignant Hyperthermia

257. Malignant hyperthermia (MH) is an inherited muscle disorder triggered by certain types of anesthesia that may cause a fast-acting, life-threatening crisis (Malignant Hyperthermia Association [MHAUS], 2015a).

258. The exact incidence of MH is unknown. The rate of occurrence has been estimated to be as frequent as one in 5,000 or as rare as one in 65,000 administrations of general anesthesia with triggering agents. The incidence varies depending on the concentration of MH-carrier families in a given geographic area. High-incidence areas in the United States include Wisconsin, Nebraska, West Virginia, and Michigan.

259. If left untreated, it can result in cardiac arrest, kidney failure, blood coagulation problems, internal hemorrhage, brain injury, and death.

260. The MH mortality rate has been reduced from as high as 70% to less than 5% with better screening, the establishment of a pharmacologic basis for MH, sophisticated monitoring techniques, and the use of dantrolene sodium. Dantrolene sodium is a skeletal muscle relaxant that blocks the release of calcium from the sarcoplasmic reticulum, which in turn decreases muscle contractions.

261. In patients who experience malignant hyperthermia, the sarcoplasmic reticulum (the calcium-storing membrane of the muscle cell) is unable to regulate calcium within the muscle cell in the presence of certain anesthetic agents.

262. When malignant hyperthermia occurs, intracellular calcium increases, and the result is sustained contracture of skeletal muscle. These contractions cause muscles to consume higher than normal amounts of oxygen, in a process that produces lactic acid and heat. The patient's temperature rises rapidly and dramatically. Electrolytes, enzymes, and myoglobin leak from the cells. Hyperkalemia may result and lead to cardiac arrhythmias. The loss of myoglobin can result in renal failure.

263. Symptoms may be multifocal and include sudden inappropriate tachycardia with tachypnea, unstable blood pressure, generalized rigidity, masseter muscle spasm, metabolic and respiratory acidosis, increased end-tidal CO_2, fever, profuse sweating, cyanotic mottling of the skin, and dark unoxygenated blood in the field. Tachycardia and increased end-tidal CO_2 are often the first symptoms to appear and may be attributed to causes other than malignant hyperthermia.

264. The classic symptom of fever may occur after the appearance of other symptoms with body temperatures rising as high as 109.4°F (43°C). Temperature can rise as much as 1.8°F (1°C) every 5 minutes.

265. Certain inhalation agents and depolarizing muscle relaxants are known to be malignant hyperthermia triggers. The following anesthetic agents are known triggers of MH and are not safe for use in MH-susceptible patients:

   - Succinylcholine
   - Desflurane
   - Enflurane
   - Sevoflurane
   - Isoflurane (rarely used)

266. When succinylcholine is the triggering agent, a sudden severe rigidity of the jaw may be seen following administration of the drug.

267. Depending on the patient and the triggering agent, malignant hyperthermia can occur immediately or as late as 24 hours following the administration of anesthesia.

268. MH is considered a genetic disorder with an autosomal mode of inheritance; however, multiple risk factors such as Duchene's muscular dystrophy and other myopathies have also been identified.

269. The nurse should be alert for the following risk factors that can sometimes be identified during the preoperative assessment:

   - Personal or family history of malignant hyperthermia or complications arising from anesthesia
   - A family history of suspicious anesthesia experience
   - Unexplained death during surgery
   - History of unexplained muscle cramps with fever
   - Inherited skeletal muscle disorders

270. If it is suspected that the patient is susceptible to malignant hyperthermia, the surgery may need to be postponed until a skeletal muscle biopsy test is performed to confirm the diagnosis.

271. Alternatively, the surgery may proceed if none of the possible triggering agents is utilized. A total intravenous anesthesia (TIVA) is performed. Regional anesthesia might considered, or the patient may be intubated be using a nondepolarizing muscle relaxant, and amnesia and analgesia are maintained using a propofol

infusion and narcotic. No inhalation agents other than oxygen are delivered to the patient.

272. Molecular diagnostic testing is also available for diagnosing patients suspected to be susceptible to MH. Genetic testing will not detect all patients at risk, whereas a muscle biopsy test is considered definitive.

273. The nurse should prepare the operating-room table with a cooling blanket, and locate the malignant hyperthermia cart and supplies.

274. Depending on institutional policy, prophylactic administration of dantrolene sodium may be ordered.

275. If a patient experiences a malignant hyperthermia episode during surgery, *get help and get dantrolene sodium!* Traditional dantrolene sodium (Dantrium, Revonto) is supplied in 20-mg vials that require 60 mL of preservative-free sterile water to reconstitute. Hospitals are required to stock 36 vials for a potential case of MH. Ryanodex, a new presentation of dantrolene sodium released in 2015, comes in 250-mg vials reconstituted with 5 mL of sterile water. Hospitals must stock 3 vials of Ryanodex. (MHAUS, 2015b).

276. Every operating room where general anesthesia is administered should have immediate access to dantrolene sodium and a written, readily accessible protocol for the management of MH, usually contained in an emergency MH cart. Staff should be familiar with the contents and the treatment protocol (**Exhibits 10-2 and 10-3**).

277. The anesthesia circuit and CO_2 absorbent should be changed to reduce the risk from residual triggering agents. Many operating rooms have an anesthesia machine reserved for an MH episode. Immediately replace the anesthesia machine in use to save the time required to change the anesthesia circuit and replace the CO_2 absorbent on the existing machine.

278. Initial treatment is to discontinue all triggering anesthetic agents immediately, hyperventilate with 100% oxygen, administer dantrolene sodium (Dantrium), and rapidly terminate the surgery.

279. Hospitals are transitioning to Ryanodex. Dantrium and Revoto must be reconstituted with 60 mL of preservative-free sterile water for each bottle. It can take from two to four licensed individuals to reconstitute the amount required for rapid administration. A 200-pound patient would require 12 vials. Only one vial of reconstituted Ryanodex is sufficient for the same patient.

280. Glucose, insulin, and calcium should be available to treat hyperkalemia, bicarbonate to treat metabolic acidosis, and a diuretic to maintain urinary output.

281. Tests frequently performed during an MH crisis include creatinine phosphokinase (CPK), lactic dehydrogenase (LDH), and blood-clotting analysis.

282. Cooling of the patient is achieved by wound irrigation with cold saline, administration of cold intravenous solutions, surface cooling with ice or a cooling blanket, and cold gastric and rectal lavage.

283. If it is impossible to terminate surgery, anesthesia is continued with nontriggering agents.

284. Following an episode of malignant hyperthermia, the patient must be closely monitored for a possible recurrent episode. Dantrolene sodium is continued for 48 hours or more.

Section Questions

1. What patient factors are associated with the incidence of unintended intraoperative awareness? [Ref 254]

2. What procedures are more likely to be associated with unintended intraoperative awareness? [Ref 254]

3. What information can the nurse provide for a patient who is concerned about unintended intraoperative awareness? [Ref 256]

4. Which factors have helped to reduce the mortality rate of malignant hyperthermia? [Ref 260]

5. Describe the pathophysiology of MH. [Refs 261–262]

6. What are some of the symptoms of MH? [Refs 263–264]

7. Which symptoms of MH are often the first to appear? [Ref 263]

(continues)

Section Questions (continued)

8. Which types of anesthetic agents are known to be triggers for MH? [Ref 265]

9. How long does it take MH to manifest following administration of the triggering agent? [Ref 267]

10. What information should be elicited during the preoperative period? [Ref 269]

11. What decisions might be made about the surgical procedure when assessment identifies a patient at risk for MH? [Refs 270–271]

12. What is the drug of choice (the only drug) for treating MH? [Refs 274–276]

13. What is the initial treatment when MH occurs? [Ref 278]

14. How does Ryanodex improve the administration of dantrolene sodium? [Ref 279]

15. In addition to administering dantrolene sodium, what other steps are taken during an MH episode? [Ref 280]

16. Which lab tests provide important information during an MH crisis? [Ref 281]

17. What interventions can be used to bring down the patient's temperature? [Ref 282]

18. If surgery is to proceed on a patient at risk for MH, what precautions will the anesthesia provider take? [Ref 283]

19. How is the patient managed following an MH crisis? [Ref 284]

20. How will the perioperative nurse prepare for a patient at risk for MH? [Refs 273–274]

Moderate Sedation/Analgesia

Overview

285. Moderate sedation/analgesia, also known as conscious sedation or IV conscious sedation, is a drug-induced depression of consciousness. The patient is able to respond purposefully to verbal commands, either alone or accompanied by light tactile stimulation. No interventions are required to maintain a patent airway. Spontaneous ventilation is adequate.

286. Moderate sedation/analgesia is frequently used for diagnostic procedures or minor surgery (e.g., colonoscopy, incision and drainage of an abscess, excision of small mass, vascular access, vasectomy, and the reduction of a dislocation with a cast application) where the presence of an anesthesiologist is not routinely necessary.

287. Goals of moderate sedation/analgesia:
- Allay fear and anxiety
- Enhance cooperation
- Maintain consciousness and the ability to respond to verbal stimulation
- Maintain respirations unassisted
- Provide adequate analgesia

- Maintain stable vital signs
- Achieve partial amnesia
- Facilitate prompt return to activities of daily living

288. Desired outcomes of moderate sedation/analgesia include the following:
- The patient demonstrates or reports adequate pain control throughout the perioperative period.
- The patient's cardiac status is consistent with or improved from baseline levels established preoperatively.
- The patient breathes unassisted and is easily aroused, and respiratory status is consistent with or improved from baseline levels established preoperatively.
- The patient is relaxed, comfortable, and cooperative.
- The patient's protective reflexes are intact.

289. Each institution should develop criteria to identify patients who are suitable candidates for moderate sedation/analgesia. Patients classified as PS1, PS2, and medically stable PS3 are normally considered appropriate for registered nurse–administered moderate sedation (AORN, 2015, p. 554).

290. Assessment should include physiologic status, psychological maturity, and the patient's ability to tolerate and maintain the desired position for the duration of the procedure.

291. An airway assessment can determine if the patient would be difficult to intubate if necessary. Factors that could make intubation difficult include significant obesity, especially of the face, neck, and tongue; significantly recessed or protruding jaw; limited range of neck motion; protruding or missing teeth, edentulous; history of sleep apnea; and presence of stridor (AORN, 2015, p. 555).

292. Sedatives and analgesic agents are delivered intravenously. Commonly used agents include diazepam (Valium), midazolam (Versed), morphine sulfate (Duramorph), meperidine (Demerol), and fentanyl (Sublimaze).

293. Reversal agents include naloxone hydrochloride (Narcan) for narcotics and flumazenil (Romazicon) for benzodiazepines.

Nursing Responsibilities

294. The registered nurse who monitors the patient receiving moderate sedation/analgesia should have no other responsibilities during the procedure that would require leaving the patient unattended and might compromise continuous monitoring (AORN, 2015, p. 555). An additional nurse should be present to function in the circulating role.

295. At a minimum, the following knowledge and skills are necessary:
    - Patient selection and assessment criteria
    - Selection, function, and proficiency in use of physiologic monitoring equipment
    - Pharmacology of the medications used
    - Airway management
    - Continuous positive airway pressure (CPAP) use
    - Basic dysrhythmia recognition and management
    - Emergency response and management
    - Advanced cardiac life support (ACLS) and pediatric advanced life support (PALS) according to the type of patients served (Some facilities require ACLS certification for nurses who monitor patients receiving moderate sedation/analgesia.)
    - Recognition of complications associated with sedation/analgesia
    - Knowledge of anatomy and physiology (AORN, 2015, pp. 557–558)

296. In addition to the ability to perform a thorough preoperative assessment, the nurse who is monitoring the patient should have a working knowledge of resuscitation equipment and the function and use of monitoring equipment, and the ability to interpret any data that are obtained.

297. Monitoring equipment should include airway management devices (e.g., oral, nasal airways, mask ventilation devices, 316 oximeter, noninvasive blood pressure monitor, and electrocardiograph). Suction should be immediately available, turned on, and functioning. The patient should have an established intravenous line, and sedative and analgesic antagonists should be in the room and immediately available. The crash cart should be immediately available (AORN, 2015, pp. 556).

298. AORN has formulated practice recommendations for the nurse who monitors the patient receiving local anesthesia or moderate sedation/analgesia. These recommendations state that monitoring should include the following elements (AORN, 2015, pp. 556–557):
    - Heart rate and function via ECG
    - Level of consciousness (LOC)
    - Blood pressure
    - Cardiac monitoring
    - Oxygenation using pulse oximetry with audible pulse rate and alarms
    - Ventilation monitored by direct observation or auscultation

299. The patient who receives moderate sedation/analgesia must be continuously monitored for any reaction to drugs and for physiologic and psychological changes that might cause the patient to progress to a state of deep sedation.

300. Because of the rapid patient response to pharmacologic agents, it is possible for the patient to lapse into unconsciousness. Deep sedation may be characterized by extremely slurred speech, not being easily aroused, inability to independently maintain a patent airway, and nonresponsiveness to verbal commands.

301. In the event that a patient progresses to a state of deep sedation and cannot be easily aroused and cannot maintain independent ventilatory function, the nurse must be competent to provide rescue measures.

302. Patients who are discharged to another unit should be monitored for several hours to ensure the maintenance of a satisfactory level of consciousness, a patent airway, and stable vital signs.

303. Criteria for discharge may include, but are not limited to, the following:

- Return to preoperative, baseline level of consciousness
- Stable vital signs

- Sufficient time interval since the last administration of an antagonist to prevent resedation of the patient
- Use of an objective patient assessment scoring system (e.g., Aldrete score)
- Absence of protracted nausea
- Adequate pain control
- Intact protective reflexes
- Return of motor/sensory control (AORN, 2015, p. 557)

304. Patients should be given written postoperative instructions, because medications used in moderate sedation/analgesia can diminish the ability to recall information that has been given verbally.

Section Questions

1. Describe moderate sedation/analgesia. [Ref 285]

2. For which types of procedures is moderate sedation frequently used? [Ref 286]

3. What are the goals of moderate sedation? [Ref 287]

4. Identify the desired outcomes of moderate sedation. [Ref 288]

5. Which patients are considered appropriate candidates for moderate sedation? [Ref 289]

6. Describe the assessment of a patient for moderate sedation. [Ref 290]

7. What are the components of an airway assessment for moderate sedation? [Ref 291]

8. Which reversal agents are available for narcotics and benzodiazepines? [Ref 293]

9. What is important about combining circulating duties and monitoring the patient receiving moderate sedation? [Ref 294]

10. What knowledge and skills are important for the perioperative nurse who will monitor patients receiving moderate sedation? [Refs 295–296]

11. Which equipment should be available to monitor the patient receiving moderate sedation? [Ref 297]

12. What practice recommendations for the nurse monitoring patients receiving local anesthesia or moderate sedation have been made by AORN? [Refs 298–299]

13. What is the implication of deep sedation for the perioperative nurse monitoring the patient? [Refs 300–301]

14. List criteria for discharge for patients who have received moderate sedation. [Ref 303]

15. Why are written instructions important for patients who have received moderate sedation? [Ref 304]

Regional Anesthesia

Overview

305. Regional anesthesia techniques include spinal, epidural, and caudal block; intravenous block; nerve block; local infiltration; and topical administration.

306. The decision to use regional anesthesia depends upon many factors including patient condition, the surgical procedure, and surgeon/anesthesia provider/patient preference.

307. One very positive attribute of regional anesthesia is that the respiratory and cardiac systems remain relatively stable, making it suitable when general anesthetic agents are

contraindicated, such as with patients who have severe metabolic, renal, cardiac, pulmonary, or hepatic disease.

308. Regional anesthesia is also preferable for patients who require emergency surgery, have a full stomach, and do not need to be unconscious for the procedure.

309. It is important to avoid providing too much sedation in addition to the regional anesthetic because of the potential for aspiration.

310. Regional anesthetic may be utilized in conjunction with a general anesthetic, especially in orthopedic or major abdominal procedures to promote postoperative pain management.

311. Real-time, dynamic ultrasound imaging can increase proficiency and decrease complications of administering a regional anesthetic by facilitating the identification of the pre-puncture location of the vessel for needle insertion, wire placement, and catheter placement (ASA, 2012c; Shekelle & Dallas, 2013). Anesthesia providers' professional organizations currently recommend that no central lines be placed without ultrasound guidance.

312. For obese patients, scanning with ultrasound enhances the ability to locate the space for epidural or spinal block.

Spinal Anesthesia

313. Spinal anesthesia is used for lower abdominal, pelvic, lower extremity, and urologic procedures, and for cesarean sections.

314. Spinal anesthesia involves injecting an anesthetic agent into the cerebrospinal fluid in the subarachnoid space. Injection is made through a lumbar interspace usually between L2 and L3 or lower, so that the needle is not inserted into the spinal cord, which normally ends at L1 to L2.

315. As the anesthetic is absorbed by the nerve fibers, nerve transmission is blocked. Spread of the anesthetic agent and the subsequent level of anesthesia are determined by cerebrospinal pressure; the injection site; the amount, concentration, and specific gravity of the anesthetic solution; the speed of injection; and the position of the patient during and immediately following the injection.

316. Spinal anesthetic solutions are generally a mixture of local anesthetic and dextrose. These solutions settle by gravity. The block can be directed upward, downward, or to one side of the spinal cord by adjusting the patient's position. After 10 or 15 minutes, the block is set and does not extend farther.

317. Agents frequently used for spinal anesthesia include lidocaine (Xylocaine), tetracaine (Pontocaine), and bupivacaine (Marcaine). A narcotic may also be added to the injection.

318. The administration of spinal anesthesia requires patient cooperation. Proper positioning is the key to successful placement of the anesthetic injection. Nursing interventions focus on helping to position the patient, assisting the anesthesia provider as needed, and reassuring and providing support for the patient during the procedure.

319. Injection of the anesthetic is done with the patient in a sitting or lateral decubitus position. In the sitting position, the patient sits on the operating table with the legs over the side and feet on a stool high enough to raise the patient's knees above the level of the waist. The patient should be encouraged to lower the chin to the chest and arch the back (**Figure 10-4**).

320. The patient in the lateral decubitus position is very close to the edge of the table, and safety measures to prevent falling are necessary (**Figure 10-5**). The patient's hips, back, and shoulders are parallel to the edge of the table. The patient's knees are flexed toward the chest, and the head and neck are flexed toward the chest. This position spreads the vertebrae and exposes the desired interspaces to facilitate correct needle insertion. The perioperative nurse should remain close to the patient and ensure that the patient feels secure.

321. When administering spinal anesthesia, strict attention to asepsis is important to prevent entry of pathogens that can cause meningitis into the subarachnoid space.

322. Other complications of spinal anesthesia include a rapid drop in blood pressure, nausea and vomiting, total spinal anesthesia, postdural headache, and neurological or integumentary positioning injury.

323. Sudden hypotension is caused by vasodilation when the anesthetic blocks sympathetic nerves that control vasomotor tone. If peripheral pooling, decreased venous return, and decreased cardiac output should occur, ephedrine may be administered to restore normotension.

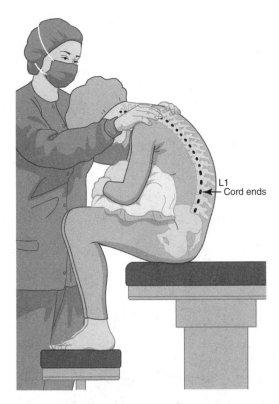

Figure 10-4 Sitting position for spinal anesthesia.

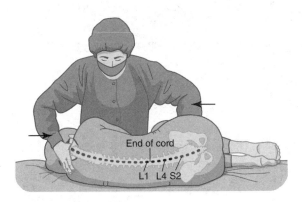

Figure 10-5 Lateral position for spinal anesthesia.

324. Nausea and vomiting can occur as a result of hypotension or as a reaction to sedation medication. Keep suction, an emesis basin, and a wet towel immediately available.

325. Total spinal anesthesia occurs when the level of anesthesia becomes high enough to paralyze the respiratory muscles causing respiratory distress. This is an emergency situation. Ventilation must be supported, and intubation may be required.

326. Patients may experience headache ("spinal headache") 24 to 48 hours following spinal

anesthesia if the dura at the site of injection does not seal itself off and cerebrospinal fluid leaks into the epidural space. Headache is caused by the loss of cerebrospinal fluid that decreases cerebrospinal pressure and leaves less fluid to cushion the brain.

327. In most cases, treatment of the headache consists of hydration, intravenous or oral caffeine, sedation, and bed rest. If symptoms persist longer than 24 hours, a blood patch of the patient's blood may be administered at the puncture site to seal the epidural leak.

328. Neurological or integumentary injuries can occur with improper positioning, because the patient's sensory pathways are blocked and the patient cannot detect or respond to the situation.

Epidural and Caudal Anesthesia

329. Epidural anesthesia is achieved by injection of the anesthetic agent into the epidural space (**Figure 10-6**). The agent is usually injected through the interspaces of the lumbar vertebrae; however, depending on the surgical site, the injection site might be thoracic or cervical.

330. Lumbar epidural anesthesia is useful for anorectal, vaginal, and perineal procedures and for obstetric surgery. It is also combined with a general anesthetic for orthopedic procedures and urologic procedures.

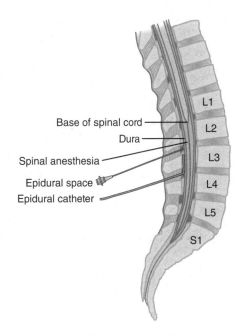

Figure 10-6 Regional anesthesia sites.

331. Thoracic epidural anesthesia will cover the surgical site for abdominal and thoracic surgeries.

332. For caudal anesthesia, the anesthetic is injected into the epidural space through the caudal canal in the sacrum. Caudal anesthesia is used in obstetrics and in small children for circumcisions.

333. Commonly used epidural and caudal anesthetic agents include lidocaine hydrochloride (Xylocaine), bupivacaine (Marcaine), ropivacaine, and chloroprocaine (Nesacaine). A narcotic agent is often added to the local anesthetic to enhance the analgesic effects.

334. Epidural anesthesia can be delivered as a single dose, or a small catheter can be left in place for continuous infusion. Continuous infusion is useful for pain management in the postoperative period.

335. Anesthetic agents that are injected into the epidural space are not as affected by positioning as in spinal anesthesia.

336. The following complications of epidural anesthesia are possible:

    • Dural puncture—postdural headache
    • Inadvertent subarachnoid injection—total spinal anesthesia
    • Inadvertent intravascular injection—extreme hypotension and cardiac arrest

Section Questions

1. List the types of available regional anesthesia techniques. [Ref 305]

2. What factors are considered when deciding whether to use regional anesthesia? [Ref 306]

3. What makes regional anesthesia a good choice for patients with severe metabolic, renal, cardiac, pulmonary, or hepatic disease? [Ref 307]

4. Why might regional anesthesia be used in conjunction with general anesthesia for orthopedic or major abdominal procedures? [Ref 310]

5. How does ultrasound increase proficiency and decrease complications when administering regional anesthesia? [Ref 311]

6. For what procedures is spinal anesthesia appropriate? [Ref 313]

7. For spinal anesthesia, where is the anesthetic injected? [Ref 314]

8. How is the level of anesthesia determined? [Ref 315]

9. What is the perioperative nurse's responsibility in assisting with spinal anesthesia? [Ref 318]

10. Describe the positions that are appropriate for administering spinal anesthesia. [Refs 319–320]

11. Why is strict aseptic technique important during the administration of spinal anesthesia? [Ref 321]

12. Describe the potential complications of spinal anesthesia. [Refs 322–324]

13. What is "total spinal anesthesia," and what are the implications of its use? [Ref 325]

14. Explain the etiology of headaches that might occur following spinal anesthesia. [Ref 326]

15. How can post-spinal anesthesia headaches be managed? [Ref 327]

16. What kind of patient injuries can result when spinal anesthesia is used? [Ref 328]

17. Contrast epidural anesthesia with spinal anesthesia. [Refs 314, 329]

18. For which procedures can epidural anesthesia be used? [Refs 330–332]

19. When is a continuous infusion of epidural anesthesia useful? [Ref 334]

20. What complications can be associated with epidural anesthesia? [Ref 336]

Intravenous Block (Bier Block)

337. A Bier block is used most often for surgeries of the upper extremities that last an hour or less.

338. A Bier block involves the injection of a local anesthetic agent into the vein of a tourniquet-occluded extremity. The procedures is conducted as follows:

   • An intravenous catheter is inserted into the operative extremity.

   • A double-cuffed tourniquet is placed on the extremity.

   • The extremity is exsanguinated by tightly wrapping an Esmarch bandage from the distal extremity to the tourniquet.

   • The proximal bladder of the tourniquet is inflated, and a fixed amount of anesthetic agent—lidocaine (Xylocaine)—is injected. The anesthetic agent infiltrates the extremity and is confined to the tissues that are distal to the tourniquet.

   • To alleviate tourniquet pain, the distal bladder is inflated after the anesthetic agent has taken effect and the proximal cuff is deflated.

339. After the procedure, the tourniquet is released slowly to control the escape of the anesthetic agent into the general circulation. Rapid release can result in cardiovascular collapse or central nervous system toxicity.

Nerve Block

340. Nerve blocks can be used for purposes of surgical intervention but are more commonly used for sustained relief in patients with chronic pain and to increase circulation in some vascular diseases.

341. Nerve blocks can be minor or major. Major blocks involve multiple nerves or a plexus. Minor blocks block a single nerve.

342. Major nerve blocks used in operative procedures include the brachial plexus block for procedures of the arm (interscalene, supraclavicular, infraclavicular, and axillary), orbital blocks for eye procedures, and cervical blocks for procedures involving the neck.

343. Common minor blocks are radial and ulnar nerve blocks for procedures of the elbow, wrist, or digits.

344. To create a nerve block, the anesthetic agent—usually lidocaine (Xylocaine)—is injected into and around a nerve or nerve group that supplies sensation to a small area of the body.

345. Ultrasound imaging can enhance nerve blocks by increasing the anesthesia provider's ability to visualize and infuse nerve fibers without cannulating adjacent vessels.

346. The perioperative nurse may assist during nerve block by aspirating the needle during placement to check for inadvertent vascular injection. Depending upon facility policy, state board of nursing regulations, and demonstrated competency, the nurse may also be asked to inject the local anesthetic while the anesthesia provider secures the placement of the needle.

Local Anesthetic Infiltration

347. Local infiltration involves the injection of the anesthetic agent into subcutaneous tissue at, or close to, the anticipated incision site.

348. Local infiltration is useful for minor, superficial procedures.

349. The most frequently used local anesthetic is lidocaine (Xylocaine). Depending upon the location, epinephrine may be added to the lidocaine to cause vasoconstriction, reduce bleeding, and slow absorption of the drug.

350. During local anesthesia, the perioperative nurse should monitor the patient's blood pressure, cardiac rate and rhythm, respiratory rate, oxygen saturation, level of consciousness, pain level, skin temperature and color, amount and local anesthetic administered, and response to medications.

351. Toxic reactions to local anesthetics can occur with too rapid an absorption from a vascular site or if there is an inadvertent intravascular injection. Toxic reactions include central nervous system and cardiovascular depression. The nurse must be alert to the possibility of a toxic reaction.

352. Initial signs of central nervous system toxicity include restlessness, lightheadedness, visual and auditory disturbances, dizziness, tremors, and convulsions, sometimes followed by unconsciousness, apnea, and cardiac arrest. Patients who say that they hear unusual sounds

or express a feeling of uneasiness may be experiencing a toxic reaction.

353. Initial treatment consists of establishing and maintaining an airway, assisting or controlling ventilation with oxygen, and administering sedation. It is the perioperative nurse's responsibility to ensure that resuscitation equipment is available when local anesthetics are administered.

Local Infiltration for Postoperative Pain Relief

354. Bupivacaine liposome (Exparel) is a local anesthetic comprised of bupivacaine encapsulated in a liposome, a formulation that releases the drug slowly over an extended period of time. Exparel is introduced into the wound at the end of a surgical procedure to provide postoperative pain relief that lasts approximately 24 hours.

355. Bupivacaine liposome should be injected no sooner than 20 minutes following administration of another local anesthetic, because other local anesthetics can cause an immediate release of the bupivacaine from the liposome, reducing the effectiveness of the drug and creating a possible overdose situation.

356. No other form of bupivacaine should be given at the same time as Exparel because of the potential for an overdose situation.

357. Because the liposome is metabolized by the liver, bupivacaine liposome is contraindicated in patients with severe liver disease.

358. Bupivacaine has been known to be excreted by the kidneys; hence, there is greater risk of toxicity in patients with impaired renal function.

359. The effects of Exparel have not been studied in pregnant women, nor has the drug been tested on patients under the age of 18 years. Nursing infants can be exposed to a dose of the drug via breastmilk, so a decision must be made based on the mother's need for pain relief whether to avoid using the drug while nursing, or to stop nursing for a period of time.

Topical Anesthesia

360. A topical anesthetic is applied directly to a mucous membrane or an open wound. Topical anesthetics are readily absorbed by mucous membranes and, therefore, act rapidly.

361. Topical anesthesia is often used for nasal surgery, cystoscopy, and procedures of the respiratory tract in which it is advantageous to eliminate cough and laryngeal reflex (gag reflex).

362. Sudden cardiovascular collapse is possible following the application of topical anesthetic in the respiratory tract. Resuscitation equipment should be immediately available.

363. Commonly used topical anesthetics include tetracaine (Pontocaine) for the eye, cocaine for nasal passages, and lidocaine (Xylocaine) for throat, nose, esophagus, and genitourinary tract. Lidocaine may be supplied as a liquid, liquid spray, or jelly.

Nursing Implications

364. Nursing responsibilities vary according to the type of regional anesthesia being administered.

365. Patients scheduled for regional anesthesia may be apprehensive about being awake during surgery, believing that will experience pain or will be unable to avoid observing the surgery. Provide reassurance, answer questions, and remain close to the patient to alleviate their anxiety. Even patients who are sedated should be aware that the nurse is close by and is available to provide support.

366. For some procedures, it is important that the patient be alert and able to cooperate with the surgeon to facilitate the procedure. In these circumstances, the perioperative nurse can provide encouragement, support, and information that the patient needs.

367. Conversation during the procedure should be respectful because patients receiving regional anesthesia are awake. Though they may be given supplemental tranquilizers and may sleep, they are arousable and may be startled by noise or made anxious by inappropriate conversation. Placing a sign on the door of the operating suite stating that the patient is awake will serve as a reminder to persons who enter.

368. During placement of the needle for spinal, epidural, caudal, and nerve block, the patient should be protected from unnecessary exposure to prevent embarrassment and becoming chilled. Provide pillows and blankets for patient comfort.

369. Preparation of the incision site with an antiseptic scrub may necessitate exposing the patient and may cause the awake patient

embarrassment or anxiety. It is important to reassure the patient, maintain dignity, and minimize exposure.

370. Every patient receiving some type of regional anesthesia should be monitored. The extent of monitoring and the person responsible for monitoring are determined by the anesthesia technique, the results of preoperative assessment, the surgical procedure, recognized anesthesia standards and practices, and the facility's policy.

371. During spinal, epidural, and caudal anesthesia; intravenous block; and nerve block, an anesthesia provider is present.

372. Administration of topical and local infiltration anesthetics is the surgeon's responsibility. It is unusual for an anesthesia provider to be present; hence, monitoring the patient's physiologic and psychological status is the responsibility of the perioperative nurse.

373. The nurse who monitors the patient receiving local anesthesia must be able to establish the patient's normal baseline data and recognize any changes that occur. Baseline data must include blood pressure, cardiac rate and rhythm, respirations, oxygen saturation, skin condition, and mental status.

374. The perioperative nurse is also responsible for familiarity with the drugs used and the appropriate responses to possible drug reactions.

375. During local anesthesia, the perioperative nurse should track and monitor the amount of anesthetic agent given. The maximum recommended dose of 1% lidocaine without epinephrine should not exceed 4.5 mg/kg of body weight, and the maximum total dose should not exceed 300 mg. The maximum recommended dose of lidocaine with epinephrine should not exceed 7 mg/kg, and the maximum total dose is 500 mg (Kapitanyan, 2012; RxList, 2015).

376. Lidocaine with epinephrine may jeopardize circulation if used on fingers or toes. Vasoconstriction can cause vascular compromise. Also, lidocaine should be used judiciously on patients with vascular insufficiency. The surgeon should be kept abreast of the amount infiltrated.

377. Nursing interventions for all patients who receive regional anesthesia should include preparation for toxic systemic reactions of the central nervous system and cardiovascular collapse.

378. Resuscitation equipment must be immediately available, and the perioperative nurse monitoring the patient must be able to use it competently.

379. The nurse must also be able to prepare medications appropriately and recognize their actions and untoward reactions.

380. Current cardiopulmonary resuscitation (CPR) certification is an essential requirement for the perioperative nurse.

Medication Safety

381. In recognition of the significant risk of patient injury related to medication errors, one of The Joint Commission's (2015) National Patient Safety Goals relates to medication use: "Improve the safety of using medications."

382. The perioperative nurse who functions in either the scrub role or as the circulating nurse shares responsibility for achieving the desired patient outcome: "The correct patient receives the correct medication(s) in accurate doses, at the correct time, and via the correct route throughout the perioperative experience" (AORN, 2011, p. 203).

383. To avoid medication errors, TJC requires that all medications/solutions on and off the sterile field be labeled. Many operating rooms have purchased sterile labeling kits for this purpose. Some kits contain printed labels; others have blank labels to use with a sterile marking pen. Items that must be labeled include the following:

    - Syringes
    - Basins
    - Medicine cups
    - Bowls
    - Other containers

384. Before dispensing a medication, the circulating nurse should confirm that the medication is not contraindicated because of patient allergy or interaction with other substance(s) the patient may be taking. The healthcare facility pharmacist should be consulted if any question arises regarding the appropriateness of the medication.

385. Whenever a medication is delivered to the sterile field, the scrub person and the circulating nurse should visually, verbally, and concurrently confirm the medication name, strength, dose, concentration, and expiration date.

386. If the scrub person or circulating nurse is relieved, the hand-off report given to the relieving personnel should include verification of all medications. Any unlabeled medications or solutions should be discarded.

387. It is not uncommon for verbal medication orders to be given to the circulating nurse during surgery. It is critical that the circulating nurse confirm the order. The operating room can be a busy place with multiple distractions. Surgical masks that muffle sound, background noise from activity, talking, telephone and beeper rings, equipment alarms, monitoring equipment sounds, and music can all interfere with communication and result in a misunderstood verbal medication order. When a verbal order is given, it is essential to ensure clear communication, validate understanding of the order, and prevent any misunderstanding.

388. At a minimum, the verbal order should be repeated and confirmed. Ideally, the verbal order should be written on a dry-erase board and read back to the person who issued the order. Verbal confirmation, coupled with visual confirmation, can decrease the risk of error and prevent injury to the patient.

389. The perioperative nurse should ensure that the patient's medication list is readily available and visible. This list should be checked for completeness—medication history, medication, dose, and schedule. Responsibility for medication reconciliation may vary according to facility and department. It is the responsibility of the perioperative nurse to know the facility policy for medication reconciliation and his or her related responsibilities.

Section Questions

1. For what procedures is a Bier block most frequently used? [Ref 337]

2. Describe the process of creating a Bier block. [Ref 338]

3. What is the purpose of deflating the tourniquet slowly? [Ref 339]

4. How are nerve blocks most commonly used? [Ref 340]

5. Differentiate between major and minor nerve blocks. [Refs 341–343]

6. How are nerve blocks created? [Ref 344]

7. How can ultrasound enhance the process of creating a nerve block? [Ref 345]

8. How does the perioperative nurse assist the anesthesia provider during nerve blocks? [Ref 346]

9. Describe local infiltration of an anesthetic agent. [Ref 347]

10. What is the purpose of epinephrine when added to lidocaine for a local infiltration? [Ref 349]

11. What does the perioperative nurse monitor during local infiltration of anesthetic? [Ref 350]

12. How can toxic reactions to local infiltration occur? [Ref 351]

13. What are the symptoms of toxic infiltration? [Ref 352]

14. What is the perioperative nurse's responsibility in case of a toxic reaction? [Ref 353]

15. What is the intended outcome of using bupivacaine liposome? [Ref 354]

16. What length of time must separate the administration of bupivacaine liposome and any other local anesthetic? [Ref 355]

17. What can happen if bupivacaine liposome and another local anesthetic agent are administered at the same time? [Ref 355]

18. In what patient population is bupivacaine liposome contraindicated? [Ref 357]

19. When is topical anesthesia most frequently used? [Ref 361]

20. What adverse outcome is associated with topical anesthetic use in the respiratory tract? [Ref 362]

(continues)

21. How can the perioperative nurse allay the fear of a patient who worries about being awake during a procedure being performed with regional anesthesia? [Ref 365]

22. What is important about conversation during a procedure where the patient is receiving regional anesthesia? [Ref 367]

23. What factors determine the extent of monitoring, and who will do the monitoring when regional anesthesia is used? [Ref 370]

24. Who is primarily responsible for administering topical and local anesthesia? [Ref 372]

25. When the patient is receiving a local infiltration, what will the perioperative nurse monitor? [Ref 373]

26. To prevent medication errors, what items does TJC require be labeled on and off the sterile field? [Ref 383]

27. Which precautions does the perioperative nurse take before dispensing any medication? [Ref 384]

28. How do the circulating nurse and the scrub person handle medications delivered to the sterile field? [Ref 386]

29. When personnel relieve one another, how should unlabeled medications be managed? [Ref 387]

30. What is a safe approach to verifying verbal orders? [Refs 388, 389]

References

Adriani M., & Moriber N. (2013). Preoperative forced-air warming combined with intraoperative warming versus intraoperative warming alone in the prevention of hypothermia during gynecologic surgery. *AANA Journal, 81*(6): 446–451. Retrieved from http://www.aana.com/newsandjournal/Documents/preoperative-forced-air-1213-p446-451.pdf

American Association of Nurse Anesthetists (AANA). (2015). *Anesthesia awareness fact sheet.* Retrieved from http://www.aana.com/forpatients/Pages/Anesthetic-Awareness-Fact-Sheet.aspx

American Society of Anesthesiologists (ASA). (2006). Practice advisory for intraoperative awareness and brain function monitoring. *Anesthesiology, 104*: 847–864.

American Society of Anesthesiologists (ASA). (2011). *Standards for basic anesthetic monitoring.* Retrieved from http://www.asahq.org/~/media/sites/asahq/files/public/resources/standards-guidelines/standards-for-basic-anesthetic-monitoring.pdf

American Society of Anesthesiologists (ASA). (2012a). Practice advisory for preanesthesia evaluation: An updated report by the American Society of Anesthesiologists task force on preanesthesia evaluation. *Anesthesiology, 116*(3): 1–17.

American Society of Anesthesiologists (ASA). (2012b). Practice guidelines for central venous access. *Anesthesiology, 116*(3): 539–573. Retrieved from http://www.asahq.org/~/media/sites/asahq/files/public/resources/standards-guidelines/practice-guidelines-for-central-venous-access.pdf#search=%22central%20venous%20access%22

American Society of Anesthesiologists (ASA). (2014). *ASA physical status classification system.* Park Ridge, IL: ASA. Retrieved from http://www.asahq.org/resources/clinical-information/asa-physical-status-classification-system

American Society of Anesthesiologists (ASA), Committee on Standards and Practice Parameters (ASA). (2011a). Practice guidelines for preoperative fasting and the use of pharmacologic agents to reduce the risk of pulmonary aspiration: Application to healthy patients undergoing elective procedures. *Anesthesiology, 114*(3): 495–511.

Association of periOperative Registered Nurses (AORN). (2011). *Perioperative nursing data set* (3rd ed.). Denver, CO: AORN.

Association of periOperative Registered Nurses (AORN). (2015). Guidelines for managing the Patient receiving moderation/analgesia. In *Guidelines for Perioperative Practice* (pp. 553–561). Denver, CO: AORN.

Bainbridge, D., Martin, J., Arango, M., & Cheng, D. (2012). Perioperative and anaesthetic-related mortality in developed and developing countries: A systematic review and meta-analysis. *Lancet, 380*(8947): 1075–1081.

Gan, T.J., Glass, P.S.A., Sigl, J., Sebel, P., Payne, F., Rosow, C., & Embree, P. (1999). Women emerge from general anesthesia faster than men. *Anesthesiology, 90*: 1283.

Hart, S., Bordes, B., Hart, J., Corsino, D., & Harmon, D. (2011). Unintended perioperative hypothermia. *The Oschner Journal, 11*(3): 259–270. Retrieved from http://ochsnerjournal.org/doi/pdf/10.1043/1524-5012-11.3.259

Litwack, K. (1995). *Post anesthesia nursing care.* St. Louis, MO: Mosby Year Book.

Malignant Hyperthermia Association of the United States (MHAUS). (2015). *What is MH?* Retrieved from http://www.mhaus.org/

Malignant Hyperthermia Association of the United States (MHAUS). (2015). What should be on an MH Cart? (Drugs). Retrieved from http://www.mhaus.org/faqs/stocking-an-mh-cart

National Institutes of Occupational Safety and Health (NIOSH). (2014). *Criteria for a recommended standard: Occupational exposure to waste anesthetic gases and vapors.* Washington, DC: NIOSH. Retrieved from http://www.cdc.gov/niosh/docs/1970/77-140.html

National Institutes of Occupational Safety and Health (NIOSH). (2015). *Pocket guide to chemical hazards: Nitrous oxide.* Washington, DC: NIOSH. Retrieved from http://www.cdc.gov/niosh/npg/npgd0465.html

Occupational Safety and Health Administration (OSHA). (2000). Anesthetic gases: Guidelines for workplace exposures. Retrieved from https://www.osha.gov/dts/osta/anestheticgases/index.html

Occupational Safety and Health Administration (OSHA). (2015). *Surgical suite module.* Washington, DC: OSHA. Retrieved from www.osha.gov/SLTC/etools/hospital/surgical/surgical.html

Rajagopalan, S., Mascha, E., Na, J., & Sessler, D. (2008). The effects of mild perioperative hypothermia on blood loss and transfusion requirement. *Anesthesiology, 108*(1): 71–77. Retrieved from http://www.ncbi.nlm.nih.gov/pubmed/18156884

RxList: The Internet Drug Index. (2015). *Xylocaine dosage.* Retrieved from http://www.rxlist.com/xylocaine-drug/indications-dosage.htm

Seaman, M., Wobb, J., Gaughan, J., Kulp, H., Kamel, I., & Dempsey, D.T. (2012). The effects of intraoperative hypothermia on surgical site infection. *Annals of Surgery, 255*(4): 789–795.

Sellick, B.A. (1961). Cricoid pressure to control regurgitation of stomach contents during induction of anæsthesia. *Lancet, 278*(7199): 404–406.

Shekelle, P., & Dallas, P. (2013). *Chapter 18: Use of real-time ultrasound guidance during central line insertion: Brief update review in making health care safer II: An updated critical analysis of the evidence for patient safety practices. Evidence reports/technology assessments, No. 211.* Rockville, MD: Agency for Healthcare Research and Quality (US). Retrieved from http://www.ncbi.nlm.nih.gov/pubmedhealth/PMH0055966/

Surgical Care Improvement Project (SCIP). (2015). *SCIP process and outcome measures.* Retrieved from http://www.dshs.state.tx.us/WorkArea/linkit.aspx?LinkIdentifier=id&ItemID=23895

The Joint Commission (TJC). (2004). *Sentinel event alert: Preventing and managing the impact of anesthesia awareness.* Retrieved from www.jointcommission.org/sentinel_event_alert_issue_32_preventing_and_managing_the_impact_of_anesthesia_awareness/

The Joint Commission (TJC). (2015a). *National patient safety goals effective January 1, 2015.* Retrieved from http://www.jointcommission.org/assets/1/6/2015_NPSG_HAP.pdf

The Joint Commission (TJC). (2015b). *Comprehensive accreditation manual for hospitals.* Retrieved from http://www.mitsstools.org/uploads/3/7/7/6/3776466/psc_for_web.pdf

Trissell, L. (2014). *Handbook of injectible drugs* (18th ed.). Bethesda, MD: American Society of Health-System Pharmacists.

Valdez-Lowe, C., Ghareeb, S., & Artinian, N. (2009). Pulse oximetry in adults. *American Journal of Nursing, 109*(6): 52–59. Retrieved from http://www.nursingcenter.com/cearticle?tid=864063

Wu, X. (2013). The safe and efficient use of forced-air warming systems. *AORN Journal, 97*(3): 302–308.

Post-Test

Part 1

Read each question carefully. Each question may have more than one correct response.

1. Which of the following is not considered patient injuries related to anesthesia?

    a. Untoward drug reaction

    b. Hypothermia

    c. Decreased cardiac output

    d. Dehydration

2. The Aldrete scoring system evaluates all of the following *except*

    a. activity.

    b. respiration.

    c. end tidal CO_2.

    d. circulation.

3. Anesthesia providers include all of the following *except*

    a. an anesthesiologist.

    b. a CRNFA.

    c. an AA.

    d. a CRNA.

4. The hand-off report from the circulator to the PACU nurse should include

    a. drug allergies.

    b. a surgical safety checklist.

    c. estimated blood loss.

    d. intraoperative medications.

5. Which statement(s) is/are true about preanesthesia data?

    a. Chest X-ray, urinalysis, and blood chemistry panel should be present for all preoperative patients.

    b. In healthy patients, there is no evidence that routine preoperative testing affects patient outcomes.

    c. It is important to know if a patient is taking beta-blocker medication.

    d. Guidelines may require certain preoperative tests based on the age of the patient or risk factors.

6. Smoking history is important because smokers can experience

    a. more problems with wound complications.

    b. pulmonary and cardiac complications.

    c. a need for increased anesthetic dosage.

    d. increased postoperative pain.

7. Benefits of smoking cessation can be evident in as few as _____ hours.

    a. 48

    b. 24

    c. 12

    d. 6

8. Which of the following is a correct description of the classes that the ASA uses for communicating physical status (PS):
   a. PS1—essentially healthy, mild organic disease (e.g., controlled diabetes mellitus)
   b. PS2—mild systemic disease (e.g., controlled hypertension)
   c. PS3—severe systemic disease that is a threat to life (e.g., unstable angina, symptomatic congestive heart failure, hepatorenal failure)
   d. PS6—moribund; not expected to survive

9. Which of the following is an accurate fasting recommendation for patients of all ages?
   a. Clear liquids—2 hours before surgery
   b. Light meal—10 hours before surgery
   c. Heavy meal—surgery should be canceled
   d. Infant formula—2 hours before surgery

10. Factors that are considered when selecting anesthetic agents and technique include
    a. age.
    b. patient preference.
    c. surgeon preference.
    d. anesthesia provider preference.

11. When conscious sedation is administered by an anesthesia provider, it is called
    a. AAS—anesthesia-assisted sedation.
    b. MAC—monitored anesthesia care.
    c. CSA—conscious sedation by anesthesia.
    d. ADS—anesthesia-delivered sedation.

12. Regional anesthesia is anesthesia delivered
    a. to a section of the body, such as a limb or the lower half of the body.
    b. as a single injection or over a long period of time.
    c. via mask induction.
    d. by both central and peripheral techniques.

13. Which statement(s) is/are true about preoperative medications/protocols?
    a. Most IV agents are administered 30–60 minutes prior to surgery.
    b. Midazolam (Versed) and diazepam (Valium) reduce anxiety and provide some amnesia.
    c. Valium is used infrequently because of its short duration of action.
    d. Metoclopramide (Reglan) is an antisialagogue given to reduce oral secretions.

14. Anticholinergics are
    a. given routinely to all patients.
    b. useful in preventing postoperative nausea.
    c. useful with patients who salivate excessively.
    d. appropriate for toddlers and children.

15. Which of the following preoperative antibiotics must be started before the 1-hour window?
    a. Kefzol
    b. Ancef
    c. Vancomycin
    d. Mefoxin

16. Patients who receive narcotics must be observed closely because

    a. narcotics provide relief from pain.

    b. narcotics can be abused.

    c. it is not uncommon for patients to have adverse reactions to narcotics.

    d. all narcotics are associated with a dose-related respiratory depression and can cause nausea and vomiting.

17. Minimum monitoring for all surgical patients should include

    a. oxygenation.

    b. ventilation.

    c. circulation.

    d. temperature.

18. The choice of monitoring device is determined by

    a. the procedure.

    b. the anesthesia provider's and surgeon's judgment.

    c. the patient's history and state of health.

    d. anticipated postoperative management.

19. Which statement(s) is/are true about pulse oximetry?

    a. Pulse oximetry measures the oxygen saturation of venous hemoglobin.

    b. O_2 saturation readings should be near 100%.

    c. O_2 saturation readings less than 95% are usually indicative of hypoxemia.

    d. Dark nail polish and acrylic nails must be removed because they obscure pulse oximetry readings.

20. Which statement(s) is/are true about hypothermia?

    a. Hypothermia is defined as body temperature less than 34°C.

    b. Hypothermia is linked to shivering, which increases oxygen consumption.

    c. Hypothermia is linked to extended recovery and surgical site infection.

    d. Hypothermia can result in increased perioperative blood loss.

21. The best approach to warming the surgical patient is

    a. warm blankets.

    b. warmed irrigating fluids.

    c. raising the room temperature.

    d. a forced-air warming blanket.

22. The greatest change in patient temperature during surgery occurs within the first

    a. 30 minutes.

    b. 60 minutes.

    c. 90 minutes.

    d. 120 minutes.

23. Capnography is useful in detecting

    a. hypoventilation.

    b. respiratory insufficiency.

    c. esophageal intubation.

    d. a disconnected circuit.

24. The effects of general anesthesia include
    a. amnesia.
    b. hypnosis.
    c. analgesia.
    d. skeletal muscle relaxation.

25. Which statement(s) is/are true about nitrous oxide?
    a. Nitrous oxide acts rapidly but lacks potency.
    b. Nitrous oxide is nonirritating and produces few aftereffects.
    c. Nitrous oxide diffuses readily into gas-filled spaces (e.g., stomach, lungs, colon).
    d. A high concentration of nitrous oxide can lead to hypoxia.

Part 2

1. Which statement(s) is/are true about desflurane?
   a. Desflurane is the agent of choice for obese patients because of its low fat solubility.
   b. Desflurane is rarely used in ambulatory surgery.
   c. Desflurane has a slow rate of induction and emergence.
   d. Desflurane is highly recommended for inhalation anesthesia.

2. Which statement(s) is/are true about volatile anesthetics?
   a. Sevoflurane has a pungent odor, which can cause gagging and laryngospasm.
   b. Isoflurane provides the most rapid induction and emergence.
   c. Sevoflurane is the induction inhalation of choice for children.
   d. Sevoflurane is irritating to the respiratory tract and the myocardium.

3. What are the color codes for tanks and fittings of O_2, N_2O, and air?
   a. Oxygen cylinders and fittings are green.
   b. Nitrous tanks and fittings are yellow.
   c. Compressed nitrogen tanks and fittings are white.
   d. Air tanks and fittings are blue.

4. Which statement(s) is/are true about anesthesia machines?
   a. The machine has a reservoir bag that can be compressed like an Ambu bag.
   b. Expired gases pass through a carbon dioxide absorber system.
   c. A scavenger system on the machine collects expired gases and vents them to outside air.
   d. A shutoff valve prevents delivery of nitrous oxide if the accompanying oxygen is less than 21%.

5. Which statement(s) is/are true about induction agents?
   a. Barbiturates are potent respiratory depressants, are short acting, and do not provide analgesia.
   b. Diprivan is the most popular nonbarbiturate induction agent.
   c. Etomidate is used for cardiac patients who cannot tolerate changes in blood pressure.
   d. Sodium pentothal results in a rapid progression from sedation to loss of consciousness.

6. Which statement(s) is/are true about ketamine?
   a. Ketamine produces a catatonic state; the patient may appear to be awake.
   b. Ketamine is used only for children.
   c. Patients should recover from ketamine in a quiet, darkened area.
   d. It is a myth that patients hallucinate postoperatively when ketamine is used.

7. Which statement(s) is/are true about narcotics?

    a. Fentanyl is more potent than morphine; sufentanil is more potent than fentanyl.

    b. Narcotics provide profound analgesia; they can also provide pain relief in the early postoperative period.

    c. Narcotics are respiratory stimulants.

    d. Demerol is used intraoperatively more frequently than other narcotics.

8. Which statement(s) is/are true about tranquilizers?

    a. Diazepam (Valium) and midazolam (Versed) are used intraoperatively.

    b. Using a tranquilizer intraoperatively permits the use of lower doses of other anesthetic agents.

    c. Diazepam produces amnesia and reduces anxiety.

    d. Respiratory depression from tranquilizers can be reversed with flumazenil (Romazicon).

9. What are the two primary indications for neuromuscular blockers?

    a. Prepare the patient for mask inhalation.

    b. Relax the jaw and larynx to facilitate tracheal intubation.

    c. Increase muscle relaxation to permit ease of tissue handling during surgery.

    d. Block impulses from the autonomic nervous system.

10. Conditions that put patients at risk for succinylcholine-induced hyperkalemia include

    a. cerebral stroke.

    b. hypertension.

    c. hypovolemia.

    d. Guillain-Barré syndrome.

11. Which statement(s) is/are true about the perioperative nurse's responsibilities related to preparation for anesthesia?

    a. The room should be ready when the patient arrives so the perioperative nurse can focus on the patient throughout induction.

    b. Suction should be working and available to the anesthesia provider.

    c. Talking should be kept to a minimum.

    d. The scrubbed person should work quietly at the back table.

12. Induction is the period from

    a. entering the room until the patient is asleep.

    b. moving onto the operating room table into the anesthesia provider's care until he or she is asleep.

    c. giving first anesthetic drug until the patient is stabilized at the desired level of anesthesia.

    d. placing the mask over the patient's face until the patient is intubated.

13. Which of the following is the first intervention in the sequence of induction of anesthesia?

    a. Sodium pentothal or propofol is injected.

    b. The endotracheal tube is inserted and secured.

    c. A paralyzing dose of muscle relaxant is administered.

    d. The patient breathes 100% O_2 by mask.

14. Which statement(s) is/are true about the perioperative nurse's role when the patient is given a barbiturate or hypnotic at the start of induction?

    a. Suction if the patient regurgitates to prevent aspiration.

    b. Lift the patient's head to prevent aspiration.

    c. Adjust the table to the reverse Trendelenburg position.

    d. Provide an emesis basin if the patient begins to regurgitate.

15. The Sellick maneuver
    a. involves firmly pressing the thyroid cartilage posteriorly with the thumb and forefinger.
    b. compresses the esophagus between the cricoid cartilage and the vertebral column.
    c. aids in visualization of the esophagus for intubation.
    d. is performed once the endotracheal tube is in place and the cuff has been inflated.

16. Malignant hyperthermia (MH) might present with which of the following symptoms?
    a. Unexplained rise in temperature
    b. Masseter muscle rigidity
    c. Unexplained tachycardia
    d. Metabolic alkalosis

17. MH can be triggered by which of the following anesthetic agents?
    a. Sufentanil
    b. Meperidine
    c. Sublimaze
    d. Succinylcholine

18. Risk factors for MH include a family history of
    a. MH or unexplained death from anesthesia experience.
    b. unexplained death during surgery.
    c. unexplained muscle cramps with fever.
    d. inherited skeletal muscle disorders.

19. In the event of an MH diagnosis during surgery, which of the following actions is appropriate?
    a. Get help.
    b. Reconstitute dantrolene sodium.
    c. Get the MH cart.
    d. Replace the breathing circuit or the entire anesthesia machine.

20. How long should dantrolene sodium administration be continued after an MH incident?
    a. 12 hours
    b. 24 hours
    c. 36 hours
    d. 48 hours or longer

21. Following an episode of MH
    a. the patient must be monitored closely for a recurrent episode.
    b. the prognosis for recovery is poor.
    c. the patient must be referred for genetic testing.
    d. the patient should not undergo surgery in the future.

22. What criteria are important for the nurse who is monitoring the patient receiving moderate sedation?
    a. The nurse must be able to recognize and manage basic cardiac dysrhythmias.
    b. The nurse must be certified in advanced cardiac life support (ACLS).
    c. The circulating nurse must be able to spend most of the time with the patient.
    d. The perioperative nurse should have no other responsibilities during the procedure.

23. At a minimum, which equipment should be available when the patient is receiving moderate sedation?

    a. Pulse oximeter

    b. Blood pressure monitor

    c. Temperature monitor

    d. ECG

24. Which of the following are criteria for discharge following conscious sedation?

    a. Return to baseline level of consciousness

    b. Absence of nausea and vomiting

    c. Adequate pain control

    d. Return of motor/sensory control

25. Which statement(s) is/are true about regional anesthesia?

    a. Regional anesthesia is preferable for emergency surgery when the patient has a full stomach.

    b. With regional anesthesia, the respiratory system remains relatively stable.

    c. Regional anesthesia can cause cardiac instability.

    d. Regional anesthesia can be used with patients in whom general anesthesia is contraindicated (e.g., patients with metabolic, hepatic, or renal disease).

26. Which statement(s) is/are true about spinal anesthesia?

    a. Administration of spinal anesthesia requires cooperation from the patient.

    b. Aseptic technique is essential to prevent meningitis.

    c. Anesthetic agents settle by gravity and the block is sensitive to the patient's position.

    d. Treatment of a "spinal headache" includes hydration, sedation, and bed rest.

27. Which statement(s) is/are true about a Bier block?

    a. A Bier block involves the use of a double tourniquet.

    b. Anesthetic is injected into the artery before the tourniquet is inflated.

    c. The second cuff is inflated and the first cuff is deflated to increase the circulation of the anesthetic.

    d. The tourniquet is released rapidly to release the remaining anesthetic from the extremity.

28. Major nerve blocks used in operative procedures include

    a. brachial plexus block.

    b. orbital block.

    c. spinal block.

    d. cervical block.

29. Which statement(s) is/are true about toxic reactions to local infiltration?

    a. Toxic reaction can occur if absorption from a vascular site is too rapid.

    b. Toxic reaction can occur following inadvertent intravascular injection.

    c. Cardiovascular depression can be a toxic reaction.

    d. Restlessness and visual and auditory disturbances are symptoms of central nervous system toxicity.

30. Which statement(s) is/are true about nursing responsibilities related to regional anesthesia?

    a. Every patient receiving some type of regional anesthesia should be monitored.

    b. During local anesthesia, the perioperative nurse should monitor the amount of anesthetic agent given.

    c. Resuscitation equipment should be immediately available.

    d. All medications should be labeled.

Competency Checklist: Anesthesia

Under "Observer's Initials," enter initials upon successful achievement of competency.
Enter N/A if competency is not appropriate for institution.

Name _____

	Observer's Initials	Date

Preoperative Assessment

1. Assesses patient/chart for anesthetic considerations (as applicable): _____ _____

   a. Coexisting disease _____ _____

   b. NPO status _____ _____

   c. Allergies to medications, contrast dyes, tape, latex _____ _____

   d. Current medications, including herbal and nutritional supplements _____ _____

   e. Previous surgeries _____ _____

   f. Patient/family history of anesthesia complications _____ _____

   g. Substance abuse _____ _____

   h. Pregnancy _____ _____

   i. Diagnostic testing _____ _____

   j. Response to preoperative medications _____ _____

   k. Anxiety level _____ _____

   l. Knowledge level _____ _____

   m. Previous anesthesia—complications _____ _____

   n. Other _____ _____

2. Verifies that patient is in compliance with preoperative instructions _____ _____

3. Communicates assessment data to surgical team as appropriate _____ _____

4. Provides emotional support (answers patient concerns, provides reassuring touch, etc.) to patient/family _____ _____

5. Provides information as needed to patient/family _____ _____

6. Reinforces preoperative teaching with patient/family _____ _____

General Anesthesia

7. In preparation for induction: _____ _____

   a. Checks suction and places for easy access to patient's mouth _____ _____

   b. Applies monitoring equipment (ECG leads, blood pressure cuff, pulse oximeter) _____ _____

   c. Places IV line _____ _____

   d. Applies safety strap _____ _____

   e. Limits patient exposure _____ _____

   f. Maintains quiet atmosphere _____ _____

   g. Remains at patient's side at head of table, provides reassurance _____ _____

8. At induction, assists in intubation as needed (passes endotracheal tube, applies cricoid pressure, suctions, inflates cuff, etc.) _____ _____

9. Following induction: _____ _____

   a. Checks position and pressure points and provides protective devices as needed _____ _____

   b. Applies warming devices as appropriate (lengthy procedure, large/deep incision, etc.) _____ _____

10. Monitors fluid output and replacement and irrigating fluid   _____   _____

11. During emergence and extubation: _____   _____

    a. Facilitates quiet, relaxing environment to minimize excitement   _____   _____

    b. Checks suction and places for easy access to patient's mouth   _____   _____

    c. Remains at head of operatingtable by patient   _____   _____

    d. Assists anesthesia care provider as needed (suction, Ambu, O_2, etc.)   _____   _____

12. Provides handoff report to post-anesthesia care unit (e.g., patient name and age, surgical procedure, surgeon and anesthesiologist, anesthesia technique, estimated blood loss, fluid and blood administration, urine output, response to surgery/anesthesia, lab results, chronic and acute health history, drug allergies, expected problems/suggested interventions, discharge plan, other)   _____   _____

Regional Anesthesia

13. Implements procedures to alert others that patient is awake   _____   _____

14. Assists in positioning patient for administration of regional anesthetic (e.g., provides stool for feet, instructs patient)   _____   _____

15. Provides safe environment for patient during positioning for administration of regional anesthetic (e.g., remains with patient)   _____   _____

16. Limits patient exposure during preparation for and administration of anesthesia   _____   _____

17. Monitors and reports amount of local anesthetic agent administered   _____   _____

Monitoring

18. Demonstrates ability to apply and use monitoring device and interpret data for: _____   _____

    a. Blood pressure   _____   _____

    b. Cardiac rate and rhythm   _____   _____

    c. Respiratory rate   _____   _____

    d. Oxygen saturation   _____   _____

    e. Mental status/level of consciousness   _____   _____

19. Demonstrates airway management, including use of oxygen delivery devices and equipment   _____   _____

20. Demonstrates ability to use resuscitative equipment   _____   _____

Emergency Preparations

21. Retrieves malignant hyperthermia supplies without hesitation   _____   _____

22. Explains protocol for malignant hyperthermia crisis   _____   _____

23. Ensures immediate availability of resuscitative equipment   _____   _____

IV, Conscious Sedation, and Local Procedures

24. Reports changes in patient condition and implements appropriate interventions   _____   _____

Documentation

25. Documents data as required by institutional policy   _____   _____

Anesthesia Machine

26. Identifies anesthesia machine components, oxygen flush button; monitors for ECG, blood pressure, pulse, respirations, breathing bag, carbon dioxide absorber canister, ventilator, flowmeters, scavenging system   _____   _____

27. Repeats/confirms verbal medication orders   _____   _____

28. Labels all medications   _____   _____

Additional Safety Measures

29. Verifies surgical site is marked (if appropriate to the surgery)   _____   _____

30. Participates in "time out"   _____   _____

31. Verifies presence and application of forced-air warming blanket as appropriate   _____ _____
32. Raises room temperature as appropriate   _____ _____
33. Verifies preop antibiotic order and administers when appropriate   _____ _____
34. Applies sequential compression devices when appropriate   _____ _____

Observer's Signature   Initials   Date

_____

Orientee's Signature

_____

11

Environment of Care and Life Safety

LEARNER OBJECTIVES

1. Review the elements of a safe environment of care related to patients and personnel.
2. List elements of a safety officer's responsibilities.
3. Identify chemical and physical hazards present in the operating room environment.
4. List the government organizations that publish regulations for healthcare worker safety.
5. List accrediting organizations' safety standards.
6. Define a sentinel event.
7. Define failure mode effects analysis (FMEA).
8. Discuss the most common causes of operating room fires.
9. Identify the Emergency Care Research Institute (ECRI) recommendations to decrease the chance of a fire in the operating room.
10. Define the acronyms RACE and PASS.
11. Describe the components of a fire safety plan.
12. Discuss elements of a fire drill report card.
13. Define the purpose of the line isolation monitoring (LIM) system.
14. Discuss elements of sharps safety.
15. State the guidelines for healthcare workers to follow when working in a room where radiation is present.
16. State the guidelines for healthcare workers to follow when working with lasers.
17. Discuss possible causes of low back pain in healthcare workers and the recommendations for preventing injury.
18. Describe the precautions for working with methyl methacrylate.
19. Discuss the difference between localized and systemic latex allergy reactions.
20. Discuss hazards of surgical smoke.
21. Discuss the personal protective equipment required in a perioperative setting.
22. Discuss the requirements of eyewash stations.

LESSON OUTLINE

Overview

1. Every healthcare facility has a safe environment of care (EOC) or safety plan to manage the workplace effectively and protect employees and patients from injury. The plan addresses threats to safety such as fire and disaster, and the physical, environmental, and chemical hazards that are inherent in the workplace. The plan includes injury-prevention strategies and plans for managing events effectively should they occur.

Culture of Safety—Just Culture

2. The Institute of Medicine (IOM) maintains that every patient deserves a healthcare environment that is safe, effective, efficient, patient centered, timely, and equitable. Healthcare workers, too, deserve a work environment that protects them from injury.

3. It is not unusual for an assessment of the environment to identify opportunities for improvement that require changes in structure, policy, protocols, and sometimes the facility culture itself.

4. The IOM (2001) in one of its landmark publications, *Crossing the Quality Chasm*, emphasized that meaningful change requires an investment in infrastructure and a culture shift. To create a truly safe healthcare environment, the facility's administration must be actively involved in the development of a culture that views errors as opportunities to improve the system and fosters openness, collaboration, teamwork, and learning from mistakes (IOM, 2001). This is known as a *just culture* or *culture of safety*. Without the support of the administration, no change in facility culture is sustainable.

5. A culture of safety relies on teamwork, respect for each individual as a change agent, openness and transparency, a commitment to prevention of harm, and the understanding that mistakes or near mistakes can promote long-term improvement rather than a focus for blame and punishment.

Regulations

6. Regulations have the force of law, and noncompliance can result in large financial penalties to the organization. Federal agencies that govern workplace safety include the Occupational Safety and Health Administration (OSHA) and the Environmental Protection Agency (EPA).

7. Many states have OSHA agencies as well. Standards established by state agencies are at least as effective as federal standards and may be more stringent. When OSHA gives "final approval" to a state's plan, it relinquishes its authority to cover occupational safety and health matters in that state.

8. In addition to enforcement, state agencies provide education, training, and consultation services.

Centers for Medicare and Medicaid Services (CMS) (www.cms.gov)

9. CMS is a government agency that provides both regulation and guidance in the healthcare arena.

10. Because senior citizens represent such a large percentage of the patient population, Medicare reimbursement accounts for a large portion of the revenue in most medical facilities.

11. CMS regulations such as not reimbursing for conditions that were *not present on admission (NPOA)* provide significant financial incentive to prevent healthcare-associated infections (HAIs). If an infection is acquired during a hospital stay (HAI), the CMS reimburses as though the secondary diagnosis (the HAI) was not present.

12. CMS also manages the Hospital Consumer Assessment of Healthcare Providers and Systems (HCAHPS) survey that solicits patients' perspectives of the care they received. The survey is not restricted to Medicare beneficiaries, hence the summary of responses represents a broad spectrum of hospital patients. HCAHPS scores impact CMS reimbursement.

Occupational Safety and Health Administration (OSHA) (www.osha.gov/law-regs.html)

13. OSHA, a federal agency established in 1970, has the primary responsibility for protecting the employee by publishing and enforcing legal workplace safety and health standards that are economically feasible.

14. OSHA regulations related to healthcare are printed in the Labor section (29) of the Code of Federal Regulations (CFR), Part 1910. Look at 29 CFR 1910.1030 for regulations related to bloodborne pathogens, including requirements for personal protective equipment (PPE; OSHA, 2015).

15. Under OSHA's General Duty Clause, every employee is entitled to a place of employment free from recognized hazards that are capable of causing or likely to cause death or serious physical harm.

16. Employers must create and implement an effective process that provides management support, involves employees in the plan, identifies problems, implements corrective actions, addresses employee and patient injury reports, provides periodic employee training, and evaluates ergonomics efforts.

17. OSHA can assess fines for workplace hazards and mandate changes to correct unsafe conditions.

Environmental Protection Agency (EPA) (www.epa.gov/lawsregs)

18. The EPA is a governmental agency that writes regulations and sets national standards to improve health by protecting the environment.

19. Under the EPA, the environment is protected from dumping of medical waste, medications, and emissions of pollutants into the air that would be harmful to the public.

20. Proper medical waste disposal is the responsibility of every employee, and each facility is held accountable for abiding by the laws and regulations.

21. Education on the proper disposal of all types of medical waste should be included in the facility's safety plan.

National Fire Protection Association (NFPA) (www.nfpa.org/codes-and-standards/document-information-pages)

22. The NFPA is a nonprofit organization, founded in 1896, that is devoted to eliminating death, injury, and property and economic loss due to fire, electrical, and related hazards by developing codes and standards to promote best practices.

23. The NFPA's *Fire Code* (NFPA1) and *Life Safety Code* (NFPA101) provide the basis for facilities' fire safety plans.

24. NFPA25, the standard related to fire protection systems, is the source of the rule that nothing may be stored closer to the ceiling than 18 inches, nor fewer than 18 inches below a sprinkler head.

Standards and Recommendations

25. Standards and recommendations carry the weight of community expectation, but they are not laws.

26. Organizations that provide standards for the healthcare community include federal agencies, professional organizations, and organizations that offer a voluntary accreditation process.

Centers for Disease Control and Prevention (CDC) (www.cdc.gov)

27. The CDC's mission is to keep Americans safe and healthy by tracking diseases, researching outbreaks, responding to emergencies of all kinds, and developing public health policies.

28. The CDC establishes guidelines for the prevention and management of diseases; it is not a rule-making body. However, CDC publications such as the *Guideline for Disinfection and Sterilization in Healthcare Facilities* (Rutala & Weber, 2008) and *Guidelines for Hand Hygiene in Health-Care Settings* (CDC, 2002), among others, prepared by the CDC's Healthcare Infection Control Practices Advisory Committee (HICPAC) set the standard for care in the United States.

National Institute for Occupational Safety and Health (NIOSH) (www.cdc.gov/niosh)

29. NIOSH, a federal agency also created in 1970, conducts research and recommends practical solutions to problems related to worker injury and illness, including biological hazards (bloodborne pathogens and tuberculosis), chemical hazards (ethylene oxide, glutaraldehyde, latex, laser/electrosurgical unit [ESU] plume), physical hazards (ergonomics and musculoskeletal disorders), and violence in the workplace.

30. NIOSH promotes continuous quality improvement activities that include staff participation in addition to management. Training and assessing knowledge and competence of all staff members are ongoing in an organization that supports and promotes safety.

American National Standards Institute (ANSI) (www.ansi.org)

31. ANSI was created in 1918 as a not-for-profit organization to be the voice of the U.S. marketplace for standards and to assess compliance with the standards. The organization has prepared standards that govern medical device safety and integrity and standards for aseptic processing of medical devices and supplies. ANSI works with other agencies such as the CDC, OSHA, and the Association for the Advancement of Medical Instrumentation to set and govern safety standards.

Association for the Advancement of Medical Instrumentation (AAMI) (www.aami.org)

32. AAMI was founded in 1967. A not-for-profit organization, it has become the primary resource for national and international standards for the use of safe and effective medical technology. ANSI/AAMI publication ST79, *Comprehensive Guide to Steam Sterilization and Sterility Assurance in Health Care Facilities,* provides the perioperative staff and the sterile processing department with standards for properly cleaning and reprocessing equipment and instrumentation.

Agency for Healthcare Research and Quality (AHRQ) (www.ahrq.gov)

33. AHRQ is the health services research arm of the U.S. Department of Health and Human Services (HHS). Its mission is to produce evidence to improve the quality of healthcare, to build the knowledge base for what works—and does not work—and to translate this knowledge into everyday practice and policymaking.

34. AHRQ specializes in research in the following major areas of healthcare:

- Quality improvement and patient safety
- Outcomes and effectiveness of care

- Clinical practice and technology assessment
- Healthcare organization and delivery systems
- Primary care (including preventive services)
- Healthcare costs and sources of payment

Emergency Care Research Institute (ECRI) (www.ecri.org)

35. ECRI is an international nonprofit organization whose mission is to benefit patient care by promoting the highest levels of safety, quality, and cost-effectiveness in healthcare.

36. AHRQ designated ECRI as an evidence-based practice center to systematically research the comparative effectiveness of brands, models, and procedures to improve patient safety.

Institute of Medicine (IOM) (http://iom .nationalacademies.org)

37. The Institute of Medicine (IOM), established in 1970, is an independent, nonprofit organization that provides unbiased and authoritative advice to decision makers and the public. It is a very well-respected research organization, and its reports have prompted major changes in healthcare structure and delivery in America.

38. *To Err is Human: Building a Safer Health System* (IOM, 2000) changed the focus in healthcare from patient outcomes to patient safety. *The Future of Nursing: Leading Change, Advancing Health* (IOM, 2010) has mobilized efforts in every state to prepare nurses to meet the objectives of increased access to quality healthcare and population health.

National Professional Organizations

39. Each healthcare delivery specialty has a professional organization that provides resources for best practice in that specialty and identifies standards of care that are accepted as a *community standard* throughout the country.

40. Specialty organizations that impact patient care delivered in the surgical setting include:

- American Association of Nurse Anesthetists (AANA)
- American Association of Surgical Physician Assistants (AASPA)
- American College of Surgeons (ACS)
- American Society of Anesthesiologists (ASA)

- American Society of PeriAnesthesia Nurses (ASPAN)
- Association of periOperative Registered Nurses (AORN)
- Association of Surgical Technologists (AST)

Accreditation

41. Earning accreditation demonstrates that a facility has achieved an established level of performance that is recognized by the community as above average. Each of the accrediting agencies has a slightly different focus and process, but all assess quality practice and accredit only those facilities that demonstrate excellence.

42. Acute care facilities are accredited by The Joint Commission, Healthcare Facilities Accreditation Program, or DNV GL Healthcare, while ambulatory settings may seek accreditation from The Joint Commission, Accreditation Association for Ambulatory Health Care, or the American Association for Accreditation of Ambulatory Surgery Facilities.

The Joint Commission (TJC) (www.jointcom mission.org)

43. TJC is an independent, not-for-profit organization that accredits and certifies healthcare organizations that voluntarily participate in a rigorous application process. TJC accreditation is recognized worldwide as an indication that a facility is committed to meeting acknowledged performance standards. TJC accredits 5,000 hospitals and 10,000 other types of facilities, and surveys its facilities every 3 years.

44. The Environment of Care (EC) chapter of The Joint Commission's standards addresses workplace safety. TJC expects both facility and staff to embrace the goal of fostering an environment that supports and promotes a culture of safety.

45. TJC identifies three basic elements of a safe environment:

- Building design that protects patients, visitors, and employees
- Equipment that is well maintained and safe to use on a regular basis
- People who are well informed and understand their responsibility in minimizing risks in the workplace (TJC, 2015a, pp. EC1–EC3)

46. TJC requires a safety plans that covers, at a minimum:

    - Safety and security of the building
    - Specific attention to security-sensitive areas: emergency department, children's ward, and nursery
    - Product failures or recalls
    - Smoking
    - Biohazardous materials
    - Hazardous waste, radiation, radioactive materials, medications, and harmful gases and vapors

Healthcare Facilities Accreditation Program (HFAP) (www.hfap.org)

47. HFAP has deeming authority from CMS and accredits approximately 200 hospitals and 200 other healthcare facilities, including laboratories (Meldi, Rhoades, & Gippe, 2009).

48. HFAP's physical and environmental standards include:

    - Fire drills and the equipment required in each department
    - Disaster response plans for internal and external disasters, including annual drills
    - Staff education on safety of the environment
    - Facilities maintenance program for building and equipment
    - Monitoring for compliance with safety plan
    - Actual overall safety of the building and equipment (HFAP, 2014)

DNVGL Healthcare (http://dnvglhealthcare.com)

49. DNVGL is an independent certification foundation established in Norway in 1864 as Det Norske Veritas (DNV). In 2013, DNV merged with GL making it one of the largest accrediting bodies in the world. DNVGL has been accrediting U.S. healthcare facilities since 2008. Between 2008 and 2015, the organization accredited nearly 500 hospitals across the United States (Meldi et al., 2009).

50. The DNVGL International Accreditation Standard (DIAS) integrates clinical and patient safety requirements with ISO 9001 Quality Management System principles. Like TJC accreditation, the process is voluntary.

51. DNVGL promotes a partnership relationship with facilities and surveys on an annual basis.

Accreditation Association for Ambulatory Health Care (AAAHC) (www.aaahc.org)

52. AAAHC was founded in 1979 by six member organizations as a peer-based, consultative, and educational survey process to advance patient care. Today there are 18 member organizations representing the broad spectrum of ambulatory health care. The organization currently accredits more than 6,000 facilities, including patient-centered medical homes (AAAHC, 2014).

53. In the AAAHC (2015) accreditation handbook, two chapters address the standards and expectations for a healthcare facility to meet national, state, and local standards for providing a safe environment for patients, visitors, and staff members.

American Association for Accreditation of Ambulatory Surgery Facilities (AAAASF) (www.aaaasf.org)

54. AAAASF was established in 1980 to develop an accreditation program to standardize and improve the quality of medical and surgical care in ambulatory surgery facilities.

55. AAAASF accredits more than 2,000 ambulatory surgery facilities.

Section Questions

1. What does a facility's safety plan address? [Ref 1]
2. Describe a *culture of safety*. [Ref 4]
3. What elements must be in place in an organization for a *culture of safety* to be possible? [Refs 4–5]

(continues)

Section Questions (continued)

4. Differentiate regulations from recommendations and standards. [Refs 6, 25]

5. What impact does CMS have on healthcare delivery? [Refs 9–12]

6. What is the focus of OSHA? [Ref 13]

7. What is the CFR, and what is the relationship between the CFR and OSHA? [Ref 14]

8. What role does the EPA play in healthcare? [Refs 18–21]

9. Describe the role of the NFPA. [Refs 22–24]

10. How does the CDC impact the healthcare arena? [Refs 27–28]

11. What is NIOSH? [Refs 29–30]

12. What do ANSI and AAMI do? [Refs 31–32]

13. What is the role of the AHRQ? [Refs 33–34]

14. What is the primary focus of ECRI? [Refs 35–36]

15. How does the IOM influence change in healthcare? [Ref 37]

16. What impact have two of the IOM publications had since 2000? [Ref 38]

17. What is the role of professional organizations in preparing caregivers to deliver patient care? [Refs 39–40]

18. What is the purpose of accreditation? [Ref 41]

19. What agencies accredit inpatient facilities? [Refs 43–51]

20. What agencies are available for accrediting ambulatory surgery centers? [Refs 52–55]

Facility Safety Plan

56. Every healthcare facility has at least one designated safety officer who is primarily responsible for the facility's safety plan and coordinates the efforts of others throughout the organization who are involved in providing a safe environment for patients and employees.

57. Usually, each department has a designated safety officer. In the operating room, different individuals may be assigned the responsibility for safety related to a specific challenge. For instance, the operating room may have a designated safety officer and a laser safety officer.

58. Individuals with safety training can be a valuable resource for designing and developing a safety program for the operating room. All staff are expected to be familiar with the safety plan and to participate in drills to improve the response to safety challenges.

59. Building, electrical, and fire codes developed for each state and city are part of creating a safe environment for patients and healthcare workers.

60. TJC (2015a, pp. EC1–EC3) identifies three basic elements of a safe environment:

- A building design that protects patients, visitors, and employees

- Equipment that is maintained and deemed safe to use on a regular basis

- People who enter the environment and understand the roles they play in minimizing risks in the environment

61. HFAP (2009, pp. 11–38) describes the following basic elements of a healthcare facility program:

- Fire drills and the equipment required in each department

- Disaster response plans for internal and external disasters, including annual drills

- Staff education on safety of the environment

- Facilities maintenance program for building and equipment

- Monitoring for compliance with safety plan

- Actual overall safety of the building and equipment

62. The components of a safety plan are influenced by the type of facility, the services provided, and the expectations of the organization that accredits it. Every safety plan addresses the environmental risks that pose a challenge to the safety of employees and patients:

    - Safety and security of the building and its occupants
    - Risks associates with physical, chemical, and biological hazards
    - Infection prevention
    - Product failures or recalls
    - Disaster preparedness

63. Developing a fire safety plan should include input from clinical representatives from all surgical specialties, clinical education, anesthesia, security, and the local fire and police departments. The chain of command should be clearly documented and disseminated to all departments.

64. The facility's governing body assumes ultimate responsibility for overseeing the safety plan.

65. The facility leadership team is responsible for environmental safety, which includes development of the safety plan; establishing standards of performance (which should be based on a culture of safety); education to ensure that employees can participate in the plan with competence; security of the building for protection of the patients, visitors, and staff; and monitoring for compliance.

66. The safety team and safety officer are responsible for reviewing and updating safety policies and procedures; monitoring the emergency call system; monitoring life safety; equipment safety inspections; utility safety inspections; environmental safety, including fire walls, fire doors, and safety equipment; storage and disposal of hazardous materials and waste; OSHA compliance; and compliance with the Safe Medical Devices Act. Employees must be updated on safety issues at least annually.

67. ECRI maintains a Medical Safety Device Reports (MDSR) database of incident and hazard information (www.mdsr.ecri.org). The database is updated periodically and is searchable. It is not meant to be an "alert system."

Job Safety Analysis

68. A job safety analysis identifies the safety issues associated with tasks that are performed in a particular environment. An analysis of tasks in the surgical environment should identify the following considerations:

    - The various tasks related to the care of the patient in surgery, including the steps required to accomplish the task and the supplies and equipment involved
    - Any potential hazards related to the task itself or to the supplies or equipment involved
    - Protocols that promote safety for the patient and employee
    - The communication and training needs to promote staff competency
    - The needs associated with monitoring for compliance

69. Planning for a job safety analysis in surgery should include personnel from the department and representatives from the hospital's safety program, infection control, and employee health. Biomedical engineering and radiology might also participate in the analysis.

70. Based on the analysis, the department can develop a safety plan that addresses hazards specific to its employees and patients, a plan for educating staff, and a plan for monitoring compliance.

71. A medical equipment maintenance and replacement protocol is part of the environmental safety plan. Malfunctioning electrical equipment can be a fire hazard. The plan addresses inspection and testing on a regular basis. The biomedical engineering department places an inspection sticker on every piece of inspected equipment so that all employees can participate actively in keeping all equipment in working order.

Monitoring and Training

72. Periodic rounding with a checklist of workplace safety issues identified during the analysis is an effective method both for monitoring compliance and for identifying new hazards. Ongoing monitoring also provides the opportunity to keep personnel informed of the standards and reinforces the importance of safe practice.

73. Monitoring may also identify opportunities for improvement, especially by engaging staff in conversation about safety and soliciting their input on the best way to accomplish the objectives.

74. Training on safety issues should occur at least annually, with more frequent attention to the

more challenging hazards such as fire safety and radiation safety.

75. Results of monitoring should be shared with personnel. The safety program should promote employee engagement in promoting safe practices in the department, and ownership of the results of their efforts. In a *culture of safety,* employees are rewarded for positive results—a more effective approach than penalizing them for not achieving the desired outcome.

76. Assessment results should be used to make changes in the environment to reduce risk, identify educational needs, and provide follow-up education for staff.

77. Emphasis on positive outcomes and regular safety training activities can increase employees' knowledge and promote both engagement in the program and improved compliance with standards.

Section Questions

1. What is the role of a facility or a department safety officer? [Refs 56–57]
2. What three basic elements of a safe environment does TJC identify? [Ref 60]
3. What elements of a facility safety plan have been identified by the HFAP? [Ref 61]
4. What factors influence the components of a healthcare facility's safety plan? [Ref 62]
5. Identify at least five components of a facility safety plan. [Ref 62]
6. What is involved in addressing environmental safety? [Ref 65]
7. What are the responsibilities of the safety team and the safety officer? [Ref 66]
8. What is the purpose of a job safety analysis? [Ref 68]
9. What should be addressed in a job safety analysis? [Ref 68]
10. Who should participate in a job safety analysis for the operating room? [Ref 69]
11. What is the significance of malfunctioning electrical equipment? [Ref 71]
12. Describe one method of monitoring compliance with the safety plan. [Ref 72]
13. What should be done with the results of compliance monitoring? [Ref 75]
14. How can assessment results be used? [Ref 76]
15. Describe ways to increase knowledge and promote engagement in the safety program. [Ref 77]

Physical Hazards

78. In the surgical environment, some of the most challenging physical hazards include:
    - Fire
    - Exposure to pathogenic microorganisms
    - Radiation
    - Musculoskeletal injuries
    - Slips, trips, and falls

Fire

79. ECRI (2015) estimates that 200 to 240 surgical fires occur in the United States each year. Between 10% and 20% of the fires reported result in serious patient injury. One or two events—usually tracheal tube fires—are fatal. Seventy-five percent of these fires occur in the oxygen-enriched area surrounding the patient's face (ECRI, 2015b).

80. Frequent ignition sources include electrosurgery, lasers, light sources, sparks from burrs, and defibrillators. Airway fires account for 21% of the total number of surgical fires, with 44% occurring on the face, head, neck, and chest (Healy, Cowles, & Hood, 2014).

81. A small fire in an oxygen-enriched operating room can progress to a large, life-threatening fire in seconds. Smoke can diminish visibility, and toxic fumes from burning synthetic materials can cause eye irritation or death if inhaled.

82. The Joint Commission requires adherence to the National Fire Protection Association's Fire Code and Life Safety Code (NFPA, 2015a, 2015b) for hospitals, ambulatory care centers, and other facilities. The Life Safety Code defines the requirements for facilities and procedures for safety from fire.

83. In 2003, TJC issued a "Sentinel Event Alert: Preventing Surgical Fires." TJC defines *sentinel events* or *never events* as preventable situations, not primarily related to the natural course of the patient's illness or underlying condition, that result in death, permanent harm, or severe temporary harm, and require intervention to sustain life. They are described as *sentinel* because they signal the need for immediate investigation and response and *never* because they can and should be prevented (TJC, 2014).

84. All TJC-accredited healthcare organizations are required to report any sentinel events that occur; to conduct a timely, thorough, and credible root-cause analysis; to develop an action plan to implement improvements to reduce risk; to implement the improvements; and to monitor the effectiveness of these improvements.

85. The sentinel alert on fires in the operating room requires that personnel meet the following criteria:

    - Be trained in use of firefighting equipment.
    - Know methods for rescue and escape.
    - Know the location of alarm systems and their use.
    - Know how to contact the local fire department.
    - Know the location of the medical gas shut-off valves and electrical controls.

86. The AORN (2015a) Fire Safety Tool Kit provides a Fire Risk Assessment tool for the perioperative setting.

87. A fire safety plan addresses the following issues:

    - Prevention strategies:
      - Increase awareness of factors that contribute to surgical fires
      - Disseminate surgical fire prevention tools
      - Promote the adoption of risk reduction practices throughout the healthcare community (Council on Surgery and Perioperative Safety, 2015)
    - A response plan
    - Alarm testing

    - Equipment maintenance and testing
    - Addressing employee competence through education and fire drills
    - Report cards addressing the response of staff and others during the drill

88. Each healthcare facility must plan for fire incidents:

    - Have a fire safety plan.
    - Schedule safety education programs.
    - Conduct periodic fire drills—at least one fire drill quarterly each shift.
    - Evaluate fire drills based on expected criteria in the fire safety plan.
    - Complete education of staff on an annual basis.

89. The fire safety plan should include the following elements:

    - A clear definition of responsibilities
    - Methods for training staff members
    - Scenarios for fire drills
    - Instruction in the use of fire extinguishers
    - A plan for implementation of the code requirements
    - Documents for life safety surveillance
    - An interim life safety plan for use in the event of construction
    - The equipment, packaging materials, and supplies that must be retained for the fire investigation following any operating room fire

90. Once the fire safety plan is finalized, education sessions should be scheduled to familiarize the entire staff with the plan and their roles in it. A safety officer should assume responsibility for surveillance, planning and conducting the fire drills, overseeing the required documentation, and overseeing an annual review of the plan.

91. Conducting periodic fire drills will ensure that healthcare workers know their roles, whether they are at the location of the fire or away from the area. All employees should know the process for contacting the fire department, the location of the medical gases shutoff valves, the operation of fire alarm systems, the use of fire extinguishers, the evacuation plans, and proper methods of rescue and escape.

92. Critique sessions following fire drills using different scenarios are invaluable for identifying portions of the plan that need revision or updating and the need for further education.

93. Life safety surveillance information should be collected and evaluated in a systematic way. In addition to fire safety, other life safety topics may include facility and personnel security, hazardous substances, radiation safety, emergency preparedness, utilities, and infection control.

94. The operating room is an oxygen-enriched environment that is home to many fire hazards that require close monitoring, including the following:

   - Electrical equipment
   - Alcohol-based prepping and handwashing solutions
   - Flammable chemicals
   - Cylinders of compressed gas
   - Draping materials
   - Lasers
   - Fiberoptic light sources and cables
   - Flammable patient care supplies and trash

95. Everyone on the surgical team must know the location of fire extinguishers, fire alarms, fire exits, and emergency shutoff gas valves. The locations of the alarms, extinguishers, and hoses must be posted in several sites.

96. Evacuation routes from all areas of the perioperative suite should be defined and posted in the hallways, operating room lounge, and operating rooms. Hallways should be free of clutter that could hinder an evacuation. Every perioperative nurse should be able to describe the evacuation route.

97. Fire extinguishers are not the first response to a fire in the operating room. The immediate response is to remove the ignition source and the fuel (drapes, etc.). A fire extinguisher would be needed when the fire involves materials that continue to burn after being removed from the patient or in the rare instance in which the file engulfs the patient.

98. ECRI specifically recommends a 5-lb CO_2 fire extinguisher be mounted just inside the entrance of each operating room suite.

99. ECRI recommends a 20-lb, dry-powder fire extinguisher be located outside the operating room for use as a last resort for fighting catastrophic fires. The very fine powder cannot mix with water and is therefore difficult to remove from a wound. It is also an airway and mucous membrane irritant (ECRI, 2014b).

100. Extinguishers that ECRI recommends *not* be used in the operating room include:
   - Water-based fire extinguishers (typically Class A)
     - The water used in the extinguisher is not sterile and could cause a patient infection or a toxic reaction.
     - Using one of these extinguishers could result in an electric shock to the user because the water may be electrically conductive.
   - Water-mist fire extinguishers (Class AC)
     - Water used in these extinguishers will not conduct electricity back to the user, but water that has pooled in, on, or around electrically energized devices could cause an electric shock.
     - The water is not sterile and, like the typical Class A extinguisher, can result in infection or a toxic reaction.
   - Halon-replacement fire extinguishers
     - In very hot fires the active agents break down to form toxic pyrolysis products that can cause arrhythmias if ingested or inhaled.
     - Effects of the agents when discharged onto a patient are undefined and may cause health issues such as emboli.

101. Fire safety training should include instruction in the use of fire extinguishers. The acronym PASS identifies the steps in deploying an extinguisher:
   - *P*: Pull the pin.
   - *A*: Aim the nozzle.
   - *S*: Squeeze the handle.
   - *S*: Sweep at the base of the fire.

102. Actual training sessions in a controlled area outside the building under the supervision of the local fire department can help employees gain expertise and confidence when using fire extinguishers.

103. Fire blankets should never be located in the operating room (ECRI, 2014b).
   - A fire blanket will trap the fire next to and under the patient.
   - They will burn in an oxygen-rich environment.
   - If kept in the operating room for use outside an oxygen-rich environment, staff may mistakenly use it incorrectly.

- Given the suddenness and intensity of most surgical fires, there is insufficient time to get a fire blanket, unpack it, and apply it to the patient before serious or fatal injuries are sustained.

104. The education of staff begins at new-employee orientation and is reinforced annually. Employees must demonstrate knowledge and competence in fire prevention, use of fire extinguishers, emergency response activities, and prevention of fire in the operating room.

Nursing Responsibilities

105. Prevention is the best approach to managing fires in the operating room. The perioperative nurse should assess the risk for fire before each surgical procedure. When a procedure has a heightened fire risk, it should be discussed during the Time Out so that every participant can explain the steps he or she has taken to address the risk.

106. The fire triangle represents the three critical elements that must be present for a fire to occur:

    - An ignition source (e.g., electrosurgery, laser, and fiberoptic cords)

    - Fuel (anything that can burn, e.g., drapes, sponges, the patient)

    - Oxygen

    Removing any one of the elements in the triangle will prevent a fire (**Table 11-1**).

107. The perioperative nurse must have a clear understanding of his or her responsibilities:

    - Remove burning material from the patient and smother fire.

    - Extinguish small fires with extinguisher.

    - Turn off emergency shutoff valves.

    - Identify the evacuation route.

    - Stay with the patient during evacuation.

    - Complete appropriate documentation.

    - ECRI provides a list of recommendations for perioperative nurses to consider (**Exhibit 11-1**).

108. The acronym RACE has been used to describe personnel roles and responsibilities during a fire.

    - *R*: Rescue people from flaming materials.

    - *A*: Alert others by announcing "Code Red" and the location of the fire three times. (Institutional policy may dictate a specific phone number to call in the event of a fire or disaster.)

    - *C*: Confine or contain fire and smoke. Close the doors and shut off medical gas valves when leaving the room or when going from the fire area to a safe zone.

    - *E*: Extinguish the fire. Smother a small fire with a wet sponge or towel, extinguish the fire with water or saline, or, if needed, use a fire extinguisher. If the fire is immediately extinguished, call "Code Red all clear" and notify the fire department.

    - *E*: Evacuate to a safe place beyond the smoke or fire barrier doors, or outside. Activate the fire pull station when exiting the area. Remain with the patients and others in the safe area.

109. Flammable vapors trapped under drapes provide an ignition source. Allow the surgical prep to dry and the vapors to evaporate before placing the surgical drapes.

110. Prep solutions should not be allowed to saturate the drapes or soak into the patient's hair or linens or pillow.

111. Surgery close to an oxygen source, such as around the head and neck, increases the risk for fire. If drapes are permitted to "tent," oxygen can become trapped underneath, creating an oxygen-rich environment very close to the surgical site. A spark under those circumstances could be disastrous. Draping should be done carefully to prevent pockets where oxygen can collect.

112. In certain procedures, the patient can contribute combustible material such as hair and gases in the intestinal tract (**Exhibit 11-2**).

113. ECRI (2014a) has identified electrosurgical devices as the most common cause of operating-room fires. Both the scrub person and circulating nurse must accept responsibility for promoting electrosurgery safely.

114. The scrub person should be aware of the location of the active electrode (ESU pencil) at all times. The pencil should:

    - Be stored away from the patient's airway

    - Be stored in a protective holder that is secured so it will not be dislodged during the surgical procedure

    - Not be wrapped around a metal surgical instrument to secure it to the drapes

    - Be cleaned periodically to remove buildup of eschar that might trap heat (AORN, 2015b, pp. 124)

    - Not be activated when the environment is enriched with flammable materials

Table 11-1	Fuels Commonly Encountered in Surgery
In/On Patient	Hair (face, scalp, body) GI tract gases (mostly methane)
Prepping Agents	Degreasers (ether, acetone) Aerosol adhesives Alcohol (also in suture packets) Tinctures (Hibitane [chlorhexidine digluconate], Merthiolate [thimerosal]), DuraPrep [iodophor])
Linens	Drapes (woven, nonwoven, adherent) Gowns (reusable, disposable) Masks Hoods and caps Shoe covers Instrument and equipment drapes and covers Egg-crate mattresses Mattresses and pillows Blankets
Dressings	Gauze Sponges Adhesive tape (cloth, plastic, paper) Ace bandages Stockinettes Collodion (mixture of pyroxylin, ether, and alcohol)
Ointments	Petrolatum (petroleum jelly) Tincture of Benzoin (74% to 80% alcohol) Aerosols (e.g., Aeroplast) Paraffin White wax
Equipment/Supplies	Anesthesia components (breathing circuits, masks, airways, tracheal tubes, suction catheters, pledgets) Flexible endoscopes Coverings of fiberoptic cables and wires (e.g., ESU leads, ECG leads) Gloves Blood pressure and tourniquet cuffs Stethoscope tubing Disposable packaging materials (paper, plastic, cardboard) Smoke evacuator hoses Some instrument boxes and cabinets

Emergency Care Research Institute (ECRI) (1992). ECRI Medical Device Safety Reports: The Patient Is on Fire! A surgical fires primer. Guidance; 21(1): 19–34. Online: http://www.mdsr.ecri.org/summary/detail.aspx?doc_id=8197 Accessed June 2015. Reprinted with permission, Copyright 2015, ECRI Institute. www.ecri.org. 5200 Butler Pike, Plymouth Meeting, PA 19462. 610-825-6000

115. Whenever an electrosurgical device is in use, wet towels, normal saline, or sterile water should be readily available (AORN, 2015b, pp. 125).

116. Fiberoptic cords and connectors become very hot when the light in on. Never uncouple the cable from an item on the field while the light is on, because it can ignite draping material or sponges and can burn the patient if it comes into contact with exposed skin.

117. Headlights should be removed when not in use. The hot cable can ignite the fabric of the surgeon's gown if it is uncoupled and allowed to hang loose down the surgeon's back.

Exhibit 11-1 Only YOU Can Prevent Surgical Fires.

ONLY *YOU* CAN PREVENT SURGICAL FIRES
Surgical Team Communication Is Essential

The applicability of these recommendations must be considered individually for each patient.

At the Start of Each Surgery:

▶ Enriched O_2 and N_2O atmospheres can vastly increase flammability of drapes, plastics, and hair. Be aware of possible O_2 enrichment under the drapes near the surgical site and in the fenestration, especially during head/face/neck/upper-chest surgery.

▶ Do not apply drapes until all flammable preps have fully dried; soak up spilled or pooled agent.

▶ Fiberoptic light sources can start fires: Complete all cable connections before activating the source. Place the source in standby mode when disconnecting cables.

▶ Moisten sponges to make them ignition resistant in oropharyngeal and pulmonary surgery.

During Head, Face, Neck, and Upper-Chest Surgery:

▶ Use only air for open delivery to the face if the patient can maintain a safe blood O_2 saturation without supplemental O_2.

▶ If the patient cannot maintain a safe blood O_2 saturation without extra O_2, secure the airway with a laryngeal mask airway or tracheal tube.

<u>Exceptions:</u> Where patient verbal responses may be required during surgery (e.g., carotid artery surgery, neurosurgery, pacemaker insertion) and where open O_2 delivery is required to keep the patient safe:

— At all times, deliver the minimum O_2 concentration necessary for adequate oxygenation.

— Begin with a 30% delivered O_2 concentration and increase as necessary.

— For unavoidable open O_2 delivery above 30%, deliver 5 to 10 L/min of air under drapes to wash out excess O_2.

— Stop supplemental O_2 at least one minute before and during use of electrosurgery, electrocautery, or laser, if possible. Surgical team communication is essential for this recommendation.

— Use an adherent incise drape, if possible, to help isolate the incision from possible O_2-enriched atmospheres beneath the drapes.

— Keep fenestration towel edges as far from the incision as possible.

— Arrange drapes to minimize O_2 buildup underneath.

— Coat head hair and facial hair (e.g., eyebrows, beard, moustache) within the fenestration with water-soluble surgical lubricating jelly to make it nonflammable.

— For coagulation, use bipolar electrosurgery, not monopolar electrosurgery.

During Oropharyngeal Surgery (e.g., tonsillectomy):

▶ Scavenge deep within the oropharynx with a metal suction cannula to catch leaking O_2 and N_2O.

▶ Moisten gauze or sponges and keep them moist, including those used with uncuffed tracheal tubes.

During Tracheostomy:

▶ Do not use electrosurgery to cut into the trachea.

During Bronchoscopic Surgery:

▶ If the patient requires supplemental O_2, keep the delivered O_2 below 30%. Use inhalation/exhalation gas monitoring (e.g., with an O_2 analyzer) to confirm the proper concentration.

When Using Electrosurgery, Electrocautery, or Laser:

▶ The surgeon should be made aware of open O_2 use. Surgical team discussion about preventive measures before use of electrosurgery, electrocautery, and laser is indicated.

▶ Activate the unit only when the active tip is in view (especially if looking through a microscope or endoscope).

▶ Deactivate the unit before the tip leaves the surgical site.

▶ Place electrosurgical electrodes in a holster or another location off the patient when not in active use (i.e., when not needed within the next few moments).

▶ Place lasers in standby mode when not in active use.

▶ Do not place rubber catheter sleeves over electrosurgical electrodes.

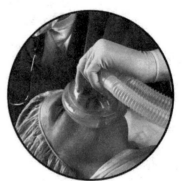

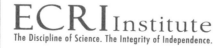
ECRI Institute
The Discipline of Science. The Integrity of Independence.

Developed in collaboration with the
Anesthesia Patient Safety Foundation.

MS09445_2

Exhibit 11-2 Recommendations for the perioperative nurse.

- Ask anesthesia if they plan to use the lowest possible concentration of oxygen for procedures on the head and neck.
- Select non-flammable preps; if flammable prep solution is required, insure sufficient drying time prior to draping the patient.
- Store alcohol-based hand rubs in an area away from ignition and heat sources
- Reduce tenting of drapes as much as possible during head & neck procedures.
- Use water-soluble lubricant to protect hair near the surgical site on head & neck procedures.
- Moisten sponges of all types used on the sterile field.
- Never silence the alarm on an electrosurgical unit
- Keep the electrosurgical pencil in an approved holster when it is not being used
- Keep ESU tip free of eschar; remove contaminated ESU pencils from the field.
- Remove foot pedals not being used to prevent unintended activation by the surgeon.
- Never keep an active fiberoptic cord on the field that has been disconnected from a lighted instrument
- Turn light source off when fiberoptic cord has been disconnected from a headlamp
- During laser procedures:
  - ❑ Place wet towels around the laser incision site.
  - ❑ Use nonreflective instrumentation.
  - ❑ Use a laser-safe endotracheal tube.
  - ❑ Keep the laser on standby when it is not being used.
  - ❑ Keep sufficient sterile water or saline on the field and additional bottles in the room

Data from ECRI (2012).

Section Questions

1. Identify ignition sources for fire in the operating room. [Ref 80]
2. What characteristic of the operating room environment places it at high risk for fire? [Ref 81]
3. What national organization is responsible for *Fire Code* standards and *Life Safety Code* standards? [Ref 82]
4. What criteria does TJC require of operating room personnel related to fire safety? [Ref 85]
5. Identify five components of a fire safety plan. [Ref 87]
6. How should a facility plan for fire incidents? [Ref 88]
7. Identify information each employee should have related to response to a fire. [Ref 91]
8. List some of the fire hazards present in the operating room environment. [Ref 94]
9. Every employee must know the location of certain items related to fire response. What are they? [Ref 95]
10. What is the immediate response expected of the nurse if a fire occurs? [Ref 97]
11. What type of fire extinguisher does ECRI recommend for the operating room? [Ref 98]
12. Explain the PASS acronym for using a fire extinguisher properly. [Ref 101]
13. What is ECRI's recommendation for fire blankets in the operating room? [Ref 103]
14. Describe the process of employee education related to fire safety. [Ref 104]
15. What are the three components of the fire triangle? [Ref 106]
16. Describe the responsibilities of the operating room nurse related to fire in the operating room. [Refs 107–108]
17. What is the significance of vapors related to a surgical procedure? [Ref 109]
18. On what part of the body are surgical procedures at highest risk for fire? [Ref 111]
19. What are the scrub person's responsibilities related to the ESU active electrode? [Ref 114]
20. What is the significance of fiberoptic cords for fire prevention? [Ref 116]

Electricity

118. Electricity is one of the primary causes of hospital fires.

119. Each piece of equipment that is used in the operating room should be checked by the facility's biomedical engineering department. Before use, the electrical outlets, switch plates, plugs, and power cords should be inspected for defects or damage. Electrical equipment that is not functioning properly can cause shock, explosion, and burns.

120. Any new equipment should be inspected by a biomedical engineer prior to use. Labels or stickers with the date of inspection and a department inventory number should be affixed to each piece of equipment. If the inspection sticker is missing, or if the inspection has expired, the equipment should not be used. Biomedical engineering personnel are also responsible for documentation of regular inspections and preventive maintenance of all electrical and mechanical equipment.

121. Electrical hazard increases with the use of inappropriate extension cords and/or equipment with frayed or faulty electrical cords.

122. Avoid the use of extension cords; extension cords are prohibited in many fire safety regulations. Equipment manufacturers must supply cords of sufficient length to allow equipment to be placed conveniently for effective use.

Alarms

123. Operating rooms are also equipped with a line isolation monitoring (LIM) system that continuously monitors ungrounded power systems that may allow leaking electricity to flow from the power system to ground. An alarm will sound if leakage exceeds the threshold for safety. The LIM system reduces the potential for electrical shock, cardiac fibrillation, or burns produced by excess electrical current flowing through the patient's body to ground.

124. In the event of an LIM alarm, the perioperative nurse should immediately unplug the piece of equipment most recently plugged in and continue this process until the alarm ceases. The equipment responsible for the alarm should be removed from service until it has been assessed and cleared by biomedical engineering.

125. In 2015, for the fourth year in a row, ECRI (2015a) placed clinical alarm hazards, most notably inadequate alarm configuration policies and practices, at the top of their list of Health Technology Hazards. ECRI has noted several deaths and other cases of severe patient harm that may have been prevented with more effective alarm policies and practices.

126. Alarm hazards are also identified by TJC (2015b) as "National Patient Safety Goal #6: Reduce the harm associated with clinical alarm systems; make improvements to ensure that alarms on medical equipment are heard and responded to on time."

Radiation

127. Many facilities today are building hybrid operating rooms that include diagnostic imaging, elevating the concern in the operating room for radiation safety.

128. The Joint Commission's (2011) Sentinel Event Alert (Issue 47) describes the dangers of diagnostic imaging: cancer, burns, and other radiation injuries.

129. Surgical procedures performed under fluoroscopy or using intraoperative X-rays are the primary sources of potential exposure to radiation for operating room staff.

130. When radiation is emitted at a constant rate, the dose received depends on the amount of exposure time and the proximity to the source.

131. The patient should be as close to the radiation source as possible to minimize radiation scatter.

132. The principles of time, distance, and shielding allow perioperative personnel to minimize their exposure to radiation. Appropriate protection is essential for personnel near the patient during radiation, and the amount of time spent during radiation should be as short as possible.

133. During fluoroscopy or other procedures involving radiation, personnel should remain as far from the radiation source as possible. Doubling the distance from the radiation source reduces the radiation intensity by a factor of four (AORN, 2015b, p. 337). Personnel should stand at least 6 feet away from the x-ray source (Phillips, 2012).

134. Non-scrubbed personnel can stand behind a mobile lead shield for protection during the emission of radiation. In rooms designed for use of radiation, there may be retractable shields mounted on the ceiling.

135. Rooms designed for procedures involving radiation exposure will have leaded walls, windows, control room, and doors.

136. Personnel should face the source of radiation. Anyone who cannot face the radiation source should wear a wrap-around lead apron to protect the back (AORN, 2015b, p. 337).

137. Personnel who must remain with the patient during radiation should wear a lead apron and thyroid shield. Additionally, leaded gloves and leaded eye protection are available when exposure will be lengthy or the individual must remain with the patient during radiation exposure.

138. In an operating room providing diagnostic radiological procedures, staff can take the following steps to prevent potential injury to patients and employees:

    - Develop a comprehensive patient safety program, including education for patients and family members.

    - Educate staff on the types of dangers to which they and their patients are exposed when performing diagnostic radiation procedures.

    - Ensure physician education and competency to include awareness of proper dose levels for each diagnostic test.

    - Provide extensive training for physicians and staff on how to use diagnostic equipment.

    - Develop clear protocols describing the maximum limit (dose) of radiation for each type of test being performed in the facility.

    - Work closely with a medical physicist to ensure staff are competent, equipment is being used properly, and the equipment is safe.

    - Communicate.

    - Ensure that staff have a safety checklist that is being used appropriately.

    - Develop policies and procedures that are detailed and can be understood by all levels of staff education.

    - Develop a culture of radiation safety (TJC, 2011).

139. Personnel who are frequently assigned to procedures in which radiation is used should be monitored for cumulative exposure. State regulations address radiation monitoring. A radiation-monitoring badge (dosimeter) consists of a strip of X-ray film encased in a plastic holder. The dosimeter should be worn outside of the lead apron in the same location each day.

140. When two dosimeters are worn, the primary dosimeter should be placed at the neck outside of the lead apron and the second under the apron (AORN, 2015b, p. 3340).

141. All pregnant personnel should wear a dosimeter at the waist and it should be read at least monthly.

142. The facility's safety officer is responsible for collecting the badges, analyzing the dosimeter readings, passing out new badges, and maintaining records according to federal and state regulations.

143. Radiation safety training should be conducted as part of new-employee orientation and periodically thereafter. The safety training should include both protection for the employee and protection for the patient based on the area of exposure.

144. Leaded aprons and thyroid shields should be stored vertically, hanging on a rack designed for this purpose, or laid flat; they should never be folded.

145. If lead aprons are not handled properly, they can develop cracks and subsequently provide inadequate protection. Lead shielding devices should be checked at regular intervals by the X-ray department, safety officer, or radiation physicist to ensure their integrity. Devices with cracks should be discarded and replaced.

146. Any healthcare facility that uses therapeutic radionuclides for patient care should identify a radiation safety officer to supervise the operation of the radiation safety program. Radionuclides are absorbed by the body, so personnel caring for those patients receiving such therapy must take radiation safety precautions in addition to standard precautions with any bodily secretions from these patients.

147. The radiation safety officer will assist perioperative personnel in complying with government safety regulations and standards. Protective measures for perioperative personnel who are caring for a patient who has received or is receiving therapeutic radionuclides include the following:

    - Using the principles of shielding, time, and distance to limit exposure to the radionuclides

- Instituting contamination control measures
- Notifying personnel caring for the patient postoperatively about the type and location of the radiation
- Observing radiation precautions when transporting the patient
- Keeping radioactive materials in a lead-lined container

- Handling radioactive needles and capsules with forceps
- Posting radiation warning signs on the doors to the operating room where the patient is located
- Documenting all protective measures on the perioperative record

Section Questions

1. How does the biomedical engineering department participate in fire safety? [Refs 119–120]

2. What is the recommendation about the use of extension cords? [Refs 121–122]

3. What is an LIM system? [Refs 123–124]

4. How does the nurse troubleshoot a problem with an LIM alarm? [Ref 124]

5. What two organizations target alarm systems as a safety issue? [Refs 125–126]

6. What procedures are the primary sourses of radiation exposure for personnel? [Ref 129]

7. What are the two factors that determine the dose of radiation received? [Ref 130]

8. What three principles allow personnel to minimize exposure to radiation? [Ref 132]

9. What distance from the X-ray tube is considered a safe distance for personnel to stand? [Ref 133]

10. What protective measures are available in surgery to protect personnel from unnecessary exposure to radiation? [Refs 133–137]

11. What steps can personnel take to prevent radiation injury for themselves and patients? [Ref 138]

12. Describe the use of a dosimeter for monitoring radiation exposure. [Refs 139–142]

13. Describe the proper way to handle and store lead aprons and other leaded shields. [Ref 144]

14. What is the danger of handling leaded protective attire improperly? [Ref 145]

15. What are protective measures for caring for patients receiving radionuclide therapy? [Refs 146–147]

Musculoskeletal Injuries

148. Musculoskeletal disorders, including back, shoulder, and knee injuries, are also called ergonomic injuries. They account for 33% of all workplace injuries and illnesses requiring time away from work (Bureau of Labor Statistics [BLS], 2013). Back injuries rate second only to the common cold as the cause of missed workdays. Most back injuries in the operating room are associated with moving patients.

149. Physical stressors in the healthcare setting (all of which occur routinely in the operating room) include:

- Forceful tasks
- Repetitive motion
- Awkward positions
- Static posture
- Moving or lifting patients and equipment
- Carrying heavy instruments and equipment
- Overexertion

150. Lifting and moving heavy pieces of equipment, instrument sets, and patients who exceed the nurse's physical capacity put excess force on the spine. Most work-related back injuries are cumulative injuries. Although the injury appears to be caused by a single incident, it is often the result of repetitive trauma over a period of time.

151. Lifting injuries include sprains and strains, acute or chronic lower back pain, and injury to the shoulder and neck.

152. Low back pain occurs more frequently in nurses than in the general population. Most back injuries are of short duration, and workers are able to return to work. However, some healthcare workers sustain back injuries that result in permanent disability and the end of a career in nursing.

153. Factors that contribute to the number of back injuries include the advancing age of the nursing workforce, staffing shortages, increasing numbers of obese patients, and sicker, less mobile patients.

154. The key to avoiding musculoskeletal injuries is to practice good body mechanics. Lifting injuries are also influenced by the height from which an item is lifted and the location and size of the item. When lifting, keep the back straight, bend the knees instead of leaning over, and hold the object close to the body. Use leg muscles, not back muscles, to lift.

155. Injuries can be caused by twisting to the side when lifting and moving heavy items and reaching for items such as instrument sets that are stored above shoulder level, rather than using a step stool.

156. Don't pull anything that you can push. Standing close to the object allows you to apply more force without straining back and shoulder muscles. Use two hands and keep your back straight.

157. An adequate number of staff members must be involved when transferring patients to and from the operatingroom table. A careful assessment of the patient will determine the number of personnel needed to maintain patient alignment, support extremities, and maintain the airway during transfer. Four is often considered the minimum number of staff needed to transfer an anesthetized adult patient. Safety devices used in the perioperative setting include slides, roller devices, and mechanical lifts.

158. When holding an extremity during prep, avoid leaning over with arms outstretched.

159. Long periods of standing in one spot, coupled with poor posture, can cause back pain. It is important for the scrubbed person to maintain good posture, stand with one foot on a standing stool, and change positions often. Standing on an anti-fatigue mat may also reduce risk of injury.

160. The following are some principles of good body mechanics:
    - Keep the back straight.
    - Bend the knees.
    - Hold the load close to the body.
    - Use the leg muscles to lift.
    - Do not turn or twist to pick up something or while carrying a heavy object.
    - Avoid reaching for items above shoulder level; reach for objects no higher than chest level, and use a ladder/stool if necessary.
    - When lifting, place the feet apart to create a wide base of support.

161. The CDC (2015a) has reported that 34.9% of adults and 17% of children in the United States are obese (have a body mass index [BMI] greater than 30%).

162. Transporting and positioning bariatric patients present special challenges. An assistive device should be used whenever a caregiver is required to lift more than 35 pounds of a patient's weight (AORN, 2015b, p. 738). Special equipment such as lateral transfer devices or mechanical lifts should be used. An air-driven mattress or friction-reducing sheet is useful.

163. Healthcare workers should participate in determining what types of equipment are necessary to serve the facility's patient population and protect the healthcare worker from injury. A needs assessment might include:
    - Lifting techniques being used in the facility
    - Type of lifting required in the facility
    - Patient positioning techniques, especially in the perioperative setting
    - Current process and content of staff education
    - Gaps between expectations and results

164. The facility safety plan should include engineering design that promotes physical conditions that protect employees from injury:
    - Heavy items placed on middle shelves
    - Step stool or ladder available when items are stored on high shelves
    - Wheels of equipment kept free of debris so that they roll freely
    - Corridors kept clear so that equipment can be moved with ease

- Employee training in correct body mechanics
- A consistent review of injury reports to identify causes of injury that might motivate work redesign or further education

165. The Washington Industrial Safety and Health Act (WISHA) provides examples of safety checklists that can be adapted for a specific facility's action plan (Washington State Department of Labor and Industries, 2015).

Slips, Trips, and Falls (STFs)

166. Workplace occupational hazards have been identified as a major contributor to nurses leaving the profession. The rate of slips, trips, and falls in hospitals is 90% greater than the average rate for all other private industries combined. STFs as a whole are the second most common cause of lost-workday injuries in hospitals. Nurses and nursing assistants had the highest injury rates of all occupations examined. Nurses accounted for 38% of the injuries reported to OSHA (CDC, 2015).

167. The most common injuries related to STFs occur to the lower extremities and include sprains, strains, dislocations, and tears. STFs are also more likely to result in fractures and multiple injuries than are other types of injuries.

168. Prevention is the best approach. OSHA recommends the following precautions:
- Keep floors clean and dry.
- Provide warning signs for wet floor areas.
- Provide safety mats where spills occur frequently, such as by sinks.
- Keep all places of employment clean and orderly.
- Maintain the integrity of flooring and stairwells; replace or repair when buckled, torn, or loose.
- Use the handrails on stairs.
- Keep aisles and passageways clear without obstructions.
- Ensure spills are reported and cleaned up immediately.
- Use nonslip floor surfaces and nonslip footwear.
- Use ladders and stepstools, not chairs or boxes, to reach high items.
- Eliminate cluttered or obstructed work areas.

- Provide adequate lighting.
- Make sure all elevators line up with floors properly when the doors open.

169. All occurrences of STFs should be investigated and causes eliminated as soon as possible.

170. In the operating room, each nurse can contribute to STF prevention:
- Place equipment, furniture, and supplies to allow for safe passage.
- Position the multiple cords and hoses of electrical and mechanical equipment out of the traffic pattern.
- Wipe up spills promptly.

Head Injury

171. Overhead operating room lights and equipment booms pose a risk for head injury. It is not uncommon for personnel to inadvertently walk into a light or boom that is positioned lower than the head. When not in use, lights should be raised above head height.

Compressed Gases

172. Modern facilities incorporate a delivery system for frequently used gases (e.g., oxygen, nitrous oxide, carbon dioxide, nitrogen, compressed air) in the building construction. These gases are accessed by connecting a hose to an outlet on a wall, a pillar, or a boom. Older facilities may still supply compressed gases in cylinders.

173. When gases are delivered in individual cylinders (e.g., portable oxygen for patient transport), they require special handling. A compressed air cylinder that is dropped or broken will behave like a missile, the escaping gas under high pressure acting as a propellant. A damaged cylinder can cause considerable damage, including death, should it strike an individual.

174. Compressed gas cylinders and portable tanks should have pressure relief devices installed and maintained (OSHA, 2015).

175. Cylinders are considered either *full* or *empty*; partially full cylinders are treated as full and subject to the same controls and storage conditions. Full and empty cylinders should be stored separately to avoid confusion. Stored cylinders and cylinders in use must be firmly secured to prevent falling or damage. Storage and use instructions are provided in a document published by the Compressed Gas Association (2015).

Section Questions

1. Describe musculoskeletal disorders. [Ref 148]

2. What are some of the stressors in the operating room that can lead to musculoskeletal disorders? [Refs 149–150]

3. What factors contribute to back injuries in the nursing population? [Ref 153]

4. What is the key to avoiding musculoskeletal injuries? [Ref 154]

5. Describe recommendations for pushing and pulling items. [Ref 156]

6. How can patient transfer contribute to employee injury? [Ref 157]

7. Describe principles of good body mechanics. [Ref 160]

8. What current epidemic in the United States contributes to the potential for musculoskeletal injury in operating room personnel? [Refs 161–162]

9. What are some elements of engineering design that can reduce the potential for musculoskeletal injury? [Ref 164]

10. What are OSHA's recommendations for preventing slips, trips, and falls? [Ref 168]

11. What can the perioperative nurse do in the operating room to prevent slips, trips, and falls? [Ref 170]

12. What piece of operating room equipment is most likely to contribute to a head injury? [Ref 171]

13. When are compressed gases in cylinders used in a healthcare facility? [Ref 172]

14. What is the danger related to compressed gas cylinders? [Ref 173]

15. How are partially empty cylinders handled? [Ref 175]

Chemical Hazards

176. OSHA requires that each employee be informed of the potential hazards of all chemicals (e.g., disinfectants, skin-prep agents, tissue preservatives, bone cement, chemotherapy agents) used in the work setting. A Safety Data Sheet (SDS—previously called Material Safety Data Sheet, or MSDS) must be available for every chemical used in the workplace.

177. The SDS is part of a required hazard communication program that also includes proper labeling of chemicals and employee training programs. The SDS has 16 sections that address the chemical composition of the product, handling, storage and disposal instructions, and postexposure first aid measures.

178. To prevent injury when employees are exposed to harmful chemicals, the employer provides appropriate personal protective equipment (PPE).

179. Employers must provide training in the use of potentially harmful chemicals. Employees must follow the label instructions closely.

180. Eyewash stations and emergency showers must be located where there is potential for exposure to corrosive materials.

Formaldehyde

181. A 37% aqueous solution of formaldehyde is used in the operating room for preservation of surgical specimens. Formaldehyde can also be combined with water and methanol to make formalin, also a preservative for specimens.

182. Formaldehyde is a carcinogen that affects the nose and upper respiratory tract. It has a strong, pungent odor that can cause watery eyes and respiratory irritation. Formaldehyde should be located in a well-ventilated area, and employees should wear gloves.

Glutaraldehyde

183. Glutaraldehyde is a toxic chemical used for high-level disinfection of heat-sensitive instruments and equipment. This chemical is also used as a fixative in pathology and histology and as a fixative for developing X-rays. With the proliferation of low-temperature sterilization technologies, high-level disinfection is no longer a common practice in most operating rooms.

184. Potential side effects of exposure include eye irritation (mild to severe) and burns to the skin if exposed to high concentrations of the

chemical. Breathing in glutaraldehyde can cause irritation of the nose, throat, and respiratory tract. Other side effects include coughing, wheezing, nausea, headaches, nosebleeds, dizziness, and drowsiness.

185. When glutaraldehyde is used, there should be at least 10 air exchanges per hour. Best practice is to provide a room that has an exhaust ventilation system such as a fume hood. Personnel should use appropriate PPE, including gloves made of butyl rubber, nitrile, or Viton, and eye protection.

Methyl Methacrylate

186. Methyl methacrylate (MMA) is an acrylic cement-type compound that combines a powder and a liquid to form a strong plastic. Its uses include securing orthopedic prostheses and neurosurgical reconstruction of cranial bone.

187. MMA can cause skin rashes, itching and watering of the eyes, headache, and respiratory tract irritation. Prolonged exposure can also damage the liver, brain, and kidney. The EPA (1994) does not consider MMA carcinogenic.

188. MMA is supplied in separate containers of a liquid and a powder that are mixed just prior to being used. The liquid is poured into the powder to prevent aerosolization. The combination forms polymethyl methacrylate (PMMA). Using a vacuum bone cement mixing system significantly reduces the emission of harmful vapors. Repeated mixing of bone cement during the day does not represent an increased health risk when vacuum mixing is used (Jelecevic, Maidanjuk, Leithner, Loewe, & Kuehn, 2014; Schlegel, Sturm, Ewerbeck, & Breusch, 2004).

189. Eye protection is required when working with MMA. Avoid wearing contact lenses, because fumes can penetrate permeable lenses, causing damage to the lens of the eye.

190. Methyl methacrylate should not come in contact with gloves until it has reached the dough stage. The outer pair of gloves should be discarded once the cement has been placed (AORN, 2015b, p. 254).

191. If a spill occurs, the area should be secured and isolated until all fumes have been exhausted and the material is cleaned up. Activated charcoal absorbent should be placed over the material. Dispose of the MMA according to state

and federal requirements, because this material is hazardous to the environment (AORN, 2015b, p. 254).

Surgical Smoke (Plume)

192. Laser and electrosurgical energy causes thermal destruction of tissue, creating a smoke byproduct referred to as surgical smoke or plume. Research has confirmed that this plume can contain toxic gases and vapors such as benzene, hydrogen cyanide, and formaldehyde; bioaerosols; dead and live cellular material (including blood fragments); and viruses (NIOSH, 1996).

193. Surgical smoke creates visual problems for the surgeon. At high concentrations, plume causes ocular and upper respiratory tract irritation. The smoke has unpleasant odors and has been shown to have mutagenic potential (NIOSH, 1996).

194. If plume is not properly evacuated, the perioperative team might experience symptoms including:

- Eye irritation
- Headache
- Nausea
- Respiratory changes
- Nasopharyngeal changes
- Neurologic issues such as weakness, fatigue, and lightheadedness

195. OSHA estimates that 500,000 healthcare workers are exposed to surgical smoke each year. Smoke evacuation recommendations for the perioperative environment are available, and perioperative nurses should be aware of these recommendations and take steps to be compliant to protect themselves and other members of the perioperative team (AORN, 2015c).

196. AORN (2015c) makes the following recommendations for smoke evacuation:

- Use a central or portable smoke evacuation system for large amounts of plume.
- Using wall suction with an inline filter for small amounts of plume is acceptable practice.
- Use a laparoscopic filtration system for laparoscopic cases.
- Wear protective equipment such as a high-filtration mask, protective eyewear, long sleeves to protect arms, and gloves to protect hands.

- Develop competencies for surgical smoke evacuation.
- Educate staff and document the education.
- Comply with all federal and state laws concerning safety in the healthcare environment.

Latex Considerations

197. Localized allergic reactions and skin irritation following contact with natural rubber latex were first reported in 1979. Reactions fall into two categories: true allergic reactions to latex protein (Type I) or chemicals used in glove manufacturing (Type IV) and contact dermatitis (Exhibit 11-3).

198. True allergic reactions to latex are less common but can be hazardous. Symptoms range from mild urticaria to anaphylaxis, and must be treated immediately.

199. A Type I allergic reaction is acute, systemic, and can lead to anaphylaxis. Severity of reactions increase with exposure to latex proteins.

200. A Type IV allergic reaction to chemicals used in the processing of latex gloves can be acute, with an immediate burning sensation and redness, to cumulative, with rash and vesicles and darkening of the skin after days or weeks of exposure.

201. Individuals with Type IV allergy can pursue alternatives such as non-latex gloves, glove liners, or changing brands of gloves. In severe cases, a temporary or permanent change of work area may be necessary. Symptoms of allergy resolve when contact with the allergen is discontinued. Individuals with Type I latex allergy must avoid latex altogether and cannot work in an environment where latex is present.

202. Contact dermatitis is the more common reaction to glove wearing. It is similar to "dishpan hands" in that it represents damage to the skin from frequent washing, inadequate drying, and the occlusive environment created by wearing gloves for long periods of time. The cure for contact dermatitis is good hand hygiene including thorough drying and moisturizing.

203. Modern healthcare facilities have created a latex-safe environment, and take extra precautions with patients who are allergic to latex.

204. The Safe Medical Devices Act requires all incidents of serious injury or death related to use of a medical device to be reported, including events involving latex allergy.

Exposure Control Plan and Personal Protective Equipment (PPE)

205. PPE was introduced in 1985 when *Universal Precautions* were recommended by OSHA and the CDC to protect healthcare workers from exposure to contaminated blood and body fluids. In 1996, the recommendations were expanded to *Standard Precautions* (CFR 1910.130 Bloodborne Pathogen Standard) mandating the use of PPE for all patient contact, because it cannot always be determined when blood and body fluids are contaminated and when they are not.

Exhibit 11-3 Reaction to Latex Gloves

Mechanical Irritation/ Contact Dermatitis	Type IV Allergy (Chemicals)	Type I Allergy (Latex Protein)
Not immunologicall mediated	T Cell-mediated	IgE-mediated; circulating antibodies
Localized to area of contact	Localized symptoms; may spread	Systemic response
Redness; itching; dry, crusted lesions	Redness; irritation; eczema; urticaria (hives)	Urticaria (hives); rhinitis; asthma-like symptoms/respiratory distress; swelling of mucous membranes; anaphylaxis
Immediate onset (worsens with continued contact)	Delayed onset (hours to days)	Immediate onset (>one hour)
Reaction to friction, chemicals in antimicrobials or gloves, or simply to occlusion	Reaction to chemicals used in glove processing	Reaction to latex protein
Uncomfortable	Significant discomfort	Can be life-threatening

206. OSHA requires employers to provide PPE for all employees in appropriate sizes for each healthcare worker and in sufficient quantities for healthcare workers to wear and to replace it appropriately.

207. Each organization must develop and implement a biohazard risk analysis covering the following issues:

    • Type of risk facing the healthcare worker

    • Type of PPE needed to protect the healthcare worker from the risk

    • The frequency with which the healthcare worker will be at risk in the area identified as high risk

208. OSHA mandates that all healthcare workers wear PPE in the areas of risk identified in the risk analysis. Wearing PPE is not optional; no healthcare worker can waive the right to wear PPE.

209. PPE appropriate for the operating room includes goggles or glasses with shields, mask, gloves, gowns, caps, and shoe covers. Appropriate PPE is selected based on the anticipated exposure to blood and body fluids.

210. All PPE must be discarded immediately after patient care. PPE cannot be worn from one setting to another.

211. Each organization must provide annual training for all healthcare workers at risk for exposure to bloodborne pathogens. Training includes the organization's risk analysis and PPE requirements, a review of the organization's policy and procedures in regard to bloodborne pathogens, and PPE as a part of the annual education program. Documentation that each employee has received the training should be kept in the employee's personnel file.

212. The facility's exposure control plan developed from the risk analysis should be updated annually. This plan should identify the following elements:

    • The location of safety equipment such as PPE, spill kits, and eyewash stations

    • The responsibilities of the safety officer

    • Hazardous chemicals used and their locations

    • Location of safety policies and procedures

    • Location of SDSs for all hazardous material used in the organization

    • Instructions for reporting an exposure or injury

213. The exposure control plan should also address exposure risks based on job description, the facility's education plan, and vaccination and immunization requirements.

Sharps Safety

214. Sharps safety should be addressed by each facility either in the exposure control plan or separately.

215. In the operating room, the two sharps most frequently involved in injuries are suture needles and scalpel blades.

216. The two components of a sharps safety plan are engineering controls and safe clinical practice.

217. Clinical practices that reduce the likelihood of a sharps injury include:

    • Double-gloving

    • Use of the neutral zone, when appropriate, to avoid hand-to-hand passage of sharps

    • No-touch technique; no recapping of hypodermic needles

    • Clear communication among team members when passing sharps

218. Engineering controls include:

    • Blunt-tip suture needles when possible

    • Safety scalpels

    • Puncture-resistant collection and disposal containers

    • Protective caps on sharp instruments

219. AORN (2015d) and the CDC (2015b) have excellent tools for developing a sharps safety plan and educating employees.

Disaster Planning

220. The facility disaster plan identifies the type of personnel, equipment, and supplies needed for each type of disaster the facility might experience, as well as a mechanism for communicating with employees (TJC, 2015a, pp. EC5–EC24):

    • Severe weather (hurricane, tornado, flood)

    • Massive trauma (transportation, bombing, fire)

    • Terrorist attack (biological, chemical exposure)

Safety Compliance

221. Compliance with safety regulations, standards, and recommendations is not optional. Noncompliance places healthcare workers, patients, and potentially the entire facility at risk for serious injury including deaths.

222. Auditing for compliance with organizational policy and procedures, plans, rules, regulations, standards, and recommendations is essential. Auditing should be done quarterly at a minimum.

223. An audit in the operating room should address at least the following:

    • PPE attire and safety

    • Hand hygiene (washing and wearing of exam gloves and sterile gloves appropriately)

    • Safety (sharps safety, patient safety, sterile field)

    • Safe medication practices

    • Fire prevention and response

    • Safe use of lasers and electrosurgery, including smoke evacuation

    • Time-out (three phases: before induction, before the incision is made, debrief following the procedure)

224. Issues identified through an audit must be addressed immediately. Policy and/or protocol changes might be necessary. It is likely that staff and/or indivdual education will be needed.

Section Questions

1. What is a safety data sheet? [Refs 176–177]

2. In addition to PPE, what must be made available in case of emergency exposure to hazardous chemicals? [Ref 180]

3. What potentially harmful chemicals are used in the operating room? [Refs 181, 183, 186]

4. How should methyl methacrylate be mixed for patient use? [Refs 188, 190]

5. What implications might methyl methacrylate have for contact lens wearers? [Ref 189]

6. What are some of the harmful components that have been identified in surgical smoke? [Ref 192]

7. Identify the AORN recommendations for surgical smoke evacuation. [Ref 196]

8. Distinguish among Type I and Type IV allergy to latex and contact dermatitis. [Refs 197, 199–200, 202]

9. Identify which of the reactions to latex is the most threatening and give your rationale. [Refs 199, 201]

10. What is OSHA's position on hospital's providing PPE for employees? [Ref 206, 208]

11. What elements are addressed in a risk analysis? [Ref 207]

12. What are the components of an exposure control plan that it based on a risk analysis? [Ref 212]

13. Describe both clinical practice and engineering control approaches to sharps safety. [Refs 217–218]

14. What types of disasters must a hospital prepare for? [Ref 220]

15. What practices should be addressed in a safety audit? [Ref 223]

References

Accreditation Association for Ambulatory Health Care (AAAHC). (2014). *2012 Setting standards, improving lives*. Skokie, IL: Author.

Accreditation Association for Ambulatory Health Care (AAAHC). (2015). *2012 Accreditation handbook for ambulatory health care*. Skokie, IL: Author.

American National Standards Institute (ANSI)/Association for the Advancement of Medical Instrumentation (AAMI) (2001). *Processing CJD: Contaminated patient care equipment and environmental surfaces*. ST79: 2013 & A1:2010 & A2:2011 Annex C. Washington, DC: ANSI/AAMI.

Association of periOperative Registered Nurses (AORN). (2015a). *Fire safety tool kit*. Retrieved from http:///www.aorn.org/Secondary.aspx?id=20877#axzz1z8QgEJqQ

Association of periOperative Registered Nurses (AORN). (2015b). *Guidelines for perioperative practice*. Denver, CO: Author.

Association of periOperative Registered Nurses (AORN). (2015c). *Management of surgical smoke toolkit.* Retrieved from http://www.aorn.org/toolkits/surgicalsmoke/

Association of periOperative Registered Nurses (AORN). (2015d). *Sharps safety tool kit.* Retrieved from http://www.aorn.org/toolkits/sharpssafety/

Bureau of Labor Statistics (BLS). (2013). *Nonfatal occupational injuries and illnesses requiring days away from work: Table 18.* Retrieved from http://www.bls.gov/news.release/osh2.nr0.htm

Centers for Disease Control and Prevention (CDC). (2002). Guideline for hand hygiene in health-care settings. *Morbidity and Mortality Weekly Report, 51*(RR-16), 1–56. Retrieved from http://www.cdc.gov/mmwr/PDF/rr/rr5116.pdf

Centers for Disease Control and Prevention (CDC). (2015). Occupational traumatic injuries among workers in health care facilities—United States, 2012–2014. *Morbidity and Mortality Weekly Report, 64*(15), 405–410. Retrieved from http://www.cdc.gov/mmwr/preview/mmwrhtml/mm6415a2.htm

Centers for Disease Control and Prevention (CDC). (2015a). *Overweight and obesity: Data and statistics.* Retrieved from http://www.cdc.gov/obesity/data/index.html

Centers for Disease Control and Prevention (CDC). (2015b). *Sharps safety for healthcare settings.* Retrieved from http://www.cdc.gov/sharpssafety/tools.html

Compressed Gas Association. (2015). CGA P-1: *Safe handling of compressed gases.* Retrieved from https://archive.org/stream/gov.law.cga.p-1.1965/cga.p-1.1965_djvu.txt

Council on Surgery and Perioperative Safety. (2015). *Preventing surgical fires.* Retrieved from http://www.cspsteam.org/TJCSurgicalFireCollaborative/preventing-surgicalfires.html

Emergency Care Research Institute (ECRI). (2014a). *ECRI Institute announces top 10 health technology hazards for 2015.* Retrieved from https://www.ecri.org/press/Pages/ECRI-Institute-Announces-Top-10-Health-Technology-Hazards-for-2015.aspx

Emergency Care Research Institute (ECRI). (2014b). *ECRI Institute recommendations for operating room fire extinguishers.* Retrieved from https://www.ecri.org/Documents/AFIG/ECRI_Institute_Recommendations_for_Operating_Room_Fire_Extinguishers.pdf

Emergency Care Research Institute (ECRI). (2015a). *2015 top 10 health technology hazards.* Retrieved from https://www.ecri.org/Pages/2015-Hazards.aspx

Emergency Care Research Institute (ECRI). (2015b). *Surgical fire prevention.* Retrieved from http://www.ecri.org/surgical_fires

Environmental Protection Agency (EPA). (1994). *Methyl methacrylate fact sheet.* Washington, DC: Author. Retrieved from http://www.epa.gov/chemfact/methy-fs.txt

Healthcare Facilities Accreditation Program (HFAP). (2014). *Accreditation requirements for healthcare facilities.* Chicago, IL: Author.

Healy, G., Cowles, C., & Hood, D. (2014). *Surgical fires: Prevention, suppression, and response.* NFPA Conference & Expo, Las Vegas, NV. Retrieved from http://www.nfpa.org/~/media/AA75771F8EA54DA5B529B39FA8D147B0.pdf

Healthcare Facilities Accreditation Program (HFAP). (2009). *Ambulatory care/office based surgery program standards manual.* Chicago, IL: Author.

Institute of Medicine (IOM). (2000). *To err is human: Building a safer health system.* Washington, DC: National Academy Press. Retrieved from http://www.nap.edu/catalog/9728/to-err-is-human-building-a-safer-health-system

Institute of Medicine (IOM). (2001). *Crossing the quality chasm: A new health system for the 21st century.* Washington, DC: National Academy Press. Retrieved from http://iom.edu/Reports/2001/Crossing-the-Quality-Chasm-A-New-Health-System-for-the-21st-Century.aspx

Institute of Medicine (IOM). (2010). *The future of nursing: Leading change, advancing health.* Washington, DC: National Academy Press. Retrieved from http://iom.nationalacademies.org/Reports/2010/The-Future-of-Nursing-Leading-Change-Advancing-Health.aspx

Jelecevic, J., Maidanjuk, S., Leithner, A., Loewe, K., & Kuehn, K. (2014). Methyl methacrylate levels in orthopedic surgery: Comparison of two conventional vacuum mixing systems. *Annals of Occupational Hygiene, 58*(4), 493–500.

The Joint Commission (TJC). (2003). *Sentinel event alert: Preventing surgical fires.* Issue 29. Retrieved from http://www.jointcommission.org/assets/1/18/SEA_29.pdf

The Joint Commission (TJC). (2011). *Sentinel event alert: Radiation risks of diagnostic imaging.* Issue 47. Retrieved from http://www.jointcommission.org/assets/1/18/SEA_47.pdf

The Joint Commission (TJC). (2014). *Sentinel event policy and procedures.* Retrieved from http://www.jointcommission.org/Sentinel_Event_Policy_and_Procedures/default.aspx

The Joint Commission (TJC). (2015a). *2012 Hospital accreditation standards.* Oakbrook Terrace, IL: Author. Retrieved from http://www.jcrinc.com/2015-hospital-accreditation-standards/

The Joint Commission (TJC). (2015b). *National patient safety goals.* Retrieved from http://www.jointcommission.org/standards_information/npsgs.aspx

Meldi, D., Rhoades, F., & Gippe, A. (2009). The big three: A side by side matrix comparing hospital accrediting agencies. *Synergy*. Retrieved from http://www.namss.org/Portals/0/Regulatory/The%20Big%20Three%20A%20Side%20by%20Side%20Matrix%20Comparing%20Hospital%20Accrediting%20Agencies.pdf

National Fire Protection Agency. (2015a). *NFPA 1: Fire code*. Retrieved from http://www.nfpa.org/codes-and-standards/document-information-pages?mode=code&code=1

National Fire Protection Agency. (2015b). *NFPA 101: Life safety code®*. Retrieved from http://www.nfpa.org/codes-and-standards/document-information-pages?mode=code&code=101

National Institute for Occupational Safety and Health (NIOSH). (1996). *Control of smoke from laser/electric surgical procedures*. Retrieved from http://www.cdc.gov/niosh/docs/hazardcontrol/hc11.html

Occupational Safety and Health Administration (OSHA). (2015). *29 CFR 1910 table of contents*. Retrieved from https://www.osha.gov/pls/oshaweb/owadisp.show_document?p_table=standards&p_id=10051

Phillips, Nancymarie (ed). (2016). Berry & Kohn's Operating Room Technique, 13th Edition. Mosby/Elsevier: Philadelphia, PA

Rutala, W. A., & Weber, D. J. (2008). *Guideline for disinfection and sterilization in healthcare facilities, 2008*. Retrieved from http://www.cdc.gov/hicpac/Disinfection_Sterilization/acknowledg.html

Schlegel, U., Sturm, M., Ewerbeck, V., & Breusch, S. (2004). Efficacy of vacuum bone cement mixing systems in reducing methylmethacrylate fume exposure: Comparison of 7 different mixing devices and handmixing. *Acta OrthopaedicaScandinavica*, 75(5), 559–566.

Washington State Department of Labor and Industries. (2015). *Helpful tools for specific rules*. Retrieved from http://www.lni.wa.gov/safety/rules/helpfultools/default.asp

Post-Test

Read each question carefully. Some questions have more than one correct answer.

1. Which of the following statements *best* describes a *culture of safety*?

    a. Achieving a safe workplace requires changes in organizational structure, policy, and protocols.

    b. Mistakes made are opportunities for improvement, and no one is ever punished.

    c. The culture of the organization, starting with administration, is focused on transparency and continuous improvement.

    d. The workplace is fair, and no one is blamed for mistakes until there is enough evidence available.

2. Describe the differences between regulations and standards.

    a. Regulations are developed by government agencies and have the force of law.

    b. State agency standards can be less stringent than federal standards.

    c. Regulations are developed by state agencies, and they supersede federal regulations.

    d. Standards are set by professional organizations, government agencies, and other organizations and have the force of law.

3. Which federal organization manages the HCAHPS survey?

    a. CDC

    b. OSHA

    c. FDA

    d. CMS

4. Which of the following organizations has primary responsibility for publishing and enforcing workplace safety and health standards?

    a. OSHA

    b. NIOSH

    c. CDC

    d. EPA

5. What does CFR stand for?

    a. Center for Regulations

    b. Center for Federal Resolutions

    c. Code of Federal Regulations

    d. Code for Regulations

6. What is the CFR location of the OSHA's bloodborne pathogen standard?

    a. 29 CFR 1910.1030

    b. 1910 CFR 29

    c. 29 CFR 1030

    d. 1030 29 CFR 1910

7. Which federal organization manages the disposal of medical waste and medications?

    a. FDA

    b. EPA

    c. CDC

    d. NFPA

8. What are the two NFPA codes on which healthcare organizations base their fire safety plans?

    a. Fire Code and Safe Building Code

    b. Fire Extinguisher Code and Life Safety Code

    c. Fire Code and Life Safety Code

    d. Safe Building Code and Life Safety Code

9. Which of the following organizations conducts research and recommends practical solutions to prevent employee illness and injury?

    a. CDC

    b. NIOSH

    c. ANSI

    d. AAMI

10. Which of the following are standard-setting organizations?

    a. ECRI

    b. AORN

    c. AAMI

    d. IOM

11. What is the primary purpose of accreditation?

    a. Demonstrate that the facility is the best in the area

    b. Get higher reimbursements from the CMS

    c. Demonstrate achievement of exceptional performance

    d. Become eligible for CMS reimbursement

12. Which of the following is *not* a component of a job safety analysis?

    a. Identification of tasks related to patient care

    b. Identification of hazards in the workplace

    c. Selection of a safety officer

    d. Review of safety protocols

13. Forty-four percent of surgical fires occur

    a. because of pooled prep solution.

    b. because the active electrode wasn't contained in a holster.

    c. when lasers ignite oxygen in the endotracheal tube.

    d. in the oxygen-rich environment surrounding the patient's face.

14. Which of the following are components of the TJC's description of a sentinel event?

    a. Preventable situation

    b. Associated with the patient's illness or underlying condition

    c. Results in death or serious hard

    d. Requires intervention to sustain life

15. The fire triangle includes which of the following?

    a. Ignition source

    b. Oxygen

    c. Fire extinguisher

    d. Fuel

16. The perioperative nurse's first responsibility in case of fire is to
    a. turn off emergency shutoff valves.
    b. get the fire extinguisher.
    c. alert the front desk to the emergency.
    d. remove burning material from the patient.

17. Which of the following has the potential for starting a fire?
    a. Placing the active electrode in a puncture-proof holder
    b. Draping as soon as the prep has been completed
    c. Draping to prevent the trapping of oxygen
    d. Scraping eschar from the active electrode tip

18. The most common cause of surgical fires is
    a. the laser unit.
    b. an electrosurgical unit.
    c. vapors from prep solutions.
    d. an uncoupled fiberoptic light cable.

19. What does the "R" in RACE stand for?
    a. Rescue
    b. Report
    c. Review
    d. Respond

20. In response to an LIM alarm, the perioperative nurse should
    a. plug the last piece of electrical equipment into another outlet.
    b. send all electrical equipment to biomedical engineering for testing.
    c. unplug electrical equipment starting with the device most recently plugged in.
    d. send the electrical device that set off the alarm to biomedical engineering for testing.

21. During fluoroscopy, what is considered the minimum safe distance from the radiation source to the stand?
    a. 4 feet
    b. 6 feet
    c. 10 feet
    d. 15 feet

22. Which of the following is/are correct statements about dosimeters?
    a. A dosimeter is a strip of X-ray film encased in a lead shield.
    b. Pregnant personnel should be prohibited from working around radiation.
    c. Clip the dosimeter to the same place every time it is worn.
    d. The dosimeter should be read weekly to assess exposure.

23. Which of the following is/are correct ways to handle lead shielding devices?
    a. Hang them vertically on a fixed rack designed for them.
    b. Fold them carefully and store them in a mobile cart.
    c. Drape them over the X-ray machine.
    d. Discard them after each procedure.

24. Around one-third of back injuries suffered by nurses occur when they are
    a. lifting instrument sets.
    b. pulling items from high shelves or lifting them from low shelves.
    c. moving heavy pieces of equipment.
    d. moving a patient.

25. Factors that influence the number of back injuries include
    a. the advancing age of the nursing workforce.
    b. increasing obesity of patients.
    c. sicker, less mobile patients
    d. lack of exercise.

26. Proper body mechanics for lifting include
    a. bending at the waist.
    b. using back muscles to lift.
    c. standing close to reach for an object above shoulder level.
    d. placing the feet apart to create a wide base of support.

27. How can the scrubbed person maintain good posture?
    a. Sit on a stool when not involved in passing instruments.
    b. Find a comfortable position and maintain it.
    c. Place one foot on a stool.
    d. Lean against the operating room bed to relieve pressure on the back.

28. What is a Safety Data Sheet (SDS)?
    a. List of all hazardous chemicals in the workplace
    b. Description of hazards associated with a chemical used in the workplace
    c. Form that describes a chemical's product composition, handling, storage, disposal, and postexposure instructions
    d. Detailed contact information for reporting exposure to a hazardous chemical

29. Which of the following statements about methyl methacrylate is/are correct?
    a. Exposure can cause skin rash, itching, watering of the eyes, and headaches.
    b. Mixing bone cement many times during the day, even with a mixing system, represents an increased health risk.
    c. The EPA considers methyl methacrylate a carcinogen.
    d. Wear two pairs of gloves.

30. How can surgical smoke negatively affect healthcare personnel?
    a. Interferes with the surgeon's vision of the wound
    b. Has mutagenic potential
    c. Causes ocular and upper respiratory tract irritation
    d. Has unpleasant odors

31. Which of the following is/are recommendations for managing surgical smoke?
    a. Use a central or portable smoke evacuation system.
    b. Regular wall suction is adequate, except for large amounts of smoke.
    c. Wear a high-filtration mask and protective eyewear.
    d. Use an inline filter for small amounts of smoke.

32. Which of the following statements is/are true?
    a. Latex allergy is less common than contact dermatitis, but more hazardous.
    b. Dermatitis is caused by exposure to chemicals in glove manufacturing.
    c. Individuals with Type IV allergy should avoid exposure to latex altogether.
    d. Latex allergy symptoms resolve when contact is discontinued.

33. Which of the following statements is/are true of PPE?
    a. PPE is mandatory, not optional.
    b. OSHA requires the hospital to provide appropriate PPE for all employees.
    c. PPE can be reused if not soiled.
    d. The type of PPE required is determined by the risk of exposure to bloodborne pathogens.

34. Which of the following statements is/are true about safety compliance?
    a. Standards and recommendations are not optional.
    b. Noncompliance puts both employees and the facility at risk.
    c. An audit program can help to assure that the facility is compliant.
    d. Fire safety and the time-out process should be included in the facility audit.

35. What type(s) of disaster would you expect to be addressed in a facility's disaster plan?
    a. Multiple motor vehicle collision
    b. Weather-related disasters
    c. Exposure to a biological agent
    d. Airplane crash

Competence Checklist: Workplace Safety

Under "Observer's Initials," enter initials upon successful achievement of the competency. Enter N/A if the competency is not appropriate for the institution.

Name_____

	Observer's Initials	Date
1. Maintains active electrode in holster	_____	_____
2. Does not wrap ESU cord around metal instrument	_____	_____
3. Periodically cleans ESU active electrode tip of eschar	_____	_____
4. Moistens gauze, sponges, and other items during surgery	_____	_____
5. Prevents contact of activated fiberoptic cord with drapes and gowns	_____	_____
6. Checks electrical cords before plugging in equipment	_____	_____
7. Places cords and equipment out of the traffic pattern to prevent tripping injury	_____	_____
8. Can describe action to take if an LIM alarm occurs	_____	_____
9. Maintains an orderly environment to prevent slips, trips, and falls	_____	_____
10. Wears nonskid shoes	_____	_____
11. Identifies location of O_2 shutoff valves, LIM, fire extinguisher, and evacuation route	_____	_____
12. Can verbalize the significance of the acronyms RACE and PASS	_____	_____
13. Wears lead apron and thyroid collar when potential for radiation exposure exists	_____	_____
14. Hangs X-ray gowns vertically when not in use (does not fold)	_____	_____
15. Uses correct body mechanics when pulling, pushing, or lifting equipment or patients	_____	_____
16. Demonstrates proper use of PPE	_____	_____
17. Can locate Safety Data Sheets	_____	_____
18. When handling methyl methacrylate, double gloves, pours liquid into powder, and uses appropriate mixing system	_____	_____
19. Demonstrates proper use of glutaraldehyde (if present in operating room)	_____	_____
20. Demonstrates proper use of formaldehyde	_____	_____
21. Demonstrates appropriate management of surgical smoke	_____	_____
22. Demonstrates sharps safety practice	_____	_____
23. Demonstrates safe medication practices	_____	_____

Observer's Signature   Initials   Date

_____

Orientee's Signature

_____

Appendix:
Answers to Post–Test Questions

Chapter 1

1. Answer: D [Ref 1]
2. Answer: C [Refs 4–6]
3. Answer: B [Ref 7]
4. Answer: B [Ref 13]
5. Answer: C [Ref 15]
6. Answer: A [Ref 16]
7. Answer: C [Ref 19]
8. Answer: A, B, C, D [Refs 23–25]
9. Answer: A [Ref 26]
10. Answer: C [Ref 28]
11. Answer: D [Ref 30]
12. Answer: B [Ref 31]
13. Answer: A [Ref 32]
14. Answer: C [Ref 39]
15. Answer: D [Ref 41]
16. Answer: A, B, C, D [Ref 44]
17. Answer: B [Ref 45]
18. Answer: B [Ref 47]
19. Answer: A, B, C [Ref 56]
20. Answer: A, B, C, D [Ref 59]
21. Answer: B [Ref 63]
22. Answer: A [Ref 70]

Chapter 2

1. Answer: B [Ref 4]
2. Answer: A, B, D [Refs 8, 9]
3. Answer: A, B, C, D [Ref 17]
4. Answer: A, B [Ref 20]
5. Answer: D [Ref 23]
6. Answer: C, D [Ref 24]
7. Answer: A, B [Refs 26, 27]
8. Answer: A, B, C [Ref 31]
9. Answer: A, B, C, D [Ref 32]
10. Answer: C [Ref 33]
11. Answer: D [Ref 36]
12. Answer: A, C [Ref 44]
13. Answer: A, B, C [Ref 53]
14. Answer: A, B, C, D [Ref 54]
15. Answer: A, B, C, D [Ref 56]
16. Answer: C [Ref 57]

17. Answer: A [Ref 60]
18. Answer: A, B, C [Ref 64]
19. Answer: B, D [Ref 67]
20. Answer: B [Ref 68]
21. Answer: A, B, C, D [Ref 75]
22. Answer: A, B, C, D [Ref 80]
23. Answer: D [Ref 82]
24. Answer: D [Ref 84]
25. Answer: C [Ref 86]

Chapter 3

1. Answer: B [Ref *Definitions*]
2. Answer: A [Ref *Definitions*]
3. Answer: A, B, C, D [Refs 1, 6, 7, 144]
4. Answer: C [Ref 8]
5. Answer: A [Ref Exhibit 3-1]
6. Answer: B [Ref Exhibit 3-1]
7. Answer: D [Ref 149]
8. Answer: A [Refs *Definitions*, 151]
9. Answer: C [Ref 154]
10. Answer: B [Ref 163]
11. Answer: A, B, D [Refs 155, 162–165, 168]
12. Answer: C [Ref 169]
13. Answer: A, B [Refs 174, 177]
14. Answer: D [Ref 174]
15. Answer: D [Ref 197]
16. Answer: A, B [Refs 206, 207]
17. Answer: B [Ref 209]
18. Answer: A, B [Refs 210, 218]
19. Answer: B, C [Refs 211, 212, 220]
20. Answer: C, D [Ref 227]
21. Answer: C [Ref 225]
22. Answer: B, C [Refs 86, 93, 127, 228, 236]
23. Answer: A, B, D [Refs 237, 238, 241]
24. Answer: A, B, C, D [Refs 242, 243, 248, 252]
25. Answer: A [Refs 245]
26. Answer: A, B, C [Refs 131, 135, 258]
27. Answer: C [Ref 138]
28. Answer: A, C, D [Refs 265, 274, 278]
29. Answer: A, B, C [Refs 281, 283, 285]
30. Answer: B [Ref 290]
31. Answer: A, B, C [Refs *Definitions*, 25]

32. Answer: A, C [Ref *Definitions*]
33. Answer: A, C, D [Refs 9, 12, 13]
34. Answer: C [Ref Exhibit 3-1]
35. Answer: B [Ref 42]
36. Answer: C [Ref 27]
37. Answer: B, D [Refs 15, 16]
38. Answer: A, C, D [Refs 15, 42]
39. Answer: A, B [Refs 17, 21]
40. Answer: A, B, C [Ref 22]
41. Answer: A, C [Ref 45]
42. Answer: C [Ref 48]
43. Answer: A, B, C, D [Refs 57, 58]
44. Answer: A, B, D [Refs 28, 29]
45. Answer: B [Ref 33]
46. Answer: B, C, [Ref 67]
47. Answer: A, B [Refs 65, 72]
48. Answer: B, D [Refs 78, 80]
49. Answer: A, B, C, D [Refs 81, 82]
50. Answer: A, B, C [Refs 87, 89, 90]
51. Answer: A, B, C, D [Refs 90, 93–96]
52. Answer: A, B [Refs 97, 98]
53. Answer: A, B, D [Refs 107, 108, 112]
54. Answer: B [Ref 117]
55. Answer: D [Ref 122]
56. Answer: A, B, C, D [Refs 127, 224, 227]
57. Answer: A, B, D [Refs 238, 239, 241]
58. Answer: A, C [Ref 133]
59. Answer: D [Ref 130]
60. Answer: D [Ref 130]
61. Answer: A, B [Refs 135, 136]
62. Answer: B, C [Refs 141, 143]
63. Answer: B, D [Refs 326, 337]
64. Answer: B, C, D [Refs 331–333]
65. Answer: A [Ref 320]

Chapter 4

1. Answer: C [Ref 3]
2. Answer: C [Ref 5]
3. Answer: A [Ref 8]
4. Answer: A [Ref 8]
5. Answer: B [Ref 15]
6. Answer: B [Ref 16]
7. Answer: D [Ref 25]
8. Answer: D [Refs 29, 33, 34, 35]
9. Answer: B [Ref 30]
10. Answer: C [Ref 37]
11. Answer: A [Ref 41]
12. Answer: D [Refs 43, 44]
13. Answer: A [Ref 45]
14. Answer: D [Refs 49, 50]
15. Answer: A [Ref 51]
16. Answer: A [Ref 54]
17. Answer: C [Ref 56]
18. Answer: B [Ref 57]

19. Answer: D [Ref 59]
20. Answer: A [Ref 61]
21. Answer: B [Ref 62]
22. Answer: C [Ref 64]
23. Answer: B [Ref 65]
24. Answer: D [Ref 80]
25. Answer: B [Refs 75, 78, 82, 83]
26. Answer: B [Ref 93]
27. Answer: A [Ref 93]
28. Answer: B [Refs 96, 99,101]
29. Answer: A [Refs 107, 109, 110]
30. Answer: D [Refs 123, 124]
31. Answer: B [Ref 129]
32. Answer: C [Refs 132, 134, 137, 138]
33. Answer: A [Ref 148]
34. Answer: B [Ref 162]
35. Answer: A [Refs 168, 169, 170]
36. Answer: C [Ref 176]
37. Answer: D [Ref 180]
38. Answer: A [Ref 198]
39. Answer: B [Ref 208]
40. Answer: D [Ref 219]
41. Answer: A [Refs 226, 227, 228]
42. Answer: C [Refs 231–233]
43. Answer: B [Refs 236, 237, 238, 240]
44. Answer: D [Ref 252]
45. Answer: A [Ref 254]
46. Answer: D [Ref 255]
47. Answer: B [Ref 261]
48. Answer: C [Ref 284]
49. Answer: C [Ref 298]
50. Answer: C [Ref 301]

Chapter 5

1. Answer: B [Ref 1]
2. Answer: A, C [Ref 2]
3. Answer: A [Ref 3]
4. Answer: A, B, C, D [Ref 4]
5. Answer: C [Refs 13, 15]
6. Answer: A, C, D [Ref 14]
7. Answer: A, B, D [Ref 22]
8. Answer: D [Ref 23]
9. Answer: B [Ref 36]
10. Answer: D [Ref 40]
11. Answer: A, B [Ref 45]
12. Answer: B, C, D [Ref 55]
13. Answer: A [Refs 58–59]
14. Answer: D [Refs 60–62]
15. Answer: A, B, C [Refs 68, 72]
16. Answer: A, B, D [Ref 82]
17. Answer: B [Ref 115]
18. Answer: A, B, C [Ref 102]
19. Answer: A, C [Refs 121, 136, 192]
20. Answer: A, D [Refs 131–132]

21. Answer: A, C, D [Ref 138]
22. Answer: A, B, D [Ref 140]
23. Answer: D [Ref 145]
24. Answer: B, C, D [Refs 148, 149]
25. Answer: A, C [Ref 150]
26. Answer: C [Ref 162]
27. Answer: B [Ref 171]
28. Answer: C [Ref 187]
29. Answer: A, D [Refs 186, 189]
30. Answer: B [Ref 199]
31. Answer: A, B, D [Ref 203]
32. Answer: A, B, C, D [Refs 210, 211, 215]
33. Answer: A, B, C, D [Refs 218–222]
34. Answer: A, C, D [Ref 226]
35. Answer: A, B, C, D [Ref 231]

Chapter 6

1. Answer: C [Ref *Definitions*]
2. Answer: A [Ref 1]
3. Answer: A, C [Ref 1]
4. Answer: A [Ref 5]
5. Answer: A, B, C, D [Ref 9]
6. Answer: B, D [Ref 8]
7. Answer: B, C, D [Ref 9]
8. Answer: B [Ref 14]
9. Answer: D [Ref 15]
10. Answer: C [Ref 25]
11. Answer: D [Ref 49]
12. Answer: B, C [Refs 44, 75]
13. Answer: B [Ref 56]
14. Answer: C [Ref 26]
15. Answer: D [Ref 64]
16. Answer: A [Ref 67]
17. Answer: A [Ref 71]
18. Answer: D [Refs 79, 81]
19. Answer: C [Ref 76]
20. Answer: A, B, C, D [Ref 89]

Chapter 7

1. Answer: A, B, C [Refs 1, 3, 5]
2. Answer: A, B [Refs 6, 7]
3. Answer: A, C [Refs 7, 8]
4. Answer: C, D [Refs 12, 13, 16]
5. Answer: A, B [Refs 18–21]
6. Answer: A, B, C, D [Refs 22–25]
7. Answer: A, C, D [Refs 26, 29, 31, 34]
8. Answer: A [Refs 35, 36, 59, 61]
9. Answer: B, C, D [Refs 45, 47]
10. Answer: A, C, D [Refs 46, 48, 50]
11. Answer: A, C, D [Refs 51, 56, 58]
12. Answer: A, D [Refs 64–66, 68]
13. Answer: A, D [Refs 74–76]
14. Answer: B, C [Refs 74, 78, 79]

15. Answer: A, B, C [Refs 81, 82, 84, 86]
16. Answer: A, B, C, D [Refs 89–92]
17. Answer: A, B [Refs 97–99]
18. Answer: A, C, D [Refs 92, 102, 105]
19. Answer: C, D [Refs 104–106]
20. Answer: A [Refs 111–114]
21. Answer: A, D [Ref 120]
22. Answer: A, B, C, D [Ref 121]
23. Answer: C, D [Ref 120]
24. Answer: B [Refs 98, 113, 121]
25. Answer: A, C, D [Refs 129, 130, 133]

Chapter 8

1. Answer: A, B, D [Refs 1, 2, 3]
2. Answer: C [Ref 5]
3. Answer: B [Refs 14, 15]
4. Answer: C [Ref 16]
5. Answer: D [Ref 24]
6. Answer: A [Ref 27]
7. Answer: C [Ref 29]
8. Answer: C [Ref 31]
9. Answer: B [Ref 33]
10. Answer: C [Ref 35]
11. Answer: B, D [Refs 38, 39]
12. Answer: C [Ref 40]
13. Answer: D [Ref 44]
14. Answer: A [Ref 53]
15. Answer: C [Ref 54]
16. Answer: C [Ref 60]
17. Answer: B, C, D [Ref Figure 8-9]
18. Answer: D [Ref 68]
19. Answer: A [Ref 69]
20. Answer: C [Refs 73, 74]
21. Answer: A [Ref 78]
22. Answer: D [Ref 80]
23. Answer: B [Ref 84]
24. Answer: C [Refs 86, 87]
25. Answer: D [Ref 89]
26. Answer: A [Ref 94]
27. Answer: C [Ref 95]
28. Answer: B [Ref 99]
29. Answer: A [Ref 103]
30. Answer: C [Ref 105]

Chapter 9

1. Answer: B, C, D [Refs 2, 3]
2. Answer: A, B, C, D [Refs 3, 4, 5]
3. Answer: A, B [Refs 8, 9, 13]
4. Answer: B [Ref 15]
5. Answer: A, B, D [Ref 22]
6. Answer: B, D [Ref 23]
7. Answer: A, C, D [Ref 24]
8. Answer: A, D [Refs 27, 28, 29, 30]

9. Answer: A, B, D, C [Refs 32–38]
10. Answer: B, C, D [Refs 43–48]
11. Answer: B, C [Refs 51, 54, 56, 59]
12. Answer: D [Ref 64]
13. Answer: A, B, C, D [Refs 71–74]
14. Answer: A, B, D [Refs 75, 79, 80]
15. Answer: A, B, C, D [Refs 86, 87, 89, 91]
16. Answer: A, C, D [Refs 97, 100, 102]
17. Answer: A, C [Refs 104, 105]
18. Answer: A, B, C [Refs 108, 112, 115]
19. Answer: A, C [Refs 120, 123]
20. Answer: A, B, C, D [Refs 130, 131, 133, 134, 136]

Chapter 10 Post-Test Part 1

1. Answer: D [Ref 4]
2. Answer: C [Ref 8]
3. Answer: B [Ref 10]
4. Answer: A, C, D [Ref 21]
5. Answer: B, C, D [Refs 27, 30, 35]
6. Answer: A, B, C, D [Ref 38]
7. Answer: C [Ref 38]
8. Answer: B [Ref 41]
9. Answer: A [Ref 49]
10. Answer: A, B, C, D [Ref 54]
11. Answer: B [Ref 64]
12. Answer: A, B, D [Refs 58, 59, 60]
13. Answer: A, B [Refs 70, 71, 74]
14. Answer: B, C, D [Refs 76, 77]
15. Answer: C [Ref 81]
16. Answer: D [Ref 85]
17. Answer: A, B, C, D [Ref 90]
18. Answer: A, B, C, D [Ref 95]
19. Answer: B [Ref 106]
20. Answer: B, C, D [Refs 117, 120–122]
21. Answer: D [Refs 124–126]
22. Answer: B [Ref 127]
23. Answer: A, C, D [Ref 133]
24. Answer: A, B, C, D [Ref 136]
25. Answer: A, B, C, D [Refs 139, 141, 142]

Chapter 10 Post-Test Part 2

1. Answer: A [Ref 147]
2. Answer: C [Ref 150]
3. Answer: A [Ref 156]
4. Answer: A, B, C, D [Refs 159–161, 166]
5. Answer: A, B, C, D [Refs 173–175, 180]
6. Answer: A, C [Refs 182, 187]
7. Answer: A, B [Refs 189, 191, 192, 194]
8. Answer: A, B, C, D [Refs 198–200, 202]
9. Answer: B, C [Ref 204]
10. Answer: A, D [Ref 210]
11. Answer: A, B, C, D [Refs 223, 224, 226, 231]
12. Answer: C [Ref 225]
13. Answer: D [Ref 236]

14. Answer: A [Ref 243]
15. Answer: B [Ref 245]
16. Answer: A, B, C [Refs 262, 263]
17. Answer: D [Ref 265]
18. Answer: A, B, C, D [Ref 269]
19. Answer: A, B, C, D [Refs 275–277]
20. Answer: D [Ref 284]
21. Answer: A [Ref 284]
22. Answer: D [Refs 294, 295]
23. Answer: A, B, D [Ref 297]
24. Answer: A, B, C, D [Ref 303]
25. Answer: A, B, D [Refs 307, 308]
26. Answer: A, B, C, D [Refs 316 318, 321, 327]
27. Answer: A [Ref 338]
28. Answer: A, B, D [Ref 342]
29. Answer: A, B, C, D [Refs 350, 351, 352]
30. Answer: A, B, C, D [Refs 370, 375, 378, 383]

Chapter 11

1. Answer: C [Ref 4, 5]
2. Answer: A [Refs 6, 7]
3. Answer: D [Ref 12]
4. Answer: A [Ref 13]
5. Answer: C [Ref 14]
6. Answer: A [Ref 14]
7. Answer: B [Ref 19]
8. Answer: C [Ref 23]
9. Answer: B [Ref 29]
10. Answer: B, C [Refs 32, 40]
11. Answer C [Ref 41]
12. Answer: C [Ref 68]
13. Answer: D [Ref 80]
14. Answer: A, C, D [Ref 83]
15. Answer: A, B, D [Ref 106]
16. Answer: D [Ref 107]
17. Answer: B [Ref 109]
18. Answer: B [Ref 113]
19. Answer: A [Ref 108]
20. Answer: C [Ref 124]
21. Answer: B [Ref 133]
22. Answer: C [Ref 139]
23. Answer: A [Ref 144]
24. Answer: D [Ref 148]
25. Answer: A B [Ref 153]
26. Answer: D [Ref 160]
27. Answer: C [Ref 159]
28. Answer: C [Ref 177]
29. Answer: A, D [Refs 187, 188, 190]
30. Answer: A, B, C, D [Refs 193, 194]
31. Answer: A, C, D [Ref 196]
32. Answer: A, D [Refs 197, 198, 201, 202]
33. Answer: A, B, D [Refs 208, 209]
34. Answer: A, B, C, D [Refs 221, 223]
35. Answer: A, B, C, D [Ref 220]

Glossary

Active electrode: An accessory used in electrosurgery to deliver current from an electrosurgical generator to a patient for the purpose of hemostasis and/or dissecting tissue during surgery.

Aeration (ethylene oxide aeration): A process utilizing warm air circulating in an enclosed cabinet to remove residual ethylene oxide from sterilized items. The length of the process is determined by the composition of the sterilized items and the amount of residual ethylene oxide. The process generally takes from 8 to 12 hours.

Alcohol-based hand rub: A product containing alcohol intended for application to the hands for the purpose of reducing the number of microorganisms on the hands. Product is available as a rinse, gel, or foam. It is usually formulated to contain between 60% and 95% alcohol and contains emollients. Some alcohol products have been cleared by the FDA for use as a surgical hand antiseptic and may be used as a surgical scrub prior to gowning and gloving for surgery.

Aldrete postanesthesia scoring system: A scoring system used to evaluate the recovery of patients who have received general anesthesia by assessing patient activity, respiration, circulation, and oxygen saturation.

Amnestic/amnesic: An anesthetic agent that causes amnesia.

Anatomical timed scrub: A scrub procedure using a sponge/brush and an antimicrobial surgical scrub agent, allocating a specified amount of time is allocated for to scrubbing each surface of the fingers, hands, forearm to just above the elbow.

Anesthesia assistant: A person with a premedical bachelor degree who has completed a clinical program at the graduate level. An anesthesia assistant must be supervised by an anesthesiologist.

Anesthesia standby: See *Moderate sedation/analgesia*.

Antisaligogue: An agent that diminishes or arrests the flow of saliva (e.g., atropine).

Antiseptic: A germicidal agent used on skin and tissue to destroy and prevent growth of microorganisms.

Anxiolytic: A drug that relieves anxiety.

Asepsis: The absence of pathogenic microorganisms.

Aseptic practice/technique: The practices by which contamination from microorganisms is prevented.

Atraumatic suture: Suture that is attached to the needle during manufacture. The needle and suture are a continuous unit in which needle diameter and suture diameter are matched as closely as possible, thereby creating minimal trauma as the needle and strand are pulled through tissue.

Autoclave: A steam sterilizer.

Back table: Also referred to as an instrument table. A stainless steel table covered with a sterile drape on which sterile surgical instruments and supplies are arranged for use during surgery.

Bagging: Manual delivery of anesthetic agents by compressing the reservoir bag on the anesthesia machine.

Barrier (sterile): Material, such as a sterile drape or wrapper, that is used to prevent the entry or migration of microorganisms from an unsterile surface or area. Gowns, drapes, and package wrappers are examples of sterile barriers.

Bier block (intravenous block): A technique in which a local anesthetic agent is injected into a tourniquet-occluded extremity for purposes of analgesia.

Bioburden: A population of viable microorganisms on an item.

Biofilm: A collection of microscopic organisms in water, protected by a polysaccharide matrix that adheres to a surface and prevents antimicrobial agents from reaching the cells in the matrix.

Biological monitor/biological indicator: A sterilization monitor consisting of a known population of spores resistant to measurable and controlled parameters of a sterilization process.

Bonewax: Wax made from beeswax, which is used to stop bleeding from bone. It is used most often in neurosurgery and orthopedic surgery.

Bovie: Dr. William Bovie was instrumental in developing the first spark-gap vacuum tube generator that produced cutting with hemostasis. Modern electrosurgical units are still referred to as "Bovies." The more accurate term is *electrosurgical unit.*

Bowie-Dick test: A test of a steam sterilizer's ability to remove air and noncondensable gases from the chamber.

Capacitive coupling: The transfer of electrical (stray) current from the active electrode into other conductive surgical equipment. Capacitive coupling can cause a burn injury, such as bowel perforation, during laparoscopic surgery that may go unnoticed and lead to peritonitis.

Capillarity: A process that allows tissue fluid to be soaked or absorbed into suture material and carried along the strand.

Capnography: A process of monitoring the inhaled and exhaled concentration or partial pressure of carbon dioxide in respiratory gases.

Cavitation: In fluids, the process in which high-intensity sound waves generate tiny bubbles that expand until they collapse or implode, causing a negative pressure on the surfaces of the instruments that dislodges soil.

Certified registered nurse anesthetist (CRNA): A registered nurse with at least 2 additional years of anesthesia training and acute care experience.

Chemical indicator: A device used to monitor one or more process parameters in the sterilization cycle. The device responds with a chemical or physical change (usually a color change) to conditions within the sterilization chamber. It is usually supplied as a paper strip, tape, or label that changes color or as a pellet that melts when the parameter has been met. A chemical indicator reading of "acceptable" does not guarantee sterility.

- Class 1 (process indicator): Chemical indicator intended for use with individual units (e.g., packs, containers) to demonstrate that the unit has been exposed to the sterilization process and to distinguish between processed and unprocessed units.
- Class 2 (Bowie-Dick test indicator): Chemical indicator designed for use in a specific test procedure (e.g., the Bowie-Dick test is used to determine whether air removal has been adequate in a steam sterilization process).
- Class 3 (single-parameter indicator): Chemical indicator designed to react to one of the critical parameters of sterilization and to indicate exposure to a sterilization cycle at a stated value of the chosen parameter.
- Class 4 (multi-parameter indicator): Chemical indicator designed to react to two or more

of the critical parameters of sterilization and to indicate exposure to a sterilization cycle at stated values of the chosen parameters.

- Class 5 (integrating indicator): Chemical indicator designed to react to all critical parameters over a specified range of sterilization cycles and whose performance has been correlated to the performance of the stated test organism under the labeled conditions (AAMI, 2011, p. 7).
- Class 6 (emulating indicator): Cycle-specific chemical indicator that verifies the presence or the absence or a specific time and temperature during a sterilization cycle.

Circulating nurse: A perioperative nurse who is present during a surgical procedure, is not scrubbed, and is responsible for managing the nursing care of the patient and for coordinating and monitoring other activities during the procedure.

Clean contaminated wound (Class II): A wound in which the gastrointestinal, genitourinary, or respiratory tract is entered under planned, controlled means. No spillage occurs, and no infection is present. Examples of clean contaminated procedures include cholecystectomy, cystoscopy, and colon resection.

Clean wound (Class I): A wound in which the gastrointestinal, genitourinary, or respiratory tract is not entered. No inflammation is encountered, and there is no break in aseptic technique. Examples of clean surgical procedures include hernia repair, carpal tunnel repair, and total joint replacement.

Closed gloving: A method of donning sterile gloves in which the hands do not emerge from the sleeves of the gown until the gown cuff is covered by the sterile glove. Only after the glove is donned are the fingers extended beyond the gown edge and inserted into the glove's finger slots.

Conscious sedation: See *Moderate sedation/analgesia.*

Contaminated: Soiled or potentially soiled with microorganisms. All items opened for surgery, whether or not they were used, are considered to be contaminated.

Contaminated wound (Class III): A wound in which gross contamination is present but obvious infection is not. Included in this category are incisions in which nonpurulent inflammation, gross spillage from the gastrointestinal tract, a traumatic wound, or a major break in aseptic technique is encountered. Examples of contaminated procedures include a gunshot wound, rectal procedures, colon resection with GI spillage, and inflamed but not ruptured appendix.

Cottonoid: A small sponge made of compressed cotton often used in neurosurgery. Cottonoids contain a radiopaque marker and come in a variety of sizes.

Counted stroke scrub: A scrub procedure using a sponge/brush and an antimicrobial surgical scrub agent delivering a prescribed number of strokes to each surface of the fingers, hands, and arms.

Critical item: An item that penetrates a mucous membrane or into a vascular space. Critical items must be sterile.

Decontamination: A process of cleaning and disinfecting items so that that they are no longer capable of transmitting infectious particles and are safe for handling by personnel not wearing personal protective equipment. Decontaminated items are not considered sterile.

Desiccation: An electrosurgical method of coagulation, whereby an active electrode is placed in direct contact with tissue.

Dirty wound (Class IV): A wound in which there is dead tissue or an infectious process. Examples of dirty or infected procedures include colon resection for ruptured diverticulitis and amputation of a gangrenous appendage.

Disinfectant: An antimicrobial agent used on inanimate surfaces to destroy microorganisms. The composition and concentration of the disinfectant and the amount of time an item is exposed to it determine the number and types of organisms that will be killed.

- High-level disinfectants kill all bacteria, viruses, fungi, and some spores. They are used only on instruments and medical devices.
- Intermediate-level disinfectants kill vegetative bacteria, mycobacteria, viruses, and fungi. They are used on environmental surfaces.
- Low-level disinfectants that are used on environmental surfaces to kill vegetative forms of bacteria, lipid viruses, and some fungi.

Disinfection: A process that kills all living microorganisms, with the exception of high numbers of spores.

Dispersive electrode: An accessory used in electrosurgery that returns current introduced into the patient by an active electrode to the electrosurgical generator. The dispersive electrode must have sufficient contact with the patient to disperse the current to prevent a burn.

Dynamic-air-removal sterilizer: A type of sterilizer that uses a series of steam flush and pressure pulses to remove air from the chamber.

Electrosurgery: A method of hemostasis and cutting of tissue using radiofrequency electrical current. The energy is supplied from an electrosurgical generator, delivered to the patient from an active electrode, and returned to the generator either via a dispersive electrode (monopolar) or via the second tine of a forcep (bipolar).

Endogenous source of infection: A source of infection that arises from within the body.

Endotoxin: Part of the outer wall of a gram-negative bacteria.

Esmarch: A long, rolled, latex bandage used to squeeze the blood from an extremity. The extremity is elevated and the Esmarch is wrapped tightly around the arm beginning at the fingers and progressing toward the shoulder.

Ethylene oxide (EtO) sterilization: A method of sterilization that utilizes ethylene oxide gas as the sterilant. It is used primarily for items that cannot tolerate the heat and moisture of steam sterilization. There are many restrictions related to installation and use of EtO and the aeration of items processed with EtO to protect personnel and patients from exposure to the sterilant and its byproducts.

Event-related sterility: A sterile item remains sterile until an event occurs that jeopardizes the integrity of the package and exposes the contents to contamination.

Exogenous source of infection: A source of infection from the environment or from sources other than the patient himself.

Extended cycle: A sterilization cycle that requires an exposure time greater than the more common cycle of 4 minutes at 270°F to 275°F (132°C to 135°C).

Fasciculation: Skeletal muscle contractions that occur when groups of muscles that are innervated by the same neuron contract simultaneously. The contractions appear as twitching. Fasciculation following administration of depolarizing muscle relaxants progresses in a cephalocaudal sequence.

Flash sterilization: See *Immediate-use steam sterilization.*

Fluid proof: Prevents the penetration of fluids through an intact barrier.

Fluid resistant: Resistant to the penetration of fluids. Over time, fluids will penetrate.

Fulguration: An electrosurgical method of coagulation whereby sparking is used to coagulate large bleeders. The active electrode does not contact tissue. Sparks contact the tissue, causing superficial coagulation followed by deep necrosis. The purpose of this process is to destroy tissue.

Gelatin sponge (Gelfoam): A sponge, resembling Styrofoam, made from purified gelatin solution and used for hemostasis.

Gossypiboma: Surgical complications resulting from the unintentional retention of soft goods. The term "gossypiboma" is derived from the Latin *gossypium* ("cotton wool, cotton").

H$_2$O$_2$ gas plasma: A fourth state of matter consisting of a cloud of ions, neutrons, and electrons created by the application of an electric or magnetic field. The plasma phase of the sterilization cycle creates free radicals that are reactive with almost all of the molecules essential for normal metabolism of living cells.

H$_2$O$_2$ vapor sterilization: Low-temperature sterilization using hydrogen peroxide to deactivate microorganisms.

Hand-off: The transfer of patient information from one caregiver to another, such as sharing information from the preoperative assessment with other teams members, giving report during relief and change of shift, passing along information during transfer to the postanesthesia care unit (PACU).

Hemoclip: See *Ligating clip.*

Immediate-use steam sterilization (IUSS): A steam sterilization process for items that are needed immediately. IUSS is used when there is insufficient time to process an item in the prepackaged method. IUSS-processed items cannot be stored or used at a later time. IUSS is not a substitute for insufficient inventory. Previously known as "flash sterilization."

Indicator: See *Chemical indicator.*

Induction: The period from the beginning of anesthesia through loss of consciousness.

Inhalation induction: Induction of anesthesia using only inhalation agents given by mask.

Integrator: A device used to monitor more than one process parameter of the sterilization cycle. An example is a paper product that contains a chemical that melts and travels along the paper when the desired parameters have been achieved. The results are displayed in a window along the strip. If the wicking reaches the target area, the parameters of sterilization have been met and sterilization is presumed to have been achieved.

Intraoperative: The period beginning when the patient is brought into the operating room and ending with transfer of the patient to the recovery area. Once a patient has been brought into the room, all open sterile supplies are considered "contaminated to the patient" and cannot be used for another procedure/another patient.

Intravenous block: See *Bier block.*

Intravenous induction: Induction of anesthesia using intravenous medications to induce a loss of consciousness.

Invasive procedure (as defined by the Centers for Medicare and Medicaid, 2009, p. 2): An operative procedure in which skin or mucous membranes and connective tissue are incised, or an instrument is introduced through a natural body orifice (exclusive of examinations and minor procedures such as drawing blood).

Iodophor: A complex of free iodine combined with detergent that is used to kill microorganisms.

I PASS the BATON: A communication tool (mnemonic) consisting of the following steps: introduction, patient, assessment, situation, safety concerns, background, actions, timing ownership, next.

IV conscious sedation: See *Moderate sedation/ analgesia.*

Kitner: A small roll of heavy cotton tape that is held in the jaws of a heavy clamp and used for dissection or absorption.

Laminar air flow: A high-powered unidirectional air flow of approximately 100 ft/min; the air passes through a HEPA filter that removes all particles equal to or greater than 0.3 μm, with an efficiency of 99.7%. The intended purpose is to reduce airborne contamination.

Lap pad (lap sponge; tape): A square or rectangular gauze pad with a radiopaque marker used for absorption where moderate or large amounts of blood or fluid are encountered.

Laryngeal mask airway (LMA): A tube with an inflatable cuff that is inserted into the pharynx (unlike an esophageal tube, which is inserted into the larynx). It supports spontaneous and artificial ventilation but does not protect the lungs from aspiration.

Ligating clip: A stainless steel, titanium, or tantalum clip used to permanently clamp a vessel.

Local anesthesia: A form of regional anesthesia in which only a small, localized area is infiltrated with an anesthetic agent.

Local standby: See *Moderate sedation/analgesia.*

Malignant hyperthermia (MH): An emergency complication of general anesthesia that is characterized by a rapid rise in end tidal CO_2, masseter muscle rigidity, extraordinary oxygen consumption, rapid uncontrolled muscle metabolism, and production of heat and carbon dioxide. Temperatures as high as 109.4°F [43°C] have been reported. Malignant hyperthermia is a crisis and the patient will most likely die without immediate infusion of dantrolene sodium.

Mayo stand: An over-bed stand with a removable stainless steel tray. The legs of the stand slide under the operating-room table and the tray extends over the patient and holds the instruments needed for the surgical procedure. The scrubbed person hands instruments from the Mayo stand to the surgeon during the procedure.

Memory: A characteristic that causes a material to return to the state in which it was originally folded or placed.

Microfibrillar collagen (Avitene, Instat): A fluffy, white, absorbable material made from purified bovine dermis that is used to provide hemostasis. It is applied topically on oozing or friable tissue.

Moderate sedation/analgesia: A minimally depressed level of consciousness that allows a surgical patient to maintain his airway independently and continuously, and to respond appropriately to verbal commands and physical stimulation. Medications are administered intravenously to provide sedation, systemic analgesia, and depression of the autonomic nervous system. This anesthesia technique may not require the presence of an anesthesia care provider. In the absence of an anesthesia care provider, the patient is monitored by the perioperative nurse with demonstrated competency in monitoring patients receiving moderate sedation/analgesia and who has no other responsibilities during the procedure. Also referred to as intravenous (IV) conscious sedation, monitored anesthesia care (MAC), anesthesia standby, and local standby.

Monitored anesthesia care (MAC): Moderate sedation/analgesia that is delivered with an anesthesia provider present.

Muscarinic effect: Bradycardia, reduced stroke volume of the heart, bronchiolar constriction, arteriolar dilatation, increased tone, motility and secretion in the alimentary tract, and increases in salivation and lacrimation in response to an anesthetic agent.

Nursing diagnosis: A clinical judgment about actual or potential individual, family, or community experiences/responses to health problems/life processes. A nursing diagnosis provides the basis for selection of nursing interventions to achieve outcomes for which the nurse has accountability.

Open gloving: A technique for donning sterile gloves by non-scrubbed personnel and by scrubbed personnel when the fingers extend beyond the cuff on the gown sleeve. Hands touch only the inside of the gloves.

Oxidized cellulose (Oxycel, Surgicel, and Surgicel Nu-Knit): A specially treated gauze or cotton that is applied directly to an oozing surface to control bleeding.

Passivation: A process that minimizes the potential for corrosion on the surface of surgical instruments. The instrument is immersed in a nitric acid solution that removes carbon steel particles and promotes the formation of a chromium oxide coating on the surface.

Peanut: A very small sponge approximately the size of a peanut that is held in the jaws of a sturdy clamp and used for blotting blood and for tissue dissection.

Peel pack: A see-through pouch made of plastic and paper, or plastic and Tyvek, that is used to contain items during sterilization and to maintain sterility during storage.

Perfusionist: A highly skilled technician and member of the surgical team who is responsible for operating the cardiac bypass equipment during open-heart surgery.

Perioperative: Encompasses the three phases of the surgical experience: preoperative, intraoperative, and postoperative. Perioperative nursing activities are activities that occur in any or all of the three phases.

Perioperative Nursing Data Set (PNDS): A standardized nursing vocabulary developed by the Association of periOperative Registered Nurses (AORN) that may be used to describe perioperative nursing practice. It identifies nursing diagnoses and interventions relative to care of the patient undergoing a surgical or invasive procedure.

Plasma (sterilization): Hydrogen peroxide gas plasma sterilizers use a technology consisting of hydrogen peroxide vapor and low-temperature gas plasma to rapidly sterilize medical devices. Plasma is a state of matter produced through the action of a strong electric or magnetic field. In hydrogen peroxide gas plasma sterilization, a plasma state is created by the action of electrical energy upon hydrogen peroxide vapor. Plasma sterilization is used primarily for sterilization of heat- and moisture-sensitive items.

Pledget: A small piece of felt used as a support under friable tissues.

Plume: Smoke that results from cauterizing tissue—most often from application of electrosurgery or laser.

Pneumatic sequential compression device (SCD): A device used to prevent formation of a thrombus or DVT. It is comprised of a sleeve that is wrapped around the patient's leg, attached a to machine that inflates and deflates the sleeve in sequential progression, encouraging blood flow.

Postoperative: The period beginning when the patient is transferred to the recovery room and ending with resolution of surgical sequelae.

Preoperative: The period that begins when the decision to have surgery is made and ends when the patient is brought into the operating room and transferred to the operating room bed.

Primary intention: See *Wound healing.*

Prion: An infectious proteinaceous particle that is responsible for causing Creutzfeldt-Jakob disease and other spongiform encephalopathies.

Process challenge device (PCD): A device used to assess the performance of a sterilization process by providing a challenge to the process that is equal to or greater than the challenge posed by the most difficult item routinely processed (AAMI, 2011, p. 105).

Prep: See *Surgical prep.*

Rapid-readout biological monitor: An enzyme-based biological indicator that is used to monitor the sterilization process. Enzyme activity correlates to the inactivation of spores; it provides a reading that may be obtained soon after sterilization. A biological monitor is included within the product and may be incubated for an additional reading.

Raytex (4x4): A gauze sponge folded into a 43/4- or 43/8-inch square and supplied in packages of 10 sponges. Raytec spongesare used where a small amount of blood or fluid is encountered.

Regional anesthesia: Anesthesia that blocks the conduction of pain impulses from a specific region of the body. The patient is awake but does not feel pain in that region during surgery.

Restricted area: An area within the operating-room suite where surgical procedures are performed and where sterile supplies are unwrapped. Surgical attire and hats are required apparel in this area. Masks are required when sterile supplies are open.

Ring stand: A metal stand with wheels that accommodates one or two stainless steel basins and is draped to become part of the sterile field. The basins hold water and saline.

Saturated steam: Steam that contains the greatest amount of water vapor possible.

SBAR: A communication technique that organizes information by situation, background, assessment, and recommendations.

Scrub: See *Surgical hand antisepsis.*

Scrubbed person: A nurse or surgical technician/technologist who performs a surgical scrub, dons sterile attire, stands within the sterile field, and provides sterile instruments and other items to the surgical team during surgery. The scrubbed person is a member of the sterile team.

Secondary intention: See *Wound healing.*

Secured airway: An airway with an endotracheal tube equipped with a cuff that prevents gastric contents from entering the trachea.

Sellick maneuver: Manual compression of the esophagus between the cricoid cartilage and the vertebral column, done for the purpose of visualizing the tracheal lumen and preventing regurgitation and aspiration during intubation.

Semi-critical item: An item that makes contact with an intact mucous membrane but does not penetrate the membrane or enter sterile tissue or the vascular system. Semi-critical items may be sterilized but must be at least high-level disinfected when used on patients. Examples of semi-critical items are thermometer, laryngoscope, gastrointestinal endoscope.

Semi-restricted area: An area within the operating-room department that includes scrub sinks, areas where clean and sterile supplies are stored, areas where instruments are processed, and corridors that lead to the restricted area of the operating room. Traffic is limited to authorized personnel in surgical attire and hats and to patients.

Sequential compression device: See *Pneumatic sequential compression device.*

Shelf life: The amount of time an item may be assumed to be sterile. Shelf life is related to events and not to actual time. The longer an item remains on a shelf, the greater the possibility that an event will occur to cause contamination of the item. If no contamination occurs, the item is considered sterile for an indefinite amount of time.

Single-use device: A device manufactured for one-time use; it is not intended to be reprocessed and reused. Also referred to as a disposable.

Skin prep: See *Surgical prep*.

Spore: An inactive, or dormant but viable, state of a microorganism that is difficult to kill. Sterilization methods are monitored by their ability to kill known populations of highly resistant spores.

Standard precautions: Guidelines recommended by the Centers for Disease Control and Prevention for reducing the risk of transmission of blood-borne and other pathogens in hospitals. They are the basic level of infection control precautions that are to be used, at a minimum, in the care of all patients as it is often not known when a patient harbors infectious microorganisms. Under standard precautions, blood, all body fluids, secretions, and excretions except sweat, whether or not they contain visible blood, nonintact skin, and mucous membranes, are considered potentially infectious. Infection prevention practices include hand hygiene, cough etiquette, safe injection practices, and personal protective equipment, such as gown, gloves, mask, eye protection, or face shield when there is the potential for exposure to these patient fluids.

Steam sterilization: A sterilization process that uses steam under pressure to kill all forms of microbial life, including spores.

Sterile: Free of all viable microorganisms, including spores.

Sterile field: The area immediately surrounding the patient into which only sterile items may be delivered. A sterile field is created by placing sterile barriers over nonsterile items. The sterile field includes the area around the site of the incision and may include furniture covered with sterile drapes to hold instruments and supplies. Personnel who enter the sterile field must be attired in sterile gowns and gloves and wear a head covering and mask. Any equipment introduced into the sterile field (e.g. C-arm, microscope, x-ray cassette) must be covered with a sterile drape.

Sterility assurance level (SAL): The probability of a viable microorganism being present on an item after sterilization. The SAL for medical devices is 10^{-6}, or equal to or less than one chance in 1 million that there is a viable microorganism present on a device after sterilization.

Sterilization: A process that kills all living microorganisms, including spores.

Sterilizer (steam): Any of the following sterilization devices:

- Gravity displacement: A type of steam sterilizer in which steam displaces air through an outlet port by means of gravity.
- Prevacuum: A type of dynamic-air-removal steam sterilizer in which a vacuum is created to remove air at the beginning of the cycle and prior to steam entry into the chamber.
- Pulse pressure: A type of dynamic-air-removal steam sterilizer in which a series of steam flushes and pressure pulses at above-atmospheric pressure remove air from the chamber.

Strike-through: An event that occurs when liquids soak through a barrier from a sterile area to an unsterile area, or from an unsterile area to a sterile area. Strike-through renders items contained within the barrier unsterile.

Styptic: An agent that causes blood vessel constriction. An example is epinephrine.

Superheating: Occurs when fabrics that are dehydrated are subjected to steam sterilization. The temperature of the fabric exceeds the temperature of the steam. Superheating destroys cloth fibers.

Surgical conscience: An inner commitment to strictly adhere to aseptic practice, to report any break in aseptic technique, and to correct any violation, whether or not anyone else is present or observes the violation. A surgical conscience mandates a commitment to aseptic practice at all times.

Surgical counts: The counting of sponges, sharps such as blades and needles, instruments that are opened and delivered to the field, and miscellaneous items used during surgery, such as drill bits, vessel loops, and ligating clips. Counts are performed prior to the incision, before closing a cavity within a cavity (e.g. uterus), and before closing the incision; these counts should reflect that all counted items delivered to the sterile field are accounted for at the end of the procedure. Counting is a safety mechanism intended to decrease the risk that items used during the surgery might be retained in the patient.

Surgical hand antisepsis: Antiseptic hand wash or antiseptic hand rub performed prior to surgery by surgical personnel to eliminate transient microorganisms and reduce resident hand flora. Done in preparation for gowning and gloving.

Surgical hand antiseptic: An antimicrobial product formulated to significantly reduce the number of microorganisms on skin. Products are broad spectrum and should exhibit both persistence and a cumulative effect that prevents or inhibits proliferation or survival of microorganisms. Products used in preparation for gowning and gloving for surgery must be cleared by the FDA for use as a surgical hand antiseptic.

Surgical prep: Preparation of the patient's skin at the incision site and surrounding area with an antimicrobial agent to reduce the number of microorganisms to as low a level as possible and to prevent rebound growth for as long as possible. The prep may or may not include hair removal at the incision site.

Surgical scrub: A process of cleansing the hands and arms for the purpose of removing as many microorganisms as possible from the hands and portion of the arms prior to donning a sterile gown and gloves. See also *Anatomical timed scrub*, *Counted stroke scrub*, and *Surgical hand antisepsis*.

Surgical-site infection (SSI): Any of the following types of infection occurring following a surgical procedure:

- Superficial incisional: Infection involving only the skin or subcutaneous tissue.

- Deep incisional: Infection involving deep soft tissue, such as fascia or muscle.

- Organ/space: Infection involving the visceral cavity or anatomic structures not opened during the surgery.

Suture: (noun) A strand of material used to tie a blood vessel so as to occlude the lumen or sew tissue together; (verb) to sew tissue using suture material.

Suture ligature: A tie with an attached needle that is used to anchor the tie through the vessel for purposes of hemostasis.

Tape: See *Lap pad*.

Telfa: A nonadherent wound dressing.

Tensile strength: The amount of tension or pull that a suture will withstand when knotted before it breaks. The tension or pull is expressed in pounds. Tensile strength determines the amount of wound support that the suture provides during the healing process.

Terminal sterilization: Sterilization of an item that has been processed and wrapped. Terminal sterilization permits storage of the sterilized item for later use.

Thrombin: An enzyme made from dried beef blood or human plasma that is used to control capillary bleeding. It is supplied as a white powder and may be mixed with water or saline to form a thrombin solution.

Tie: A strand of material that is tied around a vessel to occlude the lumen for purposes of hemostasis.

Tonsil sponge: Cotton-filled gauze in the shape of a ball with a long attached tape. It is used in the mouth or throat for absorption of blood. The tape extends outside the mouth to permit easy retrieval.

Transmission-based precautions: A method of infection control that is applicable to patients known or suspected to be infected or colonized with highly transmissible or epidemiologically important pathogens for which additional precautions are needed to prevent transmission. There are three types of transmission-based precautions: airborne, droplet, and contact. These are used in addition to standard precautions.

- Airborne precautions: Appropriate for protection against pathogens that are transmitted by the airborne route. Includes use of respiratory protection and special air handling and ventilation.

- Droplet precautions: Appropriate for protection against pathogens transmitted through droplets. Includes wearing a mask within 3 feet of an infected patient and positioning other patients at least 3 feet from infected patients.

- Contact precautions: Appropriate for protection against pathogens that are transmitted by direct or indirect contact. Includes wearing a gown and gloves and cleaning and disinfecting patient equipment (Siegel et al., 2007, pp. 70–71).

Tyvek: Material made from high-density polyethylene fibers. Compatible with H_2O_2 sterilization technology.

Universal precautions: A method of infection control that requires the careful management of blood and body fluid of infected humans (patients and personnel) to be considered infectious and that the same safety precautions be taken whether or not the patient is known to have a bloodborne infectious disease Universal precautions have been incorporated into standard precautions which mandate the same precautions for *all* patients as we cannot be sure which patients are infected and which are not.

Unrestricted area: An area within the operating-room department where street clothes are permitted. Locker rooms and break rooms are usually included in the unrestricted area which also includes a control point where communication between the semi-restricted and restricted areas is coordinated.

Washer-disinfector/washer-decontaminator: Automated processing units used to decontaminate instruments. Cycles within these machines vary but include washing and rinsing and may include ultrasonic cleaning. A chemical or thermal phase within the cycle destroys specific microorganisms.

Washer-sterilizer: An automated processing unit that washes instruments for the purpose of decontamination. Includes washing, rinsing, and sterilization. Instruments processed in a washer-sterilizer are not ready for patient use and must be subject to an additional sterilization process in a sterilizer.

Webril: A cotton padding used under a cast or tourniquet.

Wet pack: Condensation on the inner or outer surface of a package/device following a terminal sterilization process.

Wound dehiscence: A partial or complete separation of the wound edges after wound closure as a result of failure of the wound to heal or failure of the suture material to secure the wound during healing.

Wound evisceration: The protrusion of the abdominal viscera through the incision as a result of failure of the wound to heal or failure of suture to secure the wound during healing.

Wound healing: The restoration of an injured area.
- Primary intention: Wound healing that occurs by primary union. Wound edges are approximated. Wounds heal by primary intention when minimal tissue damage occurs, aseptic technique is maintained, tissue is handled gently, and all layers of the wound are approximated.

Wounds that heal by primary intention heal quickly and result in minimal scarring.
- Secondary intention: Wound healing that occurs by wound contraction. Wound edges are not approximated. The wound is left open and healing occurs from the bottom upward. Granulation tissue forms in the wound and gradually fills in the defect.
- Third (tertiary) intention: Wound healing that occurs when the wound is sutured several days after surgery. Wound suturing is delayed for several days to permit granulation to occur in an area where gross infection or extensive tissue was removed. The wound is closed only if there is no sign of infection.

Wrong-site surgery: Surgery performed on the wrong patient, body part, side, level, or site.

● ● ● References

Association for the Advancement of Medical Instrumentation (AAMI) (2011). *Steam Sterilization and Sterility Assurance in Health Care Facilities.* (ANSI/AAMI ST79: 2011). Arlington, VA: AAMI.

Association of periOperative Registered Nurses (AORN) (2012). *Perioperative Standards and Recommended Practices* (pp. 411–420). Denver, CO: AORN.

Centers for Medicare & Medicaid Services (CMS) (2009). National Coverage Determination (NCD) for Surgical or Other Invasive Procedure Performed on the Wrong Body Part (140.7) (p. 2). Baltimore: CMS. Available at www.cms.gov/medicare-coverage-database/details/ncd-details.aspx?NCDId=328&ncdver=1&bc=AgAAQAAA AAAA&. Accessed December 11, 2012.

North American Nursing Diagnosis Association (NANDA) (2012). *International Nursing Diagnosis Glossary of Terms.* Available at: www.nanda.org/Diagnosis Development/DiagnosisSubmission/PreparingYour Submission/GlossaryofTerms.aspx. Accessed July 2012.

Siegel, J. et al. (2007). *2007 Guideline for Isolation Precautions: Preventing Transmission of Infectious Agents in Healthcare Settings.* Atlanta, GA: CDC. Available at www.cdc.gov/hicpac/pdf/isolation/Isolation2007.pdf Accessed October, 2012.

Index

Note: Page numbers followed by *f* indicate figures; those followed by *t* indicate tables